COSMETICS IN DERMATOLOGY

SECOND EDITION

COSMETICS IN DERMATOLOGY

SECOND EDITION

ZOE DIANA DRAELOS, M.D., F.A.A.D.

Clinical Assistant Professor
Department of Dermatology
Bowman Gray School of Medicine
of Wake Forest University
Winston-Salem, North Carolina

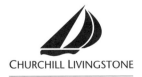

CHURCHILL LIVINGSTONE

New York, Edinburgh, London, Madrid, Melbourne, San Francisco, Tokyo

Library of Congress Cataloging-in-Publication Data

Draelos, Zoe Kececioglu.
    Cosmetics in dermatology / Zoe Diana Draelos. – 2nd ed.
        p. cm.
    Includes bibliographical references and index.
    ISBN 0-443-08965-5
    1. Cosmetics–Composition. 2. Dermatology. I. Title.
RL72.D73 1995
616.5–dc20   95-24705
                                                                                CIP

© Churchill Livingstone Inc. 1995

Distributed in the United Kingdom by Churchill Livingstone, Robert Stevenson House, 1–3 Baxter's Place, Leith Walk, Edinburgh EH1 3AF, and by associated companies, branches, and representatives throughout the world.

Accurate indications, adverse reactions, and dosage schedules for drugs are provided in this book, but it is possible that they may change. The reader is urged to review the package information data of the manufacturers of the medications mentioned.

The Publishers have made every effort to trace the copyright holders for borrowed material. If they have inadvertently overlooked any, they will be pleased to make the necessary arrangements at the first opportunity.

Acquisitions Editor: *Kerry Willis*
Production Editor: *Elizabeth Bowman-Schulman*
Production Supervisor: *Laura Mosberg Cohen*
Cover Design: *Jeannette Jacobs*

Printed in the United States of America

First published in 1995   7 6 5 4 3 2 1

To my husband, Michael Draelos, M.D.,
and my two sons, Mark and Matthew,
who fill my life with joy

Foreword

I am honored to have been asked to write the foreword to the second edition of Zoe Draelos's important, expanded textbook, *Cosmetics in Dermatology*. Zoe's contribution to the field is a major one. To this task she brings her sound credentials as a clinician scientist with a broad background ranging from engineering to medicine to dermatology. Zoe has been a private practitioner in High Point, North Carolina, since 1988 and has maintained strong academic ties with our department as a clinical assistant professor. She has been heavily involved in teaching and medical writing at the regional, national, and international levels.

The first edition of *Cosmetics in Dermatology* blazed the trail as a source of factual information for both physicians and cosmetologists interested in building a bridge between the chemical science of cosmetology, esthetics, and clinical dermatology. The first edition has been tremendously successful, but this second edition is definitely "new and improved." Zoe now presents a technical tour de force in the field with heavy use of teaching tables, extensive referencing, a doubling of pages, and many new chapters including photoaging, sunscreens, and cosmeceuticals; black skin and hair cosmetics; an approach to patients with cosmetic problems; and an approach to the patient with hair loss.

This work is most refreshing as it is written by an authority with no commercial ties to the industry and is therefore free of self-serving bias. *Cosmetics in Dermatology* remains the readable, authoritative, standard textbook in its field.

Joseph L. Jorizzo, M.D.
Professor and Chairman
Department of Dermatology
Bowman Gray School of Medicine
of Wake Forest University
Winston-Salem, North Carolina

Preface

The cosmetic and personal care industry is a large economic force in the world today. One only need stroll through department stores, mass merchandisers, drug stores, or grocery stores to realize the amount of retail space devoted to these items. Additionally, cosmetic issues comprise a large portion of the popular press. A glance at popular magazine covers and newspaper lifestyle sections invariably reveals at least one article dealing with cosmetic issues. Furthermore, prime time television frequently features advertisements for cosmetics or related products during a viewing evening.

Unfortunately, the consumer has very little background information to use in the selection and evaluation of cosmetic and personal care items. Many times purchase decisions are based on marketing claims, product packaging, or the advice of a friend. Consumers who approach cosmetic counter attendants or hair salon operators are given information that may or may not be objective or well founded. The consumer may then turn to his or her physician for medically correct, unbiased information. The purpose of this book is to provide the physician with the information required to answer patient questions intelligently and provide advice on the selection and use of cosmetics and personal care items.

The text is organized by type of cosmetic or skin care product. A general discussion of the history, formulation, application, and adverse reactions in a given cosmetic category is provided. This is intended to help the physician understand patient questions, provide timely advice, and recognize problems that may be related to cosmetic use. Every attempt has been made to insure that the information is up-to-date and correct; however, no responsibility can be accepted for inaccuracies as cosmetics companies frequently reformulate or change their product lines.

The field of cosmetics is essentially a study in the art of illusion. Cosmetics are any substances externally applied to the body to enhance beauty. A more specific definition from the Food, Drug and Cosmetic Act of 1938 defines cosmetics as "(1) articles intended to be rubbed, poured, sprinkled, or sprayed on, or introduced into, or otherwise applied to the human body or any part thereof for cleansing, beautifying, promoting attractiveness, or altering the appearance, and (2) articles intended for use as a component of any such articles; except that such term shall not include soap."[1] Their use is well founded in history.[2] Art critics frequently comment on the artist's deliberate distortion of dimensions and colors to create an image of beauty that is acceptable to the human eye. Cosmetics are used in a similar fashion by individuals to correct perceived flaws and to create an illusion of beauty that conforms to the current norms of society.

But, who defines beauty? Beauty is a concept that is defined based on an individual's background, experiences, and societal norms. This text contains recommendations based on my own concept of beauty, a concept that has been heavily influenced by experiences in my practice of dermatology, the concerns expressed by patients, my exposure to the field of cosmetology, and my perceptions as a woman. There are no absolute answers in the field of cosmetics, only personal opinions. The information presented in the pages that follow should be viewed with this understanding at all times.

It is hoped that this text will enable the physician to gain a fund of knowledge regarding the types of cosmetic products, the major ingredients in the cosmetic, the intended use of the product, possible side effects from use, and recommendations for the patient who desires cosmetic and personal care product information.

The art of cosmetics is much like the art of medicine: both are taught through textbooks, but neither can be mastered without practice. Caring for the entire patient entails ensuring inner health as well as outer health, since an individual's appearance is important to his or her emotional well-being. Physicians can more completely provide for the needs of patients by bridging the gap between medicine and cosmetology. It is hoped that this text is a step in that direction.

Zoe Diana Draelos, M.D., F.A.A.D.

References

1. 21 U.S.C. 321(i)
2. Corson R: Fashions in Makeup. Universe Books, New York, 1972

Acknowledgments

Many individuals have touched my life during the preparation of this second edition and I am grateful for their generous efforts. I am especially indebted to my husband, Michael, who provided unending computer text-editing assistance. Special appreciation goes to my practice partners: Arnold Gill, M.D., Wade Markham, M.D., Steve Uhlin, M.D., Samuel Kirby, M.D., and Brian Strauss, M.D. I also wish to thank Elizabeth Cline, who generously gave of her time to order articles and books from libraries all over the United States. And to my father, Dimitri, my mother, Lorene, and my brother, John, I am also indebted for their support.

Contents

1

Facial Foundations

Facial foundations are designed to add color, cover blemishes, and blend uneven facial color. They represent the class of cosmetics about which patients most frequently question their dermatologist. Since a foundation is usually applied to the entire face, used on a daily basis, and worn for an extended period of time, it has a dramatic effect on the skin. The variety in formulation, type, and color of facial foundations is wide and may be bewildering to physicians and patients alike. This chapter presents basic information on facial foundations, focusing on those foundations appropriate for oily, normal, combination, and dry skin and closing with a discussion on foundation selection for patients with facial scarring.

FACIAL FOUNDATIONS

History

The earliest cosmetic designed to cover facial blemishes was the beauty patch. These became popular in the 1600s to cover permanent facial scars left on those in Europe who survived smallpox epidemics. They were black silk or velvet pieces shaped like stars, moons, and hearts that were carefully placed about the face. Patch boxes, shallow metal boxes with a mirror in the cover, were carried everywhere to keep replacements handy should a patch fall off in public. The wearing of patches evolved into an unspoken language: a patch near a woman's mouth signaled flirtatiousness, a patch on a woman's right cheek indicated she was married, a patch at the corner of a woman's eye announced smoldering passion, and so forth. Patch boxes were no longer necessary after the development of the smallpox vaccination by Dr. Edward Jenner; thus they evolved into the compact used today for the application of powder and facial foundations.[1]

The modern concept of facial foundations was developed for the theater. A product used to whiten neck and arms was known as "wet white," or "French

1

White'' and consisted of face powder incorporated into a liquid vehicle.[2] This was considered an improvement over simply powdering the skin because of superior adherence. Later, ''grease paints'' were developed as pigments and fillers suspended in oily vehicles (see section on Formulation for further discussion). These products were difficult for individuals to apply and wear outside the theater. The first major breakthrough in facial foundations for the average woman came when Max Factor developed cake make-up, which he patented in 1936.[3] This product provided excellent coverage, a velvety look, and added facial color. Since that time, the variety and popularity of facial foundations have expanded tremendously.

Formulation

There are four basic facial foundation formulations: oil-based, water-based, oil-free, and water-free forms. Oil-based foundations are water-in-oil emulsions containing pigments suspended in oil, such as mineral oil or lanolin alcohol. Vegetable oils (coconut, sesame, safflower) and synthetic esters (isopropyl myristate, octyl palmitate, isopropyl palmitate) may also be incorporated. The water evaporates from the foundation following application, leaving the pigment in oil on the face. This provides facial skin with a moist feeling, especially desirable in dry, complected patients. Oil-based foundations are popular since they undergo no change in color with wearing, known as ''color drift.'' The pigment is already fully developed in oil, reducing the effect of facial sebum. These foundations are easy to apply, since the playtime (the time from application to setting) is prolonged, allowing manipulation of the pigment over the face for up to 5 minutes.

Water-based facial foundations are oil-in-water emulsions containing a small amount of oil in which the pigment is emulsified with a relatively large quantity of water. The primary emulsifier is usually a soap such as triethanolamine or a nonionic surfactant. The secondary emulsifier, present in smaller quantity, is usually glyceryl stearate or propylene glycol stearate. These popular foundations are appropriate for minimally dry to normal skin. Since the pigment is already developed in oil, this foundation type is also not subject to color drift. The playtime is shorter than with oil-based foundations, however, due to the lower oil content. These products are usually packaged in a bottle.

Oil-free facial foundations contain no animal, vegetable, or mineral oils. They may, however, contain other oily substances, such as the silicone derivatives dimethicone or cyclomethicone. These foundations are usually designed for oily skinned individuals or those with acne, since they emphasize the absence of oily substances believed to induce comedogenesis. The pigment is dissolved in water and other solvents, leaving the skin with a dry feeling resulting from the absence of oils. However, the color is more prone to drift with wearing as the pigment mixes with sebum. Foundation playtime is extremely short as the water and solvents evaporate quickly. Thus, oil-free foundations require rapid blending into one facial area at a time to prevent streaking. They can be packaged in bottles, jars, tubes, or compacts.

Water-free or anhydrous foundations are waterproof. Vegetable oil, mineral oil, lanolin alcohol, and synthetic esters form the oil phase, which may be mixed with waxes to form a cream.[4] They can be dipped from a jar, squeezed from a tube, wiped from a compact, or stroked from a stick. These foundations have a long playtime, no color drift, extended wear, and may be opaque, making them valuable for patients with facial scarring.

The coloring agents in all facial foundations are based on titanium dioxide with iron oxides, occasionally in combination with ultramarine blue. Titanium dioxide acts as both a facial concealing or covering agent and a physical sunscreen.

Facial foundations also contain talc and kaolin to function as fillers and blotters. A filler gives substance to the foundation, while a blotter functions to absorb facial secretions. Oil-control foundations contain increased concentrations of the blotters talc, kaolin, starch, or polymers to absorb facial sebum, thus preventing the development of facial shine. Oil-control foundations are not necessarily oil free, however. The oil content of a foundation can be assessed by placing a drop of the product on a sheet of 25% cotton bond paper. Oil-containing foundations will leave an oil ring on the paper, whereas oil-free foundations will not. The size of the oil ring is proportionally related to the foundation's oil concentration.[5]

Coverage

The ability of a foundation to conceal or cover the underlying skin is known as "coverage." The coverage of a foundation is directly related to the amount of titanium dioxide, zinc oxide, talc, kaolin, and precipitated chalk it contains. Sheer coverage foundations with minimal titanium dioxide are almost transparent and have a sun protection factor (SPF) around 2, moderate coverage foundations are translucent and have an approximate SPF of 4 to 5, and anhydrous high-coverage foundations with large amounts of titanium dioxide are opaque, acting as a total physical sunblock. Some foundations, known as "sportwear" or "antiaging" foundations, may contain additional chemical sunscreening agents such as PABA esters or cinnamate derivatives. A complete discussion of sun protection and sunscreens is found on pages 235 to 239.

Types

Facial foundations are available in a variety of forms: liquid, mousse, water-containing cream, soufflé, anhydrous cream, stick, cake, and shake lotion (Table 1-1).[6] Liquid formulations are most popular because they are the easiest to apply, provide sheer to moderate coverage, and create a natural appearance. As previously mentioned, they contain mainly water, oils, and titanium dioxide (TiO_2). If the liquid is aerosolized, a foam foundation known as a "mousse"

Table 1-1. Types of Facial Foundations

Type	Coverage	Wearability	Skin Type	Main Ingredients
Liquid	Sheer to moderate	Moderate	Any	Water, oil, TiO_2
Mousse	Shear	Short	Oily to normal	Aerosolized liquid formulation
Water-containing cream	Moderate	Moderate to long	Dry to normal	Water, oil, wax, TiO_2
Soufflé	Moderate	Moderate	Dry to normal	Whipped cream formulation
Anhydrous cream	Full	Long	Dry	Mineral and vegetable oils, synthetic esters, wax, TiO_2
Stick	Full	Long	Dry	Mineral oil, wax, TiO_2
Cake	Full	Moderate to long	Oily to normal	Talc, kaolin, chalk, zinc oxide, TiO_2
Shake lotion	Sheer	Short	Oily	Talc, water, solvent

See glossary for definition of terms.

Coverage: very sheer = transparent, sheer = semitransparent, moderate = translucent, heavy = semiopaque, full = opaque.

Wearability: very short = 2 hours, short = 3 hours, moderate = 4 hours, long = 8 hours.

is produced. A cream foundation has the additional ingredient of wax, which makes a thicker, occlusive, more moisturizing formula. Whipping the cream produces a soufflé foundation. An anhydrous cream with no water in its formulation provides more occlusion and superior, long-lasting coverage. Addition of increased amounts of wax to an anhydrous cream yields a product that can be extruded into a rod and packaged in a roll-up tube. These are stick foundations. Cake-type foundations, also known as ''cream/powder'' foundations, consist of talc, kaolin, precipitated chalk, zinc oxide, and titanium dioxide compressed into a cake that is applied to the skin with a dry sponge (powder) or moistened sponge (cream). Shake lotions are pigmented talc suspended in water and solvents that evaporate, leaving a thin layer of powder on the face.

Facial Foundation Finishes

Facial foundations are manufactured in a variety of finishes: matte, semimatte, moist semimatte, and shiny (Table 1-2). The finish is the surface characteristic of a cosmetic. Matte finish foundations yield a flat look with no shine and

Table 1-2. Facial Foundation Finishes

	Appearance	Formulation	Skin Type	Moisturizing Ability	
Matte	Flat, no shine	Generally oil-free	Oily	↑	Least
Semimatte	Minimal shine	Oil-free or water-based	Olly to normal		
Moist semimatte	Dewy shine	Generally water-based	Normal to dry		
Shiny	Obvious shine	Generally oil-based	Dry	↓	Most

See glossary for definition of terms.

generally are oil free. They are good for patients with oily skin, who tend to develop some shine after a foundation has been applied. Foundation finish is somewhat dictated by fashion; a matte look was popular in the late 1950s and again in the 1990s. A semimatte finish, the more popular look of the 1980s, has minimal shine and is generally an oil-free foundation or water-based foundation with minimal oil content. This finish performs well on slightly oily to normal skin. A foundation with more shine is known as a "moist" semimatte foundation and is generally water based with moderate oil content. This look was popular in the 1960s and performs well on normal to dry skin. Shiny finishes are found in oil-based foundations and are only appropriate for persons with dry skin. The shinier foundations with increased oil content also have increased moisturizing ability.

Application

The foundation selected should match the natural facial color as closely as possible. This can be difficult, however, since the nose and cheeks have redder tones than the forehead and chin. The foundation is matched to the skin along the jawline, since this is where the color must be carefully blended beneath the chin. Mismatched racial foundations generally leave a line at the jawline. A foundation color should also be selected in natural sunlight: the bright, artificial fluorescent lights used in most stores will distort color perception. This can result in selection of a dark foundation that will appear unnatural under more conventional lighting. The patient should be urged to apply a sample of foundation to the jawline in the store and then walk outside to examine the color match with a compact mirror.

In general, facial foundation should be applied with the fingertips. A dab of foundation should be placed on the forehead, nose, cheeks, and chin and then blended with a light circular motion until it is evenly spread over all the facial skin, including the lips. Finally, a puff or sponge should be used, stroking in a downward direction, to remove any streaks and to flatten vellus facial hair. Special care should be taken to rub the foundation into the hairline, over the tragus, and beneath the chin. Foundation should also be blended around the eyes and may even be applied to the entire upper eyelid if desired. The foundation should be allowed to set or dry until it can no longer be removed with light touch. If additional coverage is desired, a second layer of foundation can be applied. Makeup sponges are used to apply cake foundation, but otherwise are not recommended since they absorb a tremendous amount of foundation.

Purchase

Facial foundations can be purchased at a mass merchandiser, drug store, department store, or boutique. Less expensive, wide appeal foundations are sold by mass merchandisers and drug stores. More expensive, upscale foundations are sold by department stores, and very expensive specialty foundations are sold by elite department stores and boutiques. Physicians are frequently asked by patients if they are getting higher quality with an expensive cosmetic than a less expensive cosmetic. It is true that part of the cost of a more expensive cosmetic goes into attractive packaging and a prestige name or image. However, a wider range of colors is generally available with the more expensive product lines, and in some instances the increased cost yields superior ingredients that perform better. This especially seems to be the case with facial foundations. In general, the more expensive foundations have less color drift, better coverage, easier application, and more uniform appearance. Patients should probably be encouraged to spend the bulk of their cosmetic money on a superior foundation and then to save money by selecting good quality, less expensive moisturizers, cleansing agents, and other facial cosmetics.

Selection

The facial foundations currently available to the consumer have been arranged in table form according to skin type: acne and/or oily (Table 1-3), normal (Table 1-4), and dry (Table 1-5). The tables are presented following discussion of the foundations appropriate for each complexion. Two tables have been included under each skin type, since certain foundations are marketed only through full-service cosmetic counters at department stores and boutiques while other foundations are marketed only through drug stores, variety stores, grocery stores, and mass merchandisers.

The cosmetic counter foundations are generally more expensive than other foundations. Relative costs have been included. Coverage, the ability to cover facial blemishes, is listed on a scale from sheer to full.[7] Patients with more facial blemishes will require fuller coverage. Very sheer coverage indicates transparent, sheer coverage indicates semitransparent, moderate coverage indicates translucent, heavy coverage indicates semiopaque, and full coverage indicates opaque. Wearability, rated on a scale from short to long, refers to the length of time a foundation will remain in place on the face after application. Very short wearability is approximately 2 hours, short wearability is approximately 3 hours, moderate wearability is approximately 4 hours, and long wearability is approximately 8 hours. Patients who require that a foundation applied in the morning look presentable in the evening need a product with long wearability. Color selection is important, since not all foundations are available in a shade to match the patient's skin. Lighter complected patients require recommendations for a foundation available in fair tones while Hispanic or Oriental patients need a darker foundation. Foundations for Black skin are listed separately in Chapter 19. Foundation availability refers to the ease with which a product can be found by the patient. The foundation charts are intended to allow the physician to customize recommendations for foundations to the needs of each patient.

Table 1-3A. Cosmetic Counter Facial Foundations: Acne/Oily Skin

Name/Company	Type	Cost	Coverage	Wearability	Availability
Demi-Matte (Estee Lauder)	Liquid	+ + + +	Moderate	Moderate	Wide
Macquicontrole (Lancome)	Liquid	+ + + +	Moderate	Moderate	Wide
Pore-Minimizer (Clinique)	Shake lotion	+ + +	Very sheer	Very short	Wide
Teint Pur (Chanel)	Liquid	+ + + + + +	Sheer	Moderate	Limited
Stay-True (Clinique)	Liquid	+ + +	Sheer	Short	Wide
Makeup #3 (Prescriptives)	Liquid	+ + + +	Sheer	Moderate	Limited
Oil-Free Cream Powder (Elizabeth Arden)	Cream/ powder	+ + + +	Moderate	Moderate	Wide
Shake-It Regular Normalizer (Erno Lazlo)	Shake lotion	+ + + + + + +	Very sheer	Short	Limited
Satilane (Orlane)	Cream	+ + + + +	Sheer	Moderate	Limited
Soft Velvet Makeup (Alexandra de Markoff)	Liquid	+ + + + + +	Moderate	Moderate	Limited
Oil-Free Foundation (Mary Kay)	Liquid	+ + +	Moderate	Moderate	Sold door to door
Teint Ideal Mat (Christian Dior)	Liquid	+ + + + +	Sheer	Moderate	Limited

Cost: + = $4–5, + + = $5–10, + + + = $10–20, + + + + = $20–30, + + + + + = $30–40, + + + + + + = $40–50, + + + + + + + = $50–60.
Coverage: very sheer = only provides facial color, sheer = minimally evens facial color, moderate = conceals minor blemishes, full = conceals blemishes and minor pigmentation irregularities.
Wearability: very short = 2 hours, short = 3 hours, moderate = 4 hours, long = 8 hours.
Availability: wide = available in most department stores, limited = available in elite department stores and boutiques.

Table 1-3B. Non-Cosmetic Counter Facial Foundations: Acne and/or Oily Skin

Name/Company	Type	Cost	Coverage	Wearability	Availability
Mattique (L'Oreal)	Liquid	+ +	Moderate	Short	Wide
Springwater Makeup (Revlon)	Liquid	+ +	Moderate	Short	Wide
Shine Free (Maybelline)	Liquid	+	Very sheer	Very short	Wide
Color and Light (Max Factor)	Liquid	+ +	Sheer	Short	Wide
Oil Control Makeup (Almay)	Liquid	+ +	Sheer	Short	Wide
Clarifying Makeup (Cover Girl)	Liquid	+	Sheer	Short	Wide

Cost: + = $4–5, + + = $5–10.
Coverage: very sheer = only provides facial color, sheer = minimally evens facial color, moderate = conceals minor blemishes, full = conceals blemishes and minor pigmentation irregularities.
Wearability: very short = 2 hours, short = 3 hours, moderate = 4 hours.
Availability: wide = available in most drug stores and mass merchandisers.

Table 1-4A. Cosmetic Counter Facial Foundations: Normal Skin

Name/Company	Type	Cost	Coverage	Wearability	Availability
Maquimate Ultra Naturel (Lancome)	Liquid	+ + + +	Sheer	Moderate	Wide
Lucidity (Estee Lauder)	Liquid	+ + + +	Very sheer	Moderate	Wide
Fresh Air Makeup (Estee Lauder)	Liquid	+ + + +	Moderate	Moderate	Wide
Balanced Makeup (Clinique)	Liquid	+ + +	Moderate	Moderate	Wide
Teint Naturel (Chanel)	Liquid	+ + + + + +	Sheer	Short	Limited
Flawless Finish Mousse (Elizabeth Arden)	Mousse	+ + + +	Very sheer	Short	Wide
Makeup #2 (Prescriptives)	Liquid	+ + + +	Very sheer	Short	Limited
Cream Makeup (Alexandra de Markoff)	Cream	+ + + + + +	Moderate	Moderate	Limited
Day Radiance Liquid Foundation (Mary Kay)	Liquid	+ + +	Moderate	Moderate	Sold door to door
Teint Actuel (Christian Dior)	Soufflé	+ + + + +	Moderate	Moderate	Limited

Cost: + = $4–5, + + = $5–10, + + + = $10–20, + + + + = $20–30, + + + + + = $30–40, + + + + + + = $40–50.

Coverage: very sheer = only provides facial color, sheer = minimally evens facial color, moderate = conceals minor blemishes, full = conceals blemishes and minor pigmentation irregularities.

Wearability: very short = 2 hours, short = 3 hours, moderate = 4 hours, long = 8 hours.

Availability: wide = available in most department stores, limited = available in elite department stores and boutiques.

Table 1-4B. Non-Cosmetic Counter Facial Foundations: Normal Skin

Name/Company	Type	Cost	Coverage	Wearability	Availability
Moisture Balance Makeup (Almay)	Liquid	+ +	Sheer	Moderate	Wide
Sheer Essentials (Maybelline)	Liquid	+	Very sheer	Very short	Wide
Finish Matte (Maybelline)	Liquid	+	Sheer	Short	Wide
Airspun Powder Essence Foundation (Coty)	Liquid	+ +	Moderate	Moderate	Wide
Clean Makeup (Cover Girl)	Liquid	+	Moderate	Moderate	Wide
Active Protection Makeup (Max Factor)	Liquid	+ +	Sheer	Moderate	Wide
New Complexion Makeup (Revlon)	Liquid	+ +	Moderate	Moderate	Wide
Visuelle (L'Oreal)	Liquid	+ +	Sheer	Moderate	Wide

Cost: + = $4–5, + + = $5–10.

Coverage: very sheer = only provides facial color, sheer = minimally evens facial color, moderate = conceals minor blemishes, full = conceals blemishes and minor pigmentation irregularities.

Wearability: very short = 2 hours, short = 3 hours, moderate = 4 hours.

Availability: wide = available in most drug stores and mass merchandisers.

Table 1-5A. Cosmetic Counter Facial Foundations: Dry Skin

Name/Company	Type	Cost	Cover-age	Wear-ability	Avail-ability
Polished Performance (Estee Lauder)	Liquid	+ + + +	Sheer	Moderate	Wide
Beautiful Nutrient Makeup (Ultima II)	Cream	+ + + +	Moderate	Moderate	Wide
Country Mist (Estee Lauder)	Liquid	+ + + +	Moderate	Moderate	Wide
Liquid Perfection (Elizabeth Arden)	Liquid	+ + + +	Moderate	Moderate	Wide
Maquivelours (Lancome)	Liquid	+ + + +	Moderate	Moderate	Wide
Extra Help Makeup (Clinique)	Liquid	+ + +	Sheer	Moderate	Wide
Teint Lumiere Creme (Chanel)	Cream	+ + + + + + +	Moderate	Moderate	Limited
Makeup #1 (Prescriptives)	Liquid	+ + + +	Sheer	Moderate	Limited
B21 Foundation (Orlane)	Cream	+ + + + + + +	Moderate	Moderate	Limited
Liquid Makeup Countess Isserlyn (Alexandra de Markoff)	Shake lotion	+ + + + + + +	Moderate	Short	Limited
Day Radiance Cream Foundation (Mary Kay)	Cream	+ +	Moderate	Moderate	Sold door to door
Teint Dior (Christian Dior)	Liquid	+ + + + +	Moderate	Moderate	Limited

Cost: + = $4–5, + + = $5–10, + + + = $10–20, + + + + = $20–30, + + + + + = $30–40, + + + + + +
= $40–50, + + + + + + + = $50–60.
Coverage: very sheer = only provides facial color, sheer = minimally evens facial color, moderate = conceals minor blemishes, full = conceals blemishes and minor pigmentation irregularities.
Wearability: very short = 2 hours, short = 3 hours, moderate = 4 hours, long = 8 hours.
Availability: wide = available in most department stores, limited = available in elite department stores and boutiques.

Adverse Reactions

Facial foundations are a rare cause of allergic and irritant contact dermatitis. Usually, it is the fragrance or preservative ingredients that account for the majority of the allergic contact dermatitis cases reported. Irritant contact dermatitis is much more common since foundation is worn by patients with dermatitic skin for 8 hours or more on a daily basis. Facial foundation can be open or closed patch tested ''as is.''

Some facial foundations are labeled for ''sensitive skin.'' It is unclear exactly what this marketing claim delineates. Evaluation of these products fails to reveal avoidance of any particular chemicals or group of allergens. These products do, however, sometimes contain a substance known to soothe skin, such as allantoin. Perhaps this formulation is designed to minimize any dermatitis resulting from use of the product, allowing the patient to continue wearing the facial foundation.

Table 1-5B. Non-Cosmetic Counter Facial Foundations: Dry Skin

Name/Company	Type	Cost	Coverage	Wearability	Availability
Moisture Renew Makeup (Almay)	Liquid	+ +	Sheer	Short	Wide
Moisture Whip Makeup (Maybelline)	Liquid	+	Moderate	Moderate	Wide
Moisture Wear Cream (Cover Girl)	Cream	+	Moderate	Moderate	Wide
Whipped Cream Makeup (Max Factor)	Cream	+ +	Sheer	Short	Wide
Touch and Glow (Revlon)	Liquid	+ +	Moderate	Moderate	Wide
Hydra Perfecte (L'Oreal)	Cream	+ +	Moderate	Moderate	Wide

Cost: + = $4–5, + + = $5–10.
Coverage: very sheer = only provides facial color, sheer = minimally evens facial color, moderate = conceals minor blemishes, full = conceals blemishes and minor pigmentation irregularities.
Wearability: very short = 2 hours, short = 3 hours, moderate = 4 hours, long = 8 hours.
Availability: wide = available in most drug stores and mass merchandisers.

ACNE AND/OR OILY SKIN FACIAL FOUNDATIONS

Patients with acne and/or oily skin generally do best with matte or semimatte finish, oil-free or low oil content facial foundations (Table 1-3). While this type of foundation performs best in the long run, many patients initially are dissatisfied with such a product because oil-free or low oil foundations neither cover as well nor wear as long as oil-containing foundations. They are also more prone to collect or cake around facial blemishes, and their short playtime makes application more difficult.

The original oil-free foundations were shake lotions composed of pigmented talc in a water and solvent vehicle. Shaking was required to suspend the powder in the liquid prior to application. After the vehicle evaporated, a thin layer of powder was left on the face. The coverage of this type product is extremely sheer and the playtime is extremely short, approximately 30 seconds, thus requiring skilled application. Coverage can be improved by repeated application; however, most patients find this inconvenient. The weartime of shake lotions on an oily face is very short, approximately 1 to 2 hours. Breakdown of the thin foundation layer, known as ''separation,'' occurs commonly over the oily nose and medial cheeks as the powder foundation preferentially adheres to the pores and is wiped from the surrounding skin. A similar-appearing foundation can be made by first applying an oil-free moisturizer and then a loose transparent powder.

Patients seem to find the newer oil-free liquid foundations more appealing. These products may require minimal shaking prior to use but do not separate like a shake lotion. Oil-free foundations differ tremendously by brand in terms of coverage. Extremely sheer or transparent coverage may be appropriate for the patient with open comedones and no inflammatory papules, but the patient with more facial erythema may need more coverage with a sheer product. Moderate or translucent coverage will be required by the patient with inflammatory papules. Patients with scars may need the extremely good, heavy coverage only afforded by cake foundations with minimal oil. Unfortunately, this look can be quite theatrical.

Acne patients may apply medicated water-based creams or alcohol-based liquids under an oil-free foundation. Gel-type products that leave a film on the skin, such as topical antibiotic gels or gel sunscreens, will either change the foundation color or prevent the foundation from adhering. Any product used in this manner must be allowed to dry thoroughly before foundation is applied.

Most oil-free or low oil foundations wear longer if a loose transparent powder is applied to the face. The powder increases the weartime of the foundation by absorbing oil and increasing coverage. The loose powder should be rubbed into the foundation with the fingertips and the excess dusted away with a loose powder brush. More details are provided in Chapter 2.

NORMAL SKIN FACIAL FOUNDATIONS

Patients with normal skin and no tendencies toward acne have numerous facial foundations from which to choose (Table 1-4). These patients usually prefer a semimatte to moist semimatte finish since their facial oil production is not excessive and matte finish cosmetics will give a "floured" look. Water-based foundations perform best if a small amount of oil is included in the formulation to improve coverage, wear, and application ease. Sheer coverage can be useful in the patient who simply needs facial color. Increased coverage is required by the patient with facial telangiectasias and lentigines. The mature patient with normal skin and actinically induced dyspigmentation needs moderate coverage to deemphasize facial wrinkles.

DRY SKIN FACIAL FOUNDATIONS

Patients with dry skin need a foundation that provides all day moisturization (Table 1-5). Water-based foundations with a moderate oil content or oil-based foundations may be used. The oil content required gives the foundation a moist semimatte or shiny finish. Foundations with a substantial oil content are easy to apply because of their long playtime, cover extremely well, and are long wearing. In some cases, selection of the appropriate foundation may obviate the need for a daytime facial moisturizer. Younger patients with dry skin and no complexion problems generally prefer a moderately sheer moist semimatte finish. A more matte type finish can be achieved by applying a loose transparent powder over the foundation. Mature patients with dry skin need a moderate coverage moisturizing foundation that will not accentuate wrinkling. Patients with normal skin that has become dry due to topical medication may also need to use an oil-containing foundation.

Patients with extremely dry skin may feel that they need to use a cream of soufflé foundation. These products do contain more oils; however, they also yield a thicker appearance. If the skin surface is perfectly smooth, a thicker foundation can be attractive; if the skin surface is wrinkled or has other surface irregularities, the thicker foundation will accentuate the underlying contour. An alternative is to use a heavy cream moisturizer under the foundation followed by application of a thinner, less moisturizing foundation.

COMBINATION SKIN FACIAL FOUNDATIONS

Combination skin presents a challenge in terms of selecting a facial foundation. This is probably the most common skin type encounteed by a dermatologist. These patients are generally women between the ages of 25 and 45 who have an oily central forehead, nose, and medial cheek. This area is also known as the "T zone." Occasionally, the perioral and central chin areas are similarly affected. The more lateral facial areas are usually dry. These patients also tend to have acne, which may fluctuate with ovulation and menstruation.

No foundation has been developed to date that can supply the proper amount of moisturizing to dry areas and absorb the proper amount of sebum from oily areas. A product marketed by some cosmetic companies to deal with this problem is known as an oil-control foundation. These products contain starch, clay, polymers, or additional talc to aid in oil absorption. They usually contain a fair amount of oil and fit best under cosmetics for normal skin, since their high oil content makes them unsuitable for acne patients and their oil-absorbing capability makes them unsuitable for patients with a dry complexion. Even patients with normal skin make sebum, and oil-control foundations can wear longer than average on these individuals.

Patients with combination skin seem to do best with foundations selected from the list for patients with acne and/or oily skin (Table 1-3) that will not accentuate complexion problems. However, they must carefully prepare the face prior to application of the foundation. All oily areas should be treated with an astringent, and all dry areas should be treated with an oil-free moisturizer. The aim is to create an even oil distribution. Foundation is then applied to the entire face and a loose transparent powder applied to central facial areas. Most patients prefer a moderate coverage foundation.

Combination skin may tend to be drier in the winter and oilier in the summer. All patients should be encouraged to match their foundation to their complexion needs. Some patients may need to change foundations depending on the season, just as they change their wardrobes.

Table 1-6A. Cosmetic Counter Facial Foundations: Facial Scarring

Name/Company	Type	Cost	Coverage	Wearability	Availability
Continuous Coverage (Clinique)	Cream	+ + +	Full	Long	Wide
Dual Finish Creme/ Powder Makeup (Lancome)	Cream/ powder	+ + + +	Moderately full	Moderate	Wide
Maximum Cover (Estee Lauder)	Cream	+ + + +	Minimally full	Moderate	Wide
Ultimate Cover Makeup (Ultima II)	Cream	+ + + +	Moderately full	Moderate	Wide
Camouflage Cream (Prescriptives)	Cream	+ + +	Moderately full	Moderate	Wide
Just Perfect Cream (Estee Lauder)	Cream	+ + + +	Moderately full	Moderate	Wide
Teint Poudre (Christian Dior)	Cream/ powder	+ + + + +	Minimally full	Moderate	Limited

Cost: + = $4–5, + + = $5–10, + + + = $10–20, + + + + = $20–30, + + + + + = $30–40, + + + + + + = $40–50.
Coverage: very sheer = only provides facial color, sheer = minimally evens facial color, moderate = conceals minor blemishes, full = conceals blemishes and minor pigmentation irregularities.
Wearability: very short = 2 hours, short = 3 hours, moderate = 4 hours, long = 8 hours.
Availability: wide = available in most department stores, limited = available in elite department stores and boutiques.

FACIAL FOUNDATIONS FOR SCARRED SKIN

All of the foundations appropriate for facial scarring contain oil or a silicone derivative, since oil is required for increased coverage and extended wear (Table 1-6). It is also desirable for these foundations to be somewhat waterproof, which

Table 1-6B. Non-Cosmetic Counter Facial Foundations: Facial Scarring

Name/Company	Type	Cost	Coverage	Wearability	Availability
Pan-Stick Makeup (Max Factor)	Cream	+ +	Full	Long	Wide
Pan-Cake Makeup (Max Factor)	Cream/ powder	+ +	Full	Long	Wide
Powdercreme Makeup (Revlon)	Cream/ powder	+ +	Minimally full	Long	Wide
Creme Powder Makeup (Almay)	Cream/ powder	+ +	Minimally full	Long	Wide

Cost: + = $4–5, + + = $5–10.
Coverage: very sheer = only provides facial color, sheer = minimally evens facial color, moderate = conceals minor blemishes, full = conceals blemishes and minor pigmentation irregularities.
Wearability: very short = 2 hours, short = 3 hours, moderate = 4 hours, long = 8 hours.
Availability: wide = available in most drug stores and mass merchandisers.

necessitates a low to absent water content. These products provide increased coverage by containing higher amounts of titanium dioxide, but are not intended to be opaque. If complete occlusive coverage is desired, the section on opaque cover cosmetics should be consulted. Persons who desire an extremely long-wearing foundation or a foundation appropriate for wear while exercising or swimming should select a foundation from this group. One disadvantage of these foundations is the tendency to accentuate facial surface irregularities.

REFERENCES

1. Panati C: Extraordinary Origins of Everyday Things. Perennial Library, Harper & Row, New York, 1987
2. Schlossman ML, Feldman AJ: Fluid foundations and blush make-up. p. 741. In deNavarree MG (ed): The Chemistry and Manufacture of Cosmetics. 2nd Ed. Allured Publishing Corporation, Wheaton, IL, 1988
3. Wells FV, Lubowe II: Cosmetics and the Skin. Reinhold Publishing Corporation, New York, 1964
4. Flick EW: Cosmetic and Toiletry Formulations. 2nd Ed. Noyes Publications, Park Ridge, NJ
5. Fulton JE, Bradley S, Aqundez A, Black T: Non-comedogenic cosmetics. Cutis 17: 344, 1976
6. Fiedler JG: Foundation makeup. p. 317. In Balsam MS, Sagarin E (eds): Cosmetics, Science and Technology. 2nd Ed. Vol. 1. Wiley-Interscience, New York, 1972
7. Kimura S, Kaneda Y, Horino M, Yamamato M: Achieving uniform makeup coverage. Cosmet Toilet 107 April 1992:59, 1992

2

Facial Colored Cosmetics

Facial colored cosmetics attempt to deemphasize facial defects and to accentuate attractive facial features. Effective use of facial colored cosmetics can reshape a poorly proportioned face or minimize facial scarring. The basic facial cosmetics are powders, blushes, and rouges; bronzing gels and color washes; and cover sticks and undercover creams (Table 2-1).

FACIAL POWDERS

Facial powders provide coverage of complexion imperfections, oil control, a matte finish, and tactile smoothness to the skin. Originally, facial powder was applied over a moisturizer to function as a type of powdered foundation. Liquid foundations have largely replaced the powdered foundation, but for patients who wish sheer coverage with excellent oil control, a powdered foundation performs excellently. An appropriate moisturizer for the patient's skin type is first applied and allowed to set or dry, followed by application of a full-coverage, translucent powder.

Formulation

Full-coverage powders contain predominantly talc (hydrated magnesium silicate) and increased amounts of covering pigments. The covering pigments used in face powder, listed in order of increasing opaqueness, are titanium dioxide, kaolin, magnesium carbonate, magnesium stearate, zinc stearate, prepared chalk, zinc oxide, rice starch, precipitated chalk, and talc. It is generally accepted that the optimum opacity is achieved with a particle size of 0.25 microns. Magnesium carbonate can also be used to improve oil blotting, keep the powder fluffy, and absorb any added perfume. Kaolin (hydrated aluminium silicate)

15

Table 2-1. Facial Cosmetics

	Appearance	Coverage	Formulation	Patient Suitability
Powder	Matte or frosted	Moderate	Talc, zinc, stearate, kaolin, TiO$_2$, pigment, pearl	All
Powdered blush	Matte or frosted	Moderate	Talc, zinc stearate, TiO$_2$, pigment, pearl	All
Cream rouge	Shiny	Moderate	Petrolatum, mineral oil, pigment	Dry skin
Gel rouge	Skin stain	Sheer	Same as bronzing gels	Acne patient, male cosmetic
Bronzing gel	Skin stain	Very sheer	Water, alcohol, neutral aqueous gel, light esters, color	Acne patient, male cosmetic
Color wash	Frosted	Sheer	Petrolatum, mineral oil, pigment	Mature patient
Powdered buffer or highlighter	Frosted	Moderate	Same as powdered blush	Patient who needs facial contouring
Cover stick	Matte	Full	Mineral oil, wax, TiO$_2$, pigment	Patient with dyspigmentation
Green undercover	Matte	Full	Mineral oil, wax, TiO$_2$, pigment	Patient with red dermatosis or facial scarring
Purple undercover	Matte	Full	Mineral oil, wax, TiO$_2$, pigment	Patient with yellow skin tones
White pearlized undercover	Frosted	Moderate	Water, mineral oil, talc, TiO$_2$, pearl	Patient with shallow skin, surface irregularities, or moderate dyspigmentation

Coverage: very sheer = transparent, sheer = semitransparent, moderate = translucent, heavy = semiopaque, full = opaque.

may also function to absorb oil and perspiration. Full-coverage face powders are usually packaged in a compact and applied to the face with a puff.[1]

Transparent facial powders are more popular today to add coverage and improve oil blotting abilities of a previously applied liquid foundation. Transparent powders have the same formulation as full-coverage powders except that they contain less talc, titanium dioxide, or zinc oxide, since coverage is not a priority. Transparent facial powders commonly have a light shine, produced by nacreous pigments, such as bismuth oxychloride, mica, titanium dioxide–coated mica, or crystalline calcium carbonate.

Facial powder usually uses iron oxides as the main pigment, but other inorganic pigments such as ultramarines, chrome oxide, and chrome hydrate may also be used. These powders are designed to augment the underlying skin and foundation tones; thus transparent powders can be used by patients who have difficulty finding an appropriately tinted facial foundation. Transparent powders may also be selected in complementary colors, such as a pale bluish-green, to decrease facial erythema in rosacea, psoriasis, and systemic lupus patients.

Specialty additives to some transparent powders include partially hydrolyzed ground raw silk to improve absorbency and impart a velvety matte finish; corn silk also to impart a velvety matte finish; and treated starch and synthetic resins for increased oil absorption. Most transparent powders are packaged loose and come with an applicator brush or puff.

Application

Facial powders are removed from a compact with a puff or dusted loosely from a container with a brush. They impart a matte finish to the face. Patients who desire a shiny or moist semimatte facial appearance should avoid powder, since it will absorb the oil in the foundation, thus destroying the "dewy" look. Patients with dry complexions may also wish to avoid facial powder, since it can further dry the skin. The oil-absorbing abilities of facial powder are extremely valuable, however, for the patient with an oily complexion prone to develop a facial shine.

Adverse Reactions

The incidence of allergic contact dermatitis to facial powder itself is low; however, added fragrances may pose a problem. A more common problem with facial powders is irritant contact dermatitis due to coarse particulate matter, such as nacreous pigments, in the formulation. Inhalation of the powders may cause problems in patients with asthma or vasomotor rhinitis. Facial powder may be open or closed patch tested "as is."

FACIAL BLUSHES AND ROUGES

Facial blushes and rouges are designed to enhance rosy cheek color. In many cases, rosy cheeks simply indicate vasomotor instability or fine telangiectatic mats from actinic damage; however, cheek color remains fashionable.

Formulation

"Blush" and "rouge" are actually synonyms for a cosmetic designed to add color to the cheeks, but to many consumers blush denotes a powdered product while rouge denotes a cream product. Powdered blushes are more popular and are formulated identically to compact face powder, except more vivid pigments are added. Since color rather than coverage is desired, powdered blushes do not contain much zinc oxide. Cream rouges are formulated like anhydrous foundations, which contain light esters, waxes, mineral oil, titanium dioxide, and pigments.[2] Some patients use lipstick on the cheeks as a form of cream rouge. Lipstick-type formulations used as cream rouge are known as "facial gleamers." Powdered blushes can be easily brushed over any foundation formulation, but cream rouges will remove and smudge oil-free and low oil content foundations. Cream rouges also do not perform well if the face is powdered.

Application

For a natural appearance, cheek color should be applied beginning at a point directly beneath the pupil on the fleshy part of the cheek, sweeping upward beyond the lateral eye (Fig. 2-1).[3] This placement is designed to create or accentuate high cheek bones, which are a desired quality among women.[4]

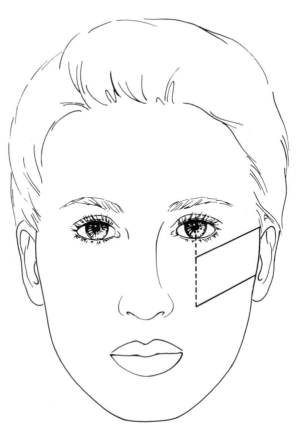

FIG. 2-1. Placement of blusher on the cheek.

Adverse Reactions

The adverse reaction concerns with blushes and rouges are identical to those for facial powders. The products can be open or closed patch tested "as is."

FACIAL BRONZING GELS AND COLOR WASHES

Facial bronzing gels and color washes are alternative products available to add facial color. If the product is intended to add color only to the cheeks, it is called a "get rouge," but if the product is designed to provide overall facial color, it is known as a "bronzing gel." Gel rouge is available in shades of red and orange, while bronzing gels, as the name suggests, are intended to give a tanned appearance.[5] Both products stain the skin and provide no coverage. They contain light esters, propylene glycol, alcohol, and water-soluble organic colors in a neutral aqueous gel. They must be applied and spread quickly, as the volatile vehicle yields a short playtime. Staining of the fingertips and clothing during application is a common problem.

Another product that provides facial color without coverage is a color wash. Color washes are liquid foundations with pigment but no titanium dioxide, frequently containing some pearl additive such as bismuth oxychloride or mica. Color washes can be worn alone or under a sheer foundation. They may not be applied over a foundation or on a powdered face. Color washes are more appropriate for patients with dry skin, while bronzing gels are more appropriate for patients with oily skin.

FACIAL BUFFERS AND HIGHLIGHTERS

Facial buffers and highlighters are formulated exactly like powdered facial blushes except that the color and amount of pearl may vary. Facial blushes are usually of an intense color, ranging from red to orange for accentuating the upper cheeks. Facial buffers, on the other hand, are usually a light pink or peach with a moderate amount of pearl. Their purpose is to blend other facial cosmetics. For example, after blush is applied to the cheek, a border forms where the color stops. Applying a facial buffer over the blush blends the edges of color into the natural skin tones. Facial buffers can also be used to blend eye shadows into the upper eyelid.

Facial highlighters are more intensely pigmented than facial blushes. They are available in deep burgundy, bronze, or brown and function to color and contour the face. For example, a bronze facial highlighter can be applied to the central forehead, nasal tip, and central chin to create the appearance of a tan since these three protuberant areas of the face generally are more deeply pigmented in a patient with recent sun exposure. Facial buffers and highlighters can be artfully used by the patient with facial defects to improve facial contour. This topic is discussed below under Corrective Facial Cosmetics.

FACIAL COVER STICKS

Facial cover sticks are intended for use under a facial foundation to cover imperfections. Facial cover sticks, also known as "under eye concealers," are matched to the skin color and applied to cover an abnormal skin color such as the redness of an acne lesion or the darkness of under eye circle.[6] These are maximum coverage products with high amounts of titanium dioxide. Other ingredients include mineral oil, waxes, pigments, and kaolin or talc. Formulations available in a roll-up stick contain more wax than cream formulations, which contain more oil. A popular packaging of the cream formulation is in a cylindrical tube with an insertable sponge tip applicator. The long-wearing, high-coverage characteristics of facial cover sticks require pigment suspended in an oil base. There are some products labeled as "oil-free"; however, they do contain silicone oils. Some cover products come in an acne medicated form and include sulfur, salicylic acid, or resorcinol.

FACIAL UNDERCOVER CREAMS

Facial undercover creams are designed to mask undesirable skin tones. They are formulated like cream foundations with oils, waxes, talc, and pigment. Undercover creams come in a variety of complementary colors and are intended to be applied under a full-coverage facial foundation. Green undercover creams are used to camouflage a reddish complexion created by such dermatologic conditions as rosacea, psoriasis, lupus, acne, or a facial nevus flammeus. The application of a green cover over underlying red skin produces a net result of brown under a foundation, since green mixed with red pigments produces a brown tone. A light purple undercover can be used by patients with a yellow complexion caused by renal failure or Oriental background to yield a pink skin tone. A peach-colored undercover can be used to mask the bluish tones of bruised skin. If the patient chooses to use an undercover cream, she must also commit herself to wearing a full line of facial cosmetics, since the cream by itself does not cover the defect. These products are more fully discussed in Chapter 7.

Another undercover product, known as a "white pearlized undercover," is an oil-based liquid makeup that contains increased amounts of titanium dioxide without any pigment. This undercover is designed for the patient with actinically damaged skin characterized by fine wrinkling, telangiectasia, and mottled pigmentation. The increased amount of titanium dioxide whitens the discolored skin, and the pearl created by bismuth oxychloride or mica minimizes the fine wrinkling.

SELF-TANNING CREAMS

Self-tanning creams produce a golden skin color overnight without sun exposure. The golden color is quite acceptable on persons with blonde or light brown hair who tend to have golden hues to their skin, but is not attractive on Mediterranean individuals with an olive complexion or extremely fair persons with pink skin tones. The active ingredient is 3% to 5% dihydroxyacetone incorporated into a glycerin and mineral oil base to form a white cream that turns the stratum corneum golden.[7] Chemically, the dihydroxyacetone acts as a sugar to interact with amino acids in the stratum corneum to produce melanoidins.[8–11] Formulations are available for the face and body, but most do not incorporate a sunscreen nor is the golden skin color protective against actinic damage. Higher concentrations of dihydroxyacetone are used to produce darker coloring of the stratum corneum.

Allergic contact dermatitis from use of the product is infrequent, but several cases of dihydroyacetone allergy have been reported.[12] Self-tanning creams can be open or closed patch tested "as is."

The color is not permanent and is lost as the stratum corneum desquamates; thus continued use is necessary. The major disadvantage of the product is that it stains all contacted skin surfaces, including the palms of the hands, if it is not removed, and will produce deeper staining of the follicular ostia, seborrheic keratosis, actinic keratosis, porokeratosis, and icthyotic skin. Many patients are not aware that they have these skin conditions until the self-tanning cream highlights the irregularity.

BRONZING POWDERS

Bronzing powders are identical in formulation to face powders except for the addition of different pigments. The powder is stroked from a compact with a powder sponge or puff and applied to the body. The product is usually dusted down the central face, neck, and shoulders to simulate a tan.[13] The powder is easily removed by rubbing and provides slight physical sun protection due to the titanium dioxide in most formulations.

TINTED MOISTURIZERS

Some moisturizers contain brown pigment that provides a sheer tanned appearance in addition to possessing emollient qualities. Technically, it is impossible to separate a tinted moisturizer from a sheer, moisturizing facial foundation.

Usually, a facial foundation contains titanium dioxide to provide coverage to underlying cutaneous pigment defects whereas a tinted moisturizer does not, but the distinction is slight.

FACIAL COSMETICS FOR ACNE PATIENTS

Facial cosmetics selection for acne patients poses a challenge for the dermatologist. The acne patient is generally self-conscious about the blemishes on her/his complexion and is anxious to apply cosmetics that will completely mask the erythema, papules, and nodules that characterize acne. This patient will generally select the facial foundation with the longest wear and highest amount of coverage. These products are inevitably oil-based and extremely occlusive, resulting in additional facial oil and follicular irritation that may aggravate the underlying acne, necessitating further cosmetic application. High-coverage foundations also create a need to use blush, lipstick, and eye shadow, since they cover not only the acne lesions but all facial contours. Unfortunately, there is no optimal solution to this problem.

Facial powder can be extremely valuable for the acne patient. It can absorb oil, thus increasing the wear of oil-free facial foundations that will rub off or separate when mixed with sebum. Powder can also increase the coverage of an oil-free foundation. To obtain maximum benefit from powder and eliminate a ''floured'' facial appearance, the powder must be properly selected and applied. A loose transparent powder is best. Transparent powders come in tones of pink, yellow, or brown, and the patient should select the tone that best matches her underlying complexion and foundation. The fingertips are then dipped in the loose powder, and it is massaged into the foundation over the entire face. Rubbing the powder into the foundation is superior to dusting the powder onto the face, since it adheres more closely to the foundation, resulting in increased foundation wearability and better oil control. Rubbing also eliminates the ''floured'' facial look and imparts a smooth feel. A fluffy brush is then used to dust away excess powder. The technique may be repeated if oily breakthrough occurs. Oily breakthrough occurs when the foundation has absorbed as much oil as possible, resulting in the development of a facial shine due to oil seeping through the layer of foundation.

Powder can also be used to increase the coverage of oil-free foundations in acne blemish areas. Foundation is dabbed onto the acne lesions with the fingertips and allowed to dry. Loose transparent powder is then massaged into the area. Another layer of foundation is then applied and the process repeated until the desired coverage is achieved. Foundation is then applied to the entire face and finished with a facial powder rub as previously described.

Loose powders usually contain less oil than pressed compact powders and are therefore recommended for the acne patient. Most loose talc-based powders will work well, except for those that contain ground particulate matter, such as walnut shell powder. These products tend to encourage the formation of closed comedones and milia. Perhaps this is due to sharp-edged particles occluding the follicle, forming closed comedones or causing epidermal damage resulting in milia.

Acne patients should also select powdered and gel facial cosmetic formulations over oily creams. This means that powdered blush should be selected over cream rouge and bronzing gels should be selected over color washes. Powdered blush can be used effectively by acne patients to absorb oil and provide a reddish color to the upper cheeks, which may aid in blending acne blemishes. For light-skinned acne patients, bronzing gels can effectively add facial color without worsening acne or creating the need to wear a full line of facial cosmetics.

FACIAL COSMETICS FOR MATURE PATIENTS

Mature patients generally have dry skin with wrinkling and other effects of actinic damage. In the presence of dry skin, oil-absorbing products such as powders should be avoided. If a powder is desired, it should be low in magnesium carbonate and zinc oxide, since these two substances have an astringent or drying effect on the face. Powder also tends to migrate into the creases, accentuating wrinkling. However, powdered blushes are still recommended over cream rouges. Cream rouge does not spread well when applied over a foundation of any type. Facial bronzing gels are also difficult to apply over furrowed skin. If increased facial color is desired, a color wash used alone or under an oil-containing foundation is preferable.

Cream undercover cosmetics perform well on mature skin because their oil base can replace a facial moisturizer. Green undercover on the upper cheeks is especially useful in the mature patient with fine facial telangiectasias. The green undercover must be covered with an oil-containing foundation. Powdered blush applied to the upper cheeks will also help to blend the telangiectasias. White pearlized undercover can be used beneath a foundation to minimize wrinkling and improve uneven facial pigmentation.

FACIAL COSMETICS FOR MEN

Facial colored cosmetics for men have been slowly gaining acceptance, but they still, for the most part, remain unpopular.[14,15] Men in the entertainment industry use cosmetics designed for women and apply the cosmetics in the same manner as women to accentuate facial color.[16] For average daily wear, facial cosmetics are impractical for men. The beard precludes even application of facial foundations, since the pigment tends to adhere to the hair shafts and prominent follicular structures. The coarse texture of male skin also is accentuated. If total facial color is required, facial foundations should be avoided in favor of bronzing gels, discussed above. This product stains the skin, thus providing color, but does not provide coverage. If coverage is required, men should select opaque cover cosmetics. Color can be effectively added to the cheeks, forehead, nose, and chin with powdered facial blushes. Facial contouring techniques with facial buffers or highlighters and facial imperfection camouflage with cover sticks are the same as for women. A transparent facial powder dusted over the entire face can minimize the appearance of large pore structures and the "five o'clock shadow" created on the cheeks by regrowth of dark facial hair after early morning shaving. No nationally distributed colored cosmetic line developed especially for men is currently available.

FACIAL COSMETICS FOR CHILDREN

Colored facial cosmetics are available for young girls to adorn the face and cheeks. Most preadolescent and early adolescent girls do not want to "look like they wear makeup," but still want to go through the motions of applying cosmetics to their face. Popular facial cosmetics for this age group include transparent facial color gels and rouges. Transparent facial color gels and teenage rouges are similar in formulation except that color gels are more lightly colored for all-over application to the face while the rouge is brightly colored and only applied to the upper cheeks. They contain light esters, propylene glycol, alcohol, and water-soluble organic colors in a neutral aqueous gel. The product must be applied evenly and quickly to avoid streaking and stains everything it contacts, including fingertips.

CORRECTIVE FACIAL COSMETICS

Corrective cosmetics for facial lesions are based on the principle that dark colors make the lesions appear smaller and to recede while light colors make the lesions look larger and appear to come forward. This concept is illustrated in Figure 2-2, where the black oval appears recessed and smaller compared with the white oval. Powdered blush-type products are best suited for this purpose. Areas of the face that need to be lightened should be brushed with a light pink or peach pearled blush or buffer. Areas of the face that need to be darkened should be brushed with a deep plum or bronze matte finish blush or highlighter.

Cosmetic facial sculpting is most successful for optimizing the shape of the face, the size of the forehead and chin, or the contour of the nose. The perfect facial shape is oval and symmetrical about the midline, as this form is most pleasing to the eye. An oval face is one and one-half times as long as it is wide and should taper gradually from its widest dimension at the forehead to its

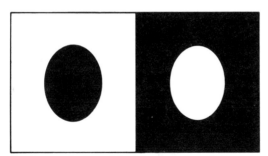

FIG. 2-2. The two fundamental rules of facial contouring: dark contours look smaller and appear to recede; light contours look larger and appear to come forward.

smallest dimension at the chin. The face should be divided into equal thirds from superior to inferior: forehead to the glabella, glabella to the subnasale, and subnasale to the base of the chin. The face should divide equally into fifths from ear to ear, with each fifth being the width of one eye.[17]

Other facial shapes are round, where the facial length is short; oblong, where the facial length is long; square, where the jaw is wide; diamond, where the forehead is small; triangular, where the cheeks are wide; and inverted triangular, where the jaw is narrow. By appropriately shading the face, the less optimal shapes described can more closely approximate a perfect oval.

For example, a round face should be shaded with a dark color along the lateral margins to deemphasize the increased width, whereas an oblong face should be shaded along the forehead and chin to deemphasize the increased length. A square face should be darkened bilaterally at the jaws. Both diamond and triangular faces should be lightened at the forehead for emphasis, and an inverted triangular face should be lightened at the chin.[18]

The same shading technique can also be used to correct a poorly formed forehead and chin. Low-set foreheads should have a light blush applied beneath the hairline, while high foreheads should have a dark blush applied here. A receding chin should have a light blush applied at the tip and sides. A double chin should be shaded with a dark blush under the entire jawbone.[19]

Facial recontouring is most useful on the nose, where hair, jewelry, or glasses cannot hide an abnormality. Figure 2-3 illustrates shading techniques. Areas to be darkened are cross-hatched, and areas to be lightened are outlined. Figure 2-3A demonstrates a broken nose that has healed crookedly with a deviation to the patient's left. The prominent upper left side of the nose is darkened, along with the lower right side and right tip. The opposite sides are lightened. A hook nose or aquiline nose (Fig. 2-3B) can also be minimized by darkening the hook along with the lateral nasal tips. A bulbous nose can be improved by shading the entire bulb on the tip and the lateral margins to the nasal root (Fig. 2-3C). Figures 2-3D and 2-3E demonstrate shading for long and short noses, respectively.[20]

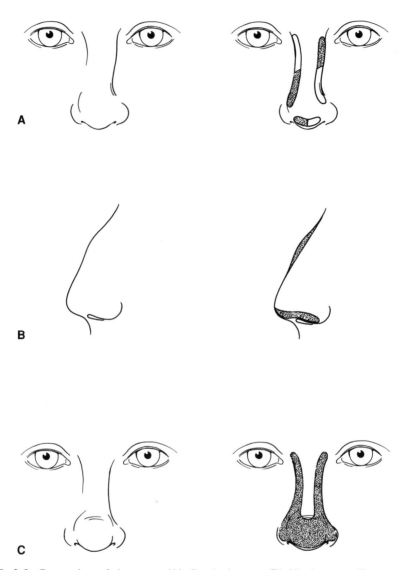

FIG. 2-3. Contouring of the nose. (**A**) Crooked nose. (**B**) Hook or aquiline nose. (**C**) Bulbous nose.

Corrective facial cosmetics are no substitute for a perfect face, and in some cases patients should be advised to consider surgical revision. These suggestions may be offered to the patient who is awaiting surgery or the patient who has not previously considered cosmetics as a way of creating the illusion of a more perfect face.

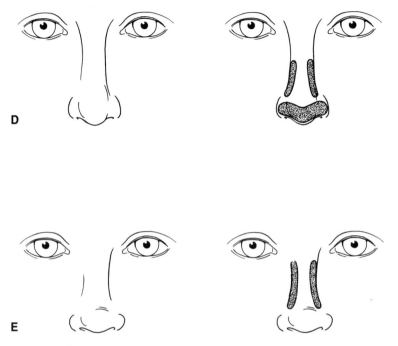

FIG. 2-3. *(continued)* **(D)** Long nose. **(E)** Short nose.

REFERENCES

1. Wetterhahn J: Loose and compact face powder. p. 921. In deNavarre MG (ed): The Chemistry and Manufacture of Cosmetics. 2nd Ed. Vol. IV. Allured Publishing Corporation, Wheaton, IL, 1988
2. Lanzet M: Modern formulations of coloring agents: facial and eye. p. 133. In Frost P, Horwitz SN (eds): Cosmetics for the Dermatologist. Mosby, St. Louis, 1982
3. Begoun P: Blue Eyeshadow Should Be Illegal. Beginning Press, Seattle, WA, 1986
4. Soldo BL, Drahos M: The Inside-Out Beauty Book. Fleming H. Revell Company, Old Tappan, NJ, 1978
5. Jackson EM: Tanning without the sun: accelerators, promoters, pills, bronzing gels, and self-tanning lotions. Am J Contact Dermatitis 5:38, 1994
6. Wesley-Hosford Z: Face Value. Bantam Books, Toronto, 1986
7. Levy SB: Dihydroxyacetone-containing sunless or self-tanning lotions. J Am Acad Dermatol 27:989, 1992
8. Maibach HI, Kligman AM: Dihydroxyacetone: a suntan-simulating agent. Arch Dermatol 35:161, 1960
9. Goldman L, Barkoff J, Blaney D et al: The skin coloring agent dihydroxyacetone. GP 12:96, 1960
10. Wittgenstein E, Berry HK: Reactions of dihydroxyacetone (DHA) with human skin callus and amino compounds. J Invest Dermatol 36:283, 1961

11. Wittgenstein E, Berry HK: Staining of skin with dihydroxyacetone. Science 132: 894, 1960
12. Morren M, Dooms-Goossens A, Heidbuchel M et al: Contact allergy to dihydroxy-acetone. Contact Dermatitis 25:326, 1991
13. Draelos ZD: Cosmetics to imitate a summer tan. Cosmet Dermatol 3:8, 1990
14. Dichter P, Fils VM: The men's product explosion. Cosmet Toilet 100 November 1985:75, 1985
15. Kavaliunas DR, Nacht S, Bogardus RE: Men's skin care needs. Cosmet Toilet 100 Novmber 1985:29, 1985
16. Draelos ZD: Cosmetics designed for men. Cosmet Dermatol 5:14, 1992
17. Powell N, Humphreys B: Proportions of the Aesthetic Face. Thieme-Stratton Inc, New York, 1984
18. Taylor P: Milady's Makeup Techniques: Milady Publishing Company, Albany, NY, 1994
19. Miller C: 8 Minute Makeovers. Acropolis Books Ltd., Washington, DC, 1984
20. Newman A, Ebenstein RS: Adrian Arpel's 851 Fast Beauty Fixes and Facts. GP Putnam's Sons, New York, 1985

3

Eyelid Cosmetics

The eyes, more than any other body part, reveal inner thoughts and emotion. Decoration of the eyelids was practiced by 4000 bc. Green powder made from malachite was heavily applied to both the upper and lower eyelids accompanied by dark kohl eyeliner paste composed of powdered antimony, burnt almonds, black copper oxide, and brown clay ocher. The eyeliner paste was stored in a pot and moistened with saliva. Eyelid glitter composed of ground beetle shells was also popular.[1] Modern colored eyelid cosmetics became popular between 1959 and 1962 (Table 3-1).[2]

EYE SHADOWS

Formulation

Eye shadows are available as pressed powders, anhydrous creams, emulsions, sticks, and pencils. Color variety is extensive, but no coal tar derivatives can be used in the eye area. Only the following purified, natural colors or inorganic pigments can be used in the United States as a result of the Food, Drug and Cosmetic Act of 1938[3]:

Iron oxides
Titanium dioxide (alone or combined with mica)
Copper, aluminum, and silver powder
Ultramarine blue, violet, and pink
Manganese violet
Carmine
Chrome oxide and hydrate
Iron blue
Bismuth oxychloride (alone or on mica or talc)
Mica

Variation in eye shadow surface texture can range from dull to a pearled shine to an iridescent finish. Titanium dioxide is used in pastel matte (dull) finish

Table 3-1. Eyelid Cosmetics

	Application Technique	Wearability	Main Ingredients
Pressed powder	Brush	Long	Talc, pigment in oily base (mineral oil, beeswax, or lanolin) with surface finish additives (titanium dioxide, bismuth oxychloride, mica, fish scale essence, ground metal particles)
Anhydrous cream	Finger	Waterproof, short	Pigment in petrolatum, cocoa butter, or lanolin
Automatic emulsion	Wand	Waterproof, moderate	Petroleum distillate, cyclomethicone, beeswax, pigment
Stick	Pencil type	Waterproof, short	Petrolatum, mineral oil, wax, pigment
Pencil	Pencil type	Waterproof, moderate	Petrolatum, wax, pigment
Unpigmented setting cream	Finger	Long	Beeswax, talc, cyclomethicone

Wearability: very short = 2 hours, short = 3 hours, moderate = 4 hours, long = 8 hours.

eye shadows to improve coverage. However, it is not found in frosted (pearled shine) finish eye shadows, since it tends to mask the desired pearled effect. Bismuth oxychloride (BiOCl), mica, and fish scale essence are the standard materials used to produce a pearly shine. A metallic (iridescent) finish is provided by copper, brass, aluminum, gold, or silver powders.

Pressed powder eye shadows are the most popular formulation and are applied to the eyelid by lightly stroking a soft sponge-tipped applicator across the skin. They are predominantly talc, with pigments and zinc or magnesium stearate used as a binder. Kaolin or chalk may be added to improve oil absorption and increase wearability. A water or oily binder system may also be used, with oily binder systems such as mineral oil, beeswax, or lanolin predominating. Powder eye shadows that are labeled ''creamy'' or ''enriched'' contain increased amounts of the oily binder.

Anhydrous cream eye shadows contain pigments in petrolatum, cocoa butter, or lanolin. These formulations are waterproof, but have a short wearing time due to their tendency to migrate into the eyelid folds, especially in patients with oily complexions or redundant eyelid skin. The product is applied with the finger and gently rubbed across the eyelid skin. Anhydrous cream eye shadows have also been formulated as an emulsion applied with a sponge-tipped applicator or wand withdrawn from a cylindrical tube and stroked across the eyelid. These products, known as ''automatic eye shadow,'' are also waterproof, with increased wear duration over the creams. They contain beeswax, cyclomethicone, and pigments in a volatile petroleum distillate vehicle.

The most popular anhydrous eye shadows are eye shadow sticks and pencils. They are composed of pigments in petrolatum, but have added waxes, such as paraffin, carnauba, or ozokerite wax, to allow extrusion of the product into a rod. Eye shadow sticks are in a roll-up tube and must be creamy to prevent drag, as they are rubbed across the eyelid skin. For this reason, eye shadow sticks tend to migrate into eyelid creases in oily complected patients or those with redundant eyelid skin. A more modern packaging is to encase the rod in wood, thus forming an eye shadow pencil that is rubbed across the eyelid. The pencil form is not as creamy as the eye shadow stick.

Application

Eye shadows are stroked or rubbed across the eyelid, depending on formulation. Selection of eye shadow color is a matter of personal preference and fashion, although colors complimentary to the natrual color of the iris are most attractive. Table 3-2 contains some basic guidelines for selecting an eye shadow color.

Adverse Reactions

The eyelid skin is the thinnest on the body and frequently affected by both irritant and allergic contact dermatitis.[4,5] The North American Contact Dermtatitis Group has determined that 12% of cosmetic reactions occur on the eyelid, but only 4% could be linked to eye makeup use.[6] Furthermore, it may be difficult to determine the etiology of the eyelid dermatitis with routine patch testing.[7] Many substances, such as nail polish, can be transferred to the eye area by the hands, complicating dermatologic evaluation.[8]

Thorough evaluation of eyelid dermatitis requires consideration of a variety

Table 3-2. Recommended Eye Shadow Colors Based on Natural Iris Color

Eye Color	Shadow Color	Effect
Blue	Brown	Intensifies blue
	Beige	Intensifies gray
	Pink	Provides contrast
	Plum	Provides contrast
Green or hazel	Charcoal	Intensifies green
	Brown	Intensifies gold
	Pink	Intensifies green
Brown	Light gray	Provides contrast
	Pink	Provides contrast
	Plum	Provides contrast

of entities. Maibach and Engasser[9] and Maibach et al.[10] have developed the concept of upper eyelid dermatitis syndrome, to include the following entities.

Mechanical rubbing
Irritant contact dermatitis
Allergic contact dermatitis
Infection
Photoirritation
Contact urticaria
Atopic dermatitis
Psoriasis
Collagen vascular disease
Conjunctivitis
Seborrheic blepharitis
Idiopathic causes

Once it has been determined that eye cosmetics are the source of the dermatitis, the distinction between irritant and allergic contact dermatitis must be made. Irritant contact dermatitis is more common than allergic contact dermatitis. Eye cosmetic ingredients associated with allergic contact dermatitis are listed in Table 3-3.[11,12]

Open or closed patch testing can be performed ''as is'' with eye shadows, but automatic emulsions should be allowed to dry throroughly prior to occlu-

Table 3-3. Cosmetic Ingredients Causing
Eyelid Allergic Contact Dermatitis

Preservatives[18]
    Parabens
    Phenyl mercuric acetate
    Imidazolidinyl urea
    Quaternium-15
    Potassium sorbate
Antioxidants
    Butylated hydroxyanisole[19]
    Butylated hydroxytoluene[19]
    Di-tert-butyl-hydroquinone[20]
Resins
    Colophony[21]
Pearlescent additives
    Bismuth oxychloride[22]
Emollients
    Lanolin[23]
    Propylene glycol[24]
Fragrances[25]
Pigment contaminants
    Nickel[26]

sion.[13] Use testing is recommended, however, for eye cosmetics: the product is placed at the corner of the eye for 5 consecutive nights and evaluated for allergic or irritant contact dermatitis.

EYE SHADOW SETTING CREAMS

Eye shadow setting creams are unpigmented and designed to provide an adherent base over which pigmented eye shadow can be applied. They increase the wearability of eye shadows and are most useful in oily complected patients or those with redundant eyelid skin who experience migration of eye shadow into eyelid creases. The setting cream is composed of beeswax, talc, and cyclomethicone. Beeswax seals the eyelid skin, while the talc provides increased adherence for the eye shadow pigment. Some newer cream eye shadows incorporate a setting cream for longer wear.

EYELID COSMETIC REMOVERS

Waterproof eye shadows must be removed with special removal products containing surfactants, such as cocamidopropyl betaine. These products may be oil-based or oil-free and can be designed to remove all eye cosmetics, including eyeliner and mascara. Allergic contact dermatitis has been linked to these eye cosmetic removers.[14]

EYELID COSMETICS FOR SENSITIVE SKIN PATIENTS AND CONTACT LENS WEARERS

Patients with sensitive skin and multiple allergies frequently have difficulty finding an eye shadow product that does not burn or itch upon application. Certainly, any eye shadow applied over broken or inflamed skin will cause discomfort. Patients with these problems should avoid all eye cosmetics until healing has occurred. They should also be evaluated for upper eyelid dermatitis syndrome, as previously discussed.

To minimize recurrence of dermatitis, allergic patients should avoid shiny, frosted, or iridescent eye shadows; the bismuth oxychloride, mica, metal powders, or fish scale essence may contribute to an irritant contact dermatitis. These substances may have sharp-edged particles that can produce pruritus. Matte finish eye shadows are therefore recommended for the sensitive skin patient. Some patients also experience more irritation with darker eye shadow colors, such as deep purple, forest green, or navy blue. Selection of a lighter shade product in peach, pink, or tan may resolve the irritancy.

Creams, sticks, and pencils may cause irritation as the product is rubbed on the eyelid. The friction from this rubbing may cause tears to develop in the eyelid skin, increasing the probability of irritation. Automatic eye shadows contain volatile vehicles, emulsifiers, and surfactants that may also be irritating. Thus, matte finish pressed powder eye shadow applied gently with a sponge applicator have the least potential for irritation.[15]

Matte finish eye shadows are also recommended for contact lens wearers because the mica, metal powders, or fish scale essence in frosted finish eye shadows may lodge under the contact lens, causing irritation or possibly corneal abrasion. It is advisable to insert the contact lense prior to application of an appropriate eye shadow and to take the lense out prior to cosmetic removal.

EYELID COSMETIC FOR ACNE PATIENTS

Cream, stick, and pencil eye shadows do not perform well on acne patients with oily complexions. Since these products are oil based, the patient's sebum mixes with the eye shadow, encouraging migration into folds. Placing an unpigmented eye shadow setting cream beneath the colored eye shadow may improve wearability slightly, but the oil-based eye shadow product may exacerbate acne or increase follicular irritation. Pressed powder eye shadows are recommended for acne patients, since the talc base has oil-control qualities and does not place additional oils on the face. For extended wear, the powder eye shadow can be applied with a moistened sponge applicator.

EYELID COSMETICS FOR MATURE PATIENTS

Mature patients should select eyelid cosmetics that minimize the appearance of redundant skin on the upper eyelid. Redundant skin encourages migration of cream, stick, and pencil eye shadows into the folds, drawing attention to the creases. Pressed powder eye shadows are recommended, even though patients may think that rich creamy eye shadows aid in moisturizing dry eyelids. Frosted finish and iridescent eye shadows also draw attention to the crepe texture of the redundant skin. Matte finish or light shine eye shadows are recommended. All eye shadows should be placed over a eye shadow setting cream in mature patients. Mature patients can also extend the wearing time of powder eye shadow by applying it with a moistened sponge applicator.

The mature skin on the upper eyelid may also demonstrate dyspigmentation from lentigines or telangiectasias. Mature patients may be tempted to select vivid, dark eye shadow colors to cover the undesirable eyelid skin color. However, vivid colors draw attention to the upper eyelid and should be avoided in favor of pastels and muted colors (pink, bluish gray, mauve, tan, peach). Dyspigmentation can be covered by applying facial foundation to the upper eyelid followed by pressed powder eye shadow. Applying facial foundation to the upper eyelid also improves eye shadow wearability.

EYE COSMETIC CAMOUFLAGE TECHNIQUES

Eye cosmetics can be used to correct the appearance of eye defects arising from surgery, congenital anomalies, or dermatoheliosis. The correction is effected by carefully selecting eye shadow colors and placing them appropriately on the eyelids.

Attractive eye placement is such that the inner canthal distance is equal to the width of one eye (Fig. 3-1). If the eyes are closer together, the patient

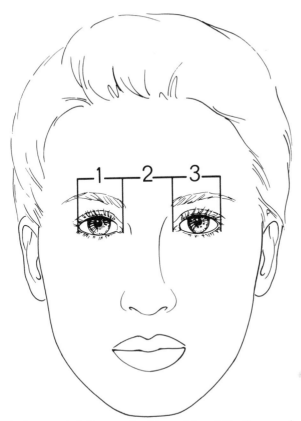

FIG. 3-1. The Intercanthal distance should equal the width of one eye in a well-proportioned face.

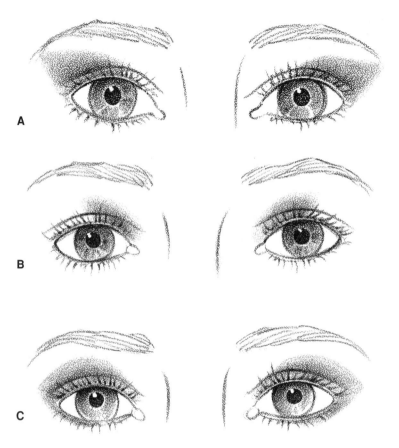

FIG. 3-2. Contouring of eyes **(A)** to make hypoteloric eyes appear more widely set, **(B)** to make hyperteloric eyes appear more closely set, **(C)** to enlarge small eyes,

appears hypoteloric; if the eyes are further apart, the patient appears hyperteloric. Abnormal intercanthal distance is congenital and may or may not be associated with other anomalies. A more pleasing appearance can be imparted to hypoteloric eyes by sweeping deeply colored eye shadow up and out from the center to outer corners of the lid (Fig. 3-2A). Hyperteloric eyes are deemphasized by placing deeply colored eye shadow from the inner canthus to the central eyelid (Fig. 3-2B). The color draws attention away from the abnormality.[16]

Deeply colored eye shadows can also be effectively used to correct the size of the eyes. Female patients who have had skin cancer on the eyelid margin may appear to have smaller eyes due to wedge resection. The eyes can be made to appear larger if deeply colored eye shadow is placed along the lateral orbital ridge and eyebrow with a small amount placed beneath the lateral lower lash line (Fig. 3-2C). A light colored eye shadow should be placed medially beneath the eyebrow. Large eyes in a female patient with exophthalmos due to hyperthy-

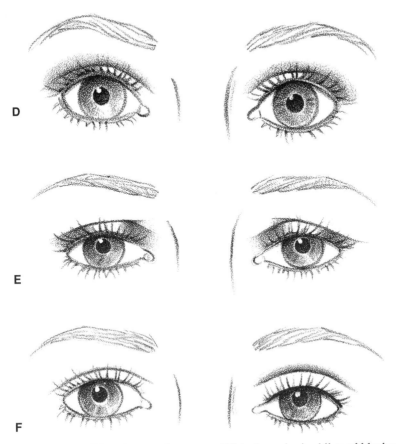

FIG. 3-2. *(continued)* (**D**) to decrease large eyes, (**E**) to deemphasize bilateral blepharochalasis, and (**F**) to deemphasize unilateral ptosis.

roidism can be made to appear smaller by applying a dark eye shadow only in the crease and on the lateral eyelid (Fig. 3-2D). A light eye shadow is then placed on the medial eyelid.[17]

Probably the most common cosmetic eye problem seen in female patients is blepharochalasis, commonly known as drooping or hooded eyelids. A drooping eyelid can be cosmetically corrected by covering the entire eyelid from the lash line to the crease with a light matte finish eye shadow (Fig. 3-2E). A complementary matte finish eye shadow two to three shades darker should be applied on the medial and lateral eyelids, leaving the area above the iris a lighter color. Sometimes unilateral ptosis develops following Bell's palsy or surgery. Normally, the upper eyelid should touch the superior border of the iris and the lower eyelid should touch the inferior border of the iris. More dramatic eye makeup should be applied to the drooping eyelid. Both eyes should be initially colored as illustrated in Figure 3-2E; however, a brown eye shadow crayon should be used on the dropping eyelid to apply a line in the crease and above the lash line (Fig. 3-2F).

Unfortunately, none of these suggestions for eye recontouring can restore the eye to its normal appearance. The intention is to provide the physician with some suggestions to share with female patients who are distraught about their appearance following surgery or as a result of the process of aging.

REFERENCES

1. Panati C: Extraordinary Origins of Everyday Things. Harper & Row Publishers, New York, 1987
2. Wells FV, Lubowe II: Rouge and eye make-up. p. 173. In: Cosmetics and the Skin. Reinhold Publishing Corporation, New York, 1964
3. Lanzet M: Modern formulations of coloring agents: facial and eye. p. 138. In Frost P, Horowitz SN (eds): Principles of Cosmetics for the Dermatologist. CV Mosby, St. Louis, 1982
4. Fisher AA: Cosmetic dermatitis of the eyelids. Cutis 34:216, 1984
5. Valsecchi R, Imberti G, Martino D, Cainelli T: Eyelid dermatitis: an evaluation of 150 patients. Contact Dermatitis 27:143, 1992
6. Adams RM, Maibach HI: A five-year study of cosmetic reactions. J Am Acad Dermatol 13:1062, 1985
7. Wolf R, Perluk H: Failure of routine patch test results to detect eyelid dermatitis. Cutis 49:133, 1992
8. Nethercott JR, Nield G, Linn Holness D: A review of 79 cases of eyelid dermatitis. J Am Acad Dermatol 21:223, 1989
9. Maibach HI, Engasser PG: Dermatitis due to cosmetics. p. 378. In Fisher AA (ed): Contact Dermatitis. 3rd Ed. Lea & Febiger, Philadelphia, 1986
10. Maibach HI, Engasser P, Ostler B: Upper eyelid dermatitis syndrome. Dermatol Clin 10:549, 1992
11. deGroot AC, Weyland JW, Nater JP: Face cosmetics. In Unwanted Effects of Cosmetics and Drugs Used in Dermatology. Elsevier, Amsterdam, 1994
12. Pascher F: Adverse reactions to eye area cosmetics and their management. J Soc Cosmet Chem 33:249, 1982
13. Van Ketel WG: Patch testing with eye cosmetics. Contact Dermatitis 5:402, 1979
14. Ross JS, White IR: Eyelid dermatitis due to cocamidopropyl betaine in an eye make-up remover. Contact Dermatitis 25:64, 1991
15. Draelos ZK: Eye cosmetics. Dermatol Clin 9:1, 1991
16. Greene A, Pomerance M: The Successful Face. Summit Books, New York, 1985
17. Arpel A: 851 Fast Beauty Fixes and Facts. GP Putnam's Sons, New York, 1985
18. Marks JG, DeLeo VA: Preservatives and vehicles. p. 107. In: Contact and Occupational Dermatology. CV Mosby, St. Louis, 1992
19. White IR, Lovell CR, Cronin E: Antioxidants in cosmetics. Contact Dermatitis, 11:265, 1984
20. Calnan CD: Ditertiary butylhydroquinone in eye shadow. Contact Dermatitis Newslett 14:402, 1973
21. Fisher AA: Allergic contact dermatitis due to rosin (colophony) in eyeshadow and mascara. Cutis 42:505, 1988

22. Eiermann HJ, Larsen W, Maibach HI, Taylor JS: Prospective study of cosmetic reactions: 1977–1980, J Am Acad Dermatol 6:909, 1982
23. Schorr WF: Lip gloss and gloss-type cosmetics. Contact Dermatitis Newslett 14: 408, 1973
24. Hannuksela M, Pirila V, Salo OP: Skin reactions to propylene glycol. Contact Dermatitis 1:112, 1975
25. Larsen WG: Cosmetic dermatitis due to a perfume. Contact Dermatitis 1:142, 1975
26. Goh CL, Ng SK, Kwok SF: Allergic contact dermatitis from nickel in eyeshadow. Contact Dermatitis 20:380, 1989

4

Eyelash Cosmetics

Eyelash cosmetics include mascaras, eyeliners, eyelash dyes, and artificial eyelashes (Table 4-1). Contact lens wearers, sensitive skin patients, acne patients, and mature patients have special eyelash cosmetic needs.

MASCARA

Mascara, whose application dates to Biblical times, is the most commonly used eyelash cosmetic. Its purpose is to darken, thicken, and lengthen the eyelashes. Since the eyelashes form a frame for the eye, luxuriant eyelashes can attract attention to this expressive facial feature. Most women consider long eyelashes a prerequisite to being attractive.

History

The original mascara worn by women of many ancient civilizations was kohl, based on antimony trisulphide. Mascara was subsequently refined into a cake composed of sodium stearate soaps and lampblack. The product was mixed with water and stroked from the cake with a brush and applied to the eyelashes. This formulation produced eye irritation on contact due to the sodium stearate and was reformulated with triethanolamine stearate. Beeswax was subsequently added to allow the product to be somewhat water-resistant.[1]

Formulation

Mascaras must be carefully formulated to allow easy and even application without smudging, irritancy, or toxicity. Coal tar colors are prohibited by the U.S. Food, Drug and Cosmetic Act for use on the eyelashes. Therefore, mascara colorants must be selected from vegetable colors or inorganic pigments and lakes. Colors employed include iron oxide to produce black, ultramarine blue

Table 4-1. Eyelash Cosmetics

Eyelash Cosmetic	Main Ingredients	Function	Adverse Reactions
Cake mascara	Soap and pigments	Darken and thicken eyelashes	Irritation due to soaps
Cream mascara	Vanishing base and pigment	Darken and thicken eyelashes	Irritant contact dermatitis
Water-based liquid mascara	Waxes, pigments, and resins	Darken and thicken eyelashes	Irritant and allergic contact dermatitis
Solvent-based liquid mascara	Petroleum distillates, pigments, and waxes	Darken and thicken eyelashes	Irritant and allergic contact dermatitis
Water/ solvent mascara	Water-in-oil or oil-in-water emulsion	Darken and thicken eyelashes	Irritant and allergic contact dermatitis
Cake eyeliner	Talc, pigment, and binders	Define eyelash line	Minimal
Liquid eyeliner	Latex or other polymers and pigment	Define eyelash line	Irritant contact dermatitis
Pencil eyeliner	Waxes and pigment	Define eyelash line	Minimal
Eyeliner tatooing	Tatoo pigments	Permanently define lash line	Minimal
Eyelash dyes	See chart in Chapter 16	Darken eyelashes	Irritant and allergic contact dermatitis
Artificial eyelashes	Human or synthetic hair fibers	Thicken eyelashes	Irritant contact dermatitis to lashes, allergic contact dermatitis to glue

to create navy, and umber (brown ochre) or burnt sienna (a mixture of hydrated ferric oxide with manganic oxide) or synthetic brown oxide to create brown.[2]

Mascaras are available in several modern formulations: cake, cream, and liquid. The liquid mascaras can be further divided into water-based, solvent-based, and a water/solvent hybrid.

Cake Mascara

Cake mascara consists of a soap and pigments compressed into a cake. The cake is stroked with a water-moistened brush and applied to the eyelashes. Unfortunately, this form is not water-resistant and smudges with tears, perspiration, or rain. Furthermore, the soaps are somewhat irritating to the eye. Less irritating soaps, such as triethanolamine stearate, and waxes have been subsequently added to make the mascara less irritating and more water-resistant.

Cake mascaras remained popular until the 1960s, when cream and liquid preparations were introduced, which provided greater ease of application. Cake mascaras are still available and may be appropriate for patients who have developed eyelid or conjunctival irritation to the newer formulations.

Cream Mascara

Cream mascaras were developed after cake mascaras, quickly becoming popular due to their lesser propensity to run with moisture contact. Additionally, they did not clump or cake as easily on the eyelashes. The product consisted of pigment suspended in a vanishing cream base that was brushed from a tube onto the eyelashes.

Liquid Mascara

Liquid mascara has largely replaced cake and thicker cream mascaras since development of the automatic mascara tube. This invention consists of a tube into which a round brush is inserted through a small aperture to remove a metered amount of product.[3]

Water-based Water-based mascaras are so named because they are formulated of waxes (beeswax, carnauba wax, synthetic waxes), in addition to pigments (iron oxides, chrome oxides, ultramarine blue, carmine, titanium dioxide) and resins dissolved in water. They are classified as oil-in-water emulsions. The water evaporates readily, creating a fast-drying product that thickens and darkens the lashes. The product is water-soluble, allowing for easy removal, but unfortunately smudges with perspiration and tearing. Some water-based mascaras are labeled ''water-resistant'' if they contain an increased amount of wax or a polymer to improve adherence of pigment to the lashes.

Water-based mascaras are easily contaminated with bacteria, which readily grow in water, and must include preservatives, usually parabens. Thus, these products may potentially cause an allergic reaction in paraben-sensitive individuals; however, water-based mascaras are generally the least sensitizing of the mascara types. Some patients may experience a contact irritancy from the emulsifiers required to maintain the pigment in solution.

Specialty additives can be incorporated into the formulation to enhance the cosmetic appearance of the lashes. These substances include hydrolyzed animal protein to condition lashes, nylon or rayon fibers to elongate lashes, and polyvinylpyrollidone (PVP) resins to decrease smudging.

Solvent-based Solvent-based mascaras are formulated with petroleum distillates to which pigments (iron oxides, chrome oxides, ultramarine blue, carmine, titanium dioxide) and waxes (candelilla wax, carnauba wax, ozokerite, hydrogenated castor oil) are added, thus making them waterproof. As a result, the product performs well with perspiration and tearing, but removal is difficult and requires an oil-based lotion or cream. Deposits can form on the lashes if the product is incompletely removed. Care must be taken to avoid smudging the product immediately after application, as solvent-based mascaras have a prolonged drying time.

Preservatives are still added, but microbial contamination is not a great problem since the petroleum-based solvent is antibacterial. Some products also contain talc or kaolin to improve lash thickening and nylon or rayon fibers to lengthen lashes. Solvent-based mascaras can be an eye irritant.

Water/solvent hybrid Some mascaras combine both solvent-based and water-based systems to form either a water-in-oil or oil-in-water emulsion. The idea is to create an optimal product that thickens with a short drying time like the water-based mascaras, but provides waterproof lash separation like a solvent-based mascara. The water in the formulation requires incorporation of a good preservative system.

Application

Modern liquid mascaras, available in a tube with a multitufted applicator brush, have virtually replaced cake and cream type mascaras. The applicator is inserted into the tube between uses, providing numerous opportunities to inoculate bacteria into the mascara. The most dangerous of these bacteria is *Pseudomonas aeruginosa*. Even though mascaras contain antibacterials, it is still wise to discard all mascara tubes after 3 months and not allow multiple persons to use the same mascara tube.[4] Persons susceptible to infection or who are known bacterial carriers should select solvent-based or disposable mascaras.

Mascaras are available in a variety of formulas to coordinate with current color and fashion styles. Color selection is wide, with various shades of blacks and browns most commonly seen, but pinks, greens, yellows, purples, and blues are also available. Even unpigmented mascara is available for those who wish to lengthen but not darken lashes.

Mascara styles, dictated by fashion, are based on the type of applicator brush employed. If thick eyelashes are fashionable, lash-thickening mascaras are used with a larger, longer bristled brush applicator to apply mascara generously. If long eyelashes are fashionable, lash-lengthening mascaras with a short bristle brush are used to apply successive thin mascara coats and increase lash separation.

Adverse Reactions

The most feared adverse reaction to mascaras is that of infection, particularly *Pseudomonas aeruginosa* corneal infections, which can permanently destroy visual acuity.[5,6] *Staphylococcus epidermidis* and *Staphylococcus aureus* organisms can also proliferate in contaminated mascaras.[7] Infections are more common if the eyeball is traumatized with the infected mascara. As mentioned previously, individuals with recurrent bacterial infections due to colonization should probably select solvent-based mascaras.[8]

Fungal organisms can also contaminate mascaras and result in eye infection.[9] This is rarer and usually found only in patients who are immunocompromised or wear contact lenses.

The pigment contained within mascaras can result in conjunctival pigmentation, if the mascara is washed into the conjunctival sac by lacrimal fluid.[10] This colored particulate matter can be observed on the upper margin of the tarsal conjunctiva. Histologically, the pigment is seen within macrophages and extracellularly with varying degrees of lymphocytic infiltrate. Electron microscopy suggests that ferritin, carbon, and iron oxides are present within the tissues.[11] Unfortunately, there is no treatment for the condition, which fortunately is usually asymptomatic.

Allergic contact dermatitis has been reported to the rosin (colophony)[12] and dihydroabietyl alcohol (Abitol)[13,14] contained in some mascaras. But waterproof eye cosmetic removal products, used to remove solvent-based mascaras, can also be a source of eyelid dermatitis.[15] Mascaras can be open or closed patch tested ''as is,'' but should be allowed to dry thoroughly prior to closed patch testing to avoid an irritant reaction from the volatile vehicle.

EYELINER

Eyeliner defines the margins of the eye. It is placed immediately outside and sometimes inside the lash line. The color and placement of eyeliner are dictated by fashion. In the 1960s, a well-defined, thin black line drawn outside the upper and lower lash line was considered appropriate; however, the 1980s look was to use a subdued gray or deep blue smudged thick line outside the lower lash line only. The look of the 1990s is a thick sharp black line surrounding the entire eye with extension beyond the lateral canthus, a look sometimes termed a ''cat eye.''

Formulation

Eyeliner is available in cake, liquid, and pencil forms. Cake eyeliner has the same composition as eye shadow, except for the addition of surfactants promoting formation of a paste when the powder is mixed with water. Cake eyeliner has largely been replaced by liquid eyeliner, which contains the same pigments premixed in a water-soluble latex base. Latex-based liquid eyeliners contain water, cellulose gum, thickeners (magnesium aluminum silicate), and styrene-butadiene latex. These products are packaged as marking pens or in the same form as mascaras, with a cylindrical tube and unitufted applicator brush. Automatic eyeliners are based on polymers, such as an ammonium acrylate copolymer, that leave a pigmented film after drying.[16]

Pencil type eyeliners are popular due to their application ease. Automatic liquid eyeliners create a defined line that requires a steady artistic hand for application, but pencil eyeliners give a smudged look and require less application skill. Pencil eyeliners contain natural and synthetic waxes combined with pigments, mineral or vegetable oils, and lanolin derivatives that are extruded into rods and encased in wood. The pencil is then sharpened to the desired tip, which can be thin or broad depending on the patient's preference. Resharpening also removes exposed eyeliner, thus decreasing contamination.

Application

The application method used for eyeliners depends largely on fashion. The cake, liquid, or pencil is stroked across the upper and/or lower eyelid in the amount and position desired.

Adverse Reactions

Eyeliners are subject to the same bacterial and fungal contamination as mascaras, especially if the liquid form is chosen. But the main adverse reaction is conjunctival pigmentation, also seen with mascaras.[17] This problem is more commonly associated with eyeliner when it is applied within the lower lid margin. Usually blue eyeliner is used in this location to create the appearance of whiter sclera. This practice is unsafe.

Open and closed patch testing can be performed ''as is,'' but liquid eyeliner should be allowed to dry prior to occlusion.

EYELINER TATTOOING

Eyeliner tattooing, practiced by ophthalmologists, dermatologists, plastic surgeons, and some beauty operators, involves the intradermal insertion of black pigment, or other colored pigments such as brown or navy blue, on or outside of the upper and lower eyelash line. The pigment is inserted into the upper dermis at a constant depth by punctures created with a specially designed needle. The black, brown, green, or navy blue pigments are of low allergenic potential, accounting for the rare incidence of side effects.

Eyeliner tattooing has gained popularity among entertainment personalities, both male and female; however, for the average patient, permanent eyeliner does not allow the fashion versatility most persons desire. Patients with permanent eyelash loss may wish to consider eyeliner tattooing, which can be applied as outlined below under Corrective Eyelash Cosmetics. The tattooing should be done in a thin line so that the patient can apply a colored eyeliner pencil, if desired, to conform to fashion trends.

Patients who elect eyeliner tatooing should recognize that the color will fade with time, and some migration of the pigment is possible. The decision should be considered carefully prior to tatooing as the pigment is exceedingly difficult to remove once inserted into the dermis.

EYELASH DYES

Eyelash dyes are used by those persons who have light-colored eyelashes due to canities, natural hair color, or dermatoses such as vitiligo. No over-the-counter eyelash dyes are available due to the risk of eye damage. The U.S. Food and Drug Administration is currently attempting to outlaw the use of eyelash dyes. Some dyeing products are imported illegally from Europe, and some salons use products intended for scalp hair on the eyelashes. Products used by professional cosmetologists may contain either paraphenylenediamine dyes or metallic dyes. Further discussion of these products is included in Chapter 16.

Eyelash dyes should not be used more than every 3 weeks, since they are extremely irritating to the eye and can cause an irritant or allergic contact dermatitis. They are patch tested in the same manner as hair dyes.

Light-colored eyelashes can be darkened nicely with repeated application of a black or brown waterproof mascara containing talc or kaolin for lash thickening.

ARTIFICIAL EYELASHES

Artificial eyelashes are most popular among those in the entertainment industry, although they can be effectively used by patients who have thinned or absent eyelashes. Human hair and synthetic nylon lashes are available in varying colors and lengths, with costs ranging from $1 to $20. The lashes are attached to existing lashes on the upper or lower eyelids with a clear or pigmented methacrylate-based glue.

Artificial eyelashes are available as lash singlets, demilashes, and complete eyelashes. If lash singlets are used, several artificial lashes are glued to the patient's existing natural eyelashes. Demilashes, which are sparse artificial lashes, and complete lashes, which are dense artificial lashes, are glued immediately above the existing lash line. The eyelashes are removed with a solvent specially designed to remove the adhesive.

Lash singlets are difficult for the novice to apply, but can be used effectively at the lateral upper lash line to minimize the appearance of overhanging eyelids. Complete lashes are only appropriate for patients who have total loss of their own eyelashes. Demilashes are appropriate for the patient with short, thinned, or partially absent lashes. Demilashes are routinely worn by television personalities and can be quite natural appearing if the length is not exaggerated. Artificial eyelashes can be easily trimmed and customized with scissors.

Artificial eyelashes may be difficult to wear since the eyelashes themselves can irritate the eye, tarsal plate, and eyelid. Both irritant and allergic contact dermatitis can develop in response to the attachment glue and removal solvent. The most adherent eyelash glues are based in methacrylate, which is a known sensitizer.

EYELASH COSMETICS FOR SPECIAL NEEDS

Certain patients within a physician's practice may require careful selection of eyelash cosmetics. These are patients with allergies and/or contact lenses, as well as patients undergoing treatment for acne. Mature patients may require special eyelash cosmetic consultation to achieve an optimal appearance.

Eyelash Cosmetics for Sensitive Patients and/or Contact Lens Wearers

Eyelash cosmetics are commonly a source of irritant or allergic contact dermatitis. Most cases represent irritant dermatitis, since the Food and Drug Administration (FDA) closely regulates the chemicals, preservatives, and pigments used in eyelash cosmetics. Many sensitive skin patients find mascaras extremely irritating to their eyes and should be advised to wear a product specifically designed for allergic patients or a water-based mascara. Unpigmented mascaras seem to cause less irritation in some patients.

Application techniques can also minimize problems. Mascara can be applied in several coats only to the eyelash tips. This emphasizes the lashes while limiting mascara contact with the eye and skin. All waterproof mascaras should be avoided since the removal solvent and the rubbing required to remove the mascara may produce irritation. Artificial eyelashes and eyelash dyeing should also be avoided.

Pencil type eyeliners are better tolerated by some sensitive skin patients, but the eyeliner should never be placed inside the lower lid margin where it is removed by tearing and washed into the eye. This is not advisable as the pigment may tatoo the conjunctiva and possibly the lower palpebral sac.

Some contact lens wearers are bothered by mascaras that cake on the lashes and flake into the eye. Water-based mascaras are more likely to cake than solvent-based mascaras. Patients wearing sort contact lenses, with a high water content, may prefer waterproof, solvent-based mascaras, since these are less likely to bind to the lens. The pigment in mascaras and eyeliners can actually stain water- and gas-permeable contact lenses.

Eyelash Cosmetics for Acne and/or Oily Complected Patients

Many dermatologists recommend water-based cosmetics for their acne patients as a general rule, including water-based mascaras. Acne patients who have oily complexions may find that water-based mascaras are easily wetted by sebum, causing running and smudging. Solvent-based mascaras should be recommended for oily complected patients. The solvent-based mascaras can smudge if not adequately allowed to dry between coats, but, once dry, they are resistant to smudging.

Patients with oily complexions may also notice that pencil type eyeliners wear poorly and smudge. This is due to poor adhesion between the cosmetic and skin caused by sebum. Pencil type eyeliners will wear longer if a foundation covered by a loose powder is placed on the eyelid prior to eyeliner application. A polymer eyeliner could also be selected as an alternative.

Eyelash Cosmetics for Mature Patients

Eyelash cosmetics are important for the mature patient. Mascara can darken lashes lightened by canities and should be applied from the base of the lash to the tips in long strokes to cover the lashes completely with pigment. However, black mascara should be avoided in patients with recessed eyes, since it will only darken already shadowed eyes. Brown or navy blue mascara is more appropriate.

Eyelash length and thickness also tend to decrease in the mature patient. Eyelash length can be maximized by using a lengthening mascara containing nylon or rayon fibers. Each successive coat should dry completely to maximize lash length. Thickening mascaras containing talc or kaolin can increase lash size with repeated applications to the tips only.

The appearance of blepharochalasis can be minimized by lengthening the eyelashes, since some of the eyelash length is covered by redundant skin. An appearance of lengthened eyelashes can be created by curling the eyelashes with an eyelash curler immediately following mascara application. The eyelashes are placed in a rubber padded holder that bends them upward at a more acute angle. This decreases the natural curl of the eyelashes, making them appear longer, but can also promote eyelash breakage. Demilashes slightly longer than the patient's natural lashes can also be used to create the appearance of longer eyelashes.

CORRECTIVE EYELASH COSMETICS

Eyelashes function cosmetically as a frame for the eye. Unfortunately, they may thin due to age, alopecia areata, or eyelid scarring secondary to surgery or infections such as herpes zoster. Thinned or absent eyelashes result in nondescript eyes and loss of the main focal point for the face.

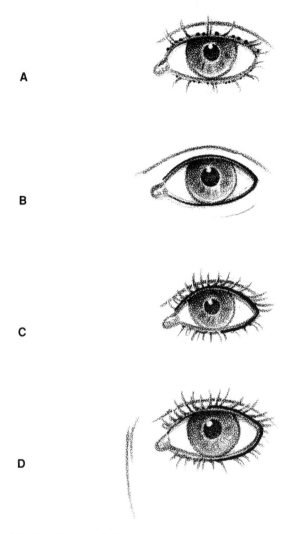

FIG. 4-1. Eye lining techniques (**A**) to reconstruct thinned or partially absent eyelashes, (**B**) to reconstruct totally absent eyelashes, (**C**) to enlarge small eyes, and (**D**) to widen hypoteloric eyes.

Eyeliner, mascara, and loose transparent face powder can be used to compensate cosmetically for thinned eyelashes. The first step is to use a liquid eyeliner to dot the upper and lower eyelid (Fig. 4-1A), creating the illusion of eyelashes. A light application of dark brown or black fibered mascara should then be applied to the remaining lashes. A powder brush is then dipped in loose powder and dusted on the wet mascara, with the eye closed to prevent powder from entering the eye. Another layer of mascara is then applied and the process repeated until the remaining lashes have been thickened to the desired degree. This technique is useful only in patients who have generalized eyelash thinning or focal areas of complete loss.

It is more difficult to reconstruct the lash line in patients who have large areas of eyelash loss or total eyelash loss. In these female patients, a brown or black liquid or pencil eyeliner should be used to rim the entire eye, except for one-quarter inch around the inner canthus on the upper and lower eyelids (Fig. 4-1B). On the normal eye, terminal hairs do not grow around the inner canthus. For female patients with more extensive loss, artificial demilashes can be applied at this point, or, for the patient with total eyelash loss, complete artificial eyelashes can be applied.

Eyeliner can also be used to contour the eyes while simultaneously reconstructing a lash line. Small eyes can be enlarged by lining the entire upper lash line and the lateral half of the lower lash line (Fig. 4-1C). Hypoteloric eyes can be widened by lining the lateral half of both the upper and lower lash lines (Fig. 4-1D).

REFERENCES

1. Rutkin P: Eye make-up. p. 712. In de Navarre MG (ed). The Chemistry and Manufacture of Cosmetics. Allured Publishing Corp., Wheaton, IL, 1988
2. Wilkinson JB, Moore RJ: Harry's Cosmeticology. 7th Ed. Chemical Publishing, New York, 1982
3. Lanzet M: Modern formulations of coloring agents: facial and eye. In Frost P, Horwitz SN (eds): Principles of Cosmetics for the Dermatologist. CV Mosby, St. Louis, 1982
4. Bhadauria B, Ahearn DG: Loss of effectiveness of preservative systems of mascaras with age. Appl Environ Microbiol 39:665, 1980
5. Wilson LA, Ahern DG. *Pseudomonas*-induced corneal ulcer associated with contaminated eye mascaras. Am J Ophthalmol 84:112, 1977
6. MMWR Reports: *Pseudomonas aeruginosa* corneal infection related to mascara applicator trauma. Arch Dermatol 126:734, 1990
7. Ahearn DG, Wilson, LA: Microflora of the outer eye and eye area cosmetics. Dev Ind Microbiol 17:23, 1976
8. Ahern DG, Wilson LA, Julian AJ et al: Microbial growth in eye cosmetics: contamination during use. Dev Ind Microbiol 15:211, 1974
9. Kuehne JW, Ahearn DG: Incidence and characterization of fungi in eye cosmetics. Dev Ind Microbiol 12:1973, 1971
10. Jervey JH: Mascara pigmentation of the conjunctiva. Arch Ophthalmol 81:124, 1969
11. Platia EV, Michaels RG, Green WR: Eye cosmetic-induced conjunctional pigmentation. Ann Ophthalmol 10:501, 1978
12. Fisher AA: Allergic contact dermatitis due to rosin (colophony) in eyeshadow and mascara. Cutis 42:507, 1988
13. Rapaport MJ: Sensitization to abitol. Contact Dermatitis 6:137, 1980
14. Dooms-Goosens A, Degreef J, Luytens E: Dihydroabietyl alcohol (Abitol), a sensitizer in mascara. Contact Dermatitis 5:350, 1979

15. Ross JS, White IR: Eyelid dermatitis due to cocamidopropyl betaine in an eye make-up remover. Contact Dermatitis 25:64, 1991
16. Lanzet M: Modern formulations of coloring agents: facial and eye. p. 143. In Frost P, Horwitz SN (eds): Principles of Cosmetics for the Dermatologist. CV Mosby, St. Louis 1982
17. Stewart CR: Conjunctival absorption of pigment from eye make-up. Am J Optometry 50:571, 1973

5

Eyebrow Cosmetics

The accepted shape and width of the eyebrows is subject to fashion trends. Eyebrows were almost completely plucked in the 1950s, with a thin pencil line drawn to connect the few remaining hairs. Unfortunately, many women who are now in their 60s and 70s can no longer grow eyebrow hairs as a result of over plucking during their younger years. This is in direct contrast to the eyebrow look of the 1960s, which was totally natural and ungroomed. The 1990s style is a compromise, with thick eyebrows considered attractive, but stray hairs beneath the brow line are plucked to give a groomed appearance.

There are several eyebrow cosmetics: pencils, sealers, dyes, and artificial eyebrows (Table 5-1).

EYEBROW PENCIL

Eyebrow pencils are used to darken light or gray eyebrows, fill in sparse or absent eyebrow hairs, and reconstruct malformed or misshapen eyebrows. Eyebrow pencils are formed by mixing pigments, petrolatum, lanolin, and synthetic or natural waxes. This formulation is similar to lipstick products, but differs in that higher melting point waxes are used to yield a firmer product. Formulations may be encased in wood to form a pencil or extruded into rods placed in a plastic holder.

Pencils are available in a variety of colors, from grays to browns to blacks. Inert, mainly inorganic pigments are used because the Federal Food, Drug and Cosmetic Act prohibits the use of coal tar colors in the eye area. They are stroked over the skin in the eyebrow region to actually color the skin and eyebrow hairs.[1]

Contact dermatitis caused by eyebrow pencils is rare. The product can be open or closed patch tested ''as is.''

EYEBROW SEALER

Eyebrow sealers are intended as a grooming agent for unruly eyebrows and a glossening agent to add shine to eyebrow hairs. Originally, white petroleum jelly was used for this purpose, but now cosmetic companies market a more

Table 5-1. Eyebrow Cosmetics

Eyebrow Cosmetic	Main Ingredients	Function	Adverse Reactions
Eyebrow pencil	Pigment, wax, petrolatum, lanolin	Darken and thicken eyebrows	Minimal
Eyebrow sealer	Synthetic polymer	Eyebrow hair grooming agent	Minimal
Eyebrow dye	Metallic dyes, stains, or permanent dyes	Darken eyebrow hairs	May be illegal and cause blindness, contact dermatitis
Artificial eyebrows	Human, synthetic, or wool hair	Replace missing eyebrow hair	Irritant contact dermatitis to hair; allergic contact dermatitis to adhesive
Eyebrow tatooing	Tatoo pigments	Replace missing eyebrows	Allergic contact dermatitis caused by tatoo pigment

elegant product. The sealer is essentially a liquid hair spray containing polymer holding agents packaged in a mascara-type tube. A brush is used to stroke the product over the eyebrow hairs.

Eyebrow sealers can be used by persons with bushy eyebrows to hold the hairs closer to the orbital ridge or by those with multidirectional eyebrow hairs who wish to hold the hairs in a more cosmetically acceptable line. The product is easily removed with soap and water.

Eyebrow sealers could be a source of irritant contact dermatitis due to the incorporation of volatile vehicles. The product can be patch tested ''as is,'' but should be thoroughly dry prior to occlusion.

EYEBROW DYE

Eyebrow hair can be dyed in the same manner as scalp hair. This service is offered at many professional salons; however, hair dye packaging specifically states that dyestuff is not to be used in the eye area and contains the following warning: ''Caution—This product contains ingredients which may cause skin irritation on certain individuals and a preliminary test according to accompanying directions should first be made. This product must not be used for dyeing the eyelashes or eyebrows; to do so may cause blindness.'' The FDA has engaged unsuccessfully in several law suits to remove eye area dyes from the market.[2]

Eyebrow dyes that are present in some salons are metallic types, stains, or permanent hair dyes. The metallic dyes, containing lead or silver, are applied over a period of weeks and cause gradual darkening of the hairs due to formation of metallic oxides and sulfides on the hair shaft, imparting a yellow brown to black color. Some salons use professional stains that are specifically manufactured for eyebrow dyeing. The stain is applied with a toothpick only to the eyebrow hairs, as skin contact will result in staining. A special product is used to remove stain from the skin. Other salons use the same dye that is applied to the scalp for dyeing the eyebrows, taking care to keep material from entering the eye.

It should be reemphasized that the FDA considers all the eyebrow dyeing products discussed here to be dangerous and illegal.

ARTIFICIAL EYEBROWS

Artificial eyebrows are available for individuals who have permanently lost a substantial amount of their natural eyebrow hair. Synthetic or natural human hair can be knotted onto a thin netting in the appropriate amount and shape for a patient's face. The netting is then glued on the superior orbital ridge with a waterproof adhesive. Salons specializing in hair replacement can provide patient assistance.

The use of crepe hair is an eyebrow replacement technique, adapted from the theater, that is more appropriate for the patient who has temporarily lost substantial eyebrow hair.[3] Crepe hair is made from wool and is available as braids in a variety of colors. The braided fibers are separated, straightened, and cut to the desired length. Adhesive is then used to glue the fibers directly to the skin. New fibers must be prepared and glued for each application.

Possible adverse reactions include irritant contact dermatitis to the eyebrow prosthesis and/or allergic contact dermatitis to the adhesive, which may contain methacrylate.

EYEBROW TATOOING

Eyebrows can be reconstructed or thickened with the use of tatoo pigment. Brown, black, gray, yellow, or orange pigments can be blended and placed within the superficial dermis to add color to the eyebrow area. Certainly, this must be done by a trained individual under hygienic conditions. Unfortunately, eyebrow tatooing is less than optimal since the overlying skin has a rather unnatural shiny appearance. Allergic contact dermatitis can result from some of the pigments.

CORRECTIVE EYEBROW COSMETICS

The structure of the eyebrows can be abnormal due to congenital deformity, surgical procedures, or acquired loss from alopecia universalis, hypothyroidism, leprosy, traumatic scarring, and other conditions. Before cosmetic reconstruc-

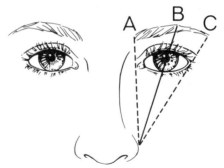

FIG. 5-1. The well-proportioned eyebrow should begin at Point A, maximally arch at point B, and end at point C.

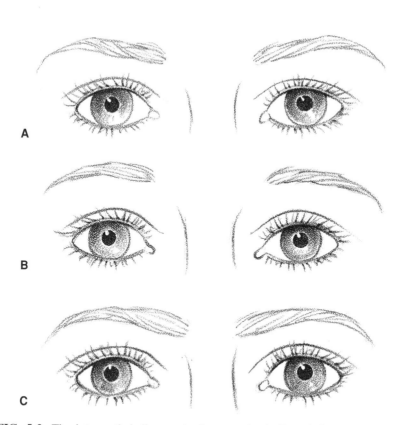

FIG. 5-2. The intercanthal distance is the same in **A, B** and **C**; however, the distance between the medial eyebrows has been changed. Note the resultant illusion of hypertelorism in **B** and hypotelorism in **C**.

tion can begin, it is important to identify the proper location of the eyebrow on the face (Fig. 5-1). The medial aspect of the eyebrow should begin at a point defined by a straight line drawn from the lateral nose upward. The eyebrow should maximally arch at a point defined by a line drawn from the lateral nose through the pupil. The eyebrow should end at a point defined by a line drawn from the lateral nose through the lateral aspect of the eyeball. Any hair removal to improve eyebrow appearance should be from the inferior aspect of the eyebrow. Hairs should never be removed from the superior border, as this will disturb the natural eyebrow contour.

Improper placement of the eyebrows can alter facial expression and the appearance of the eyes (Fig. 5-2A). Eyebrows that are placed too far apart give the impression of surprise and can make the patient appear hyperteloric (Fig. 5-2B), while eyebrows that are too close together give an angry, intense look and impart hypotelorism (Fig. 5-2C). If the eyes are improperly placed on the face, these concepts can be used to alter eyebrow position to create the illusion of properly spaced eyes.

Eyebrow pencil can be used to draw absent hairs. A more natural appearance is created if the pencil is used in short strokes rather than to draw one straight line.[4] The eyebrow pencil will adhere better if the skin is first covered with a facial foundation.

REFERENCES

1. Klarmann EG: Cosmetic Chemistry for the Dermatologist. Charles C Thomas, Springfield, IL, 1962
2. Draelos ZK: Caution: eyebrow dyeing may be illegal. Cosmet Dermatol 3:39, 1990
3. Rayner V: Clinical Cosmetology: A Medical Approach to Esthetics Procedures. Milady Publishing Company, Albany, NY, 1993
4. Allsworth J: Skin Camouflage. Stanley Thornes Ltd, Cheltenham, England, 1985

6

Lip Cosmetics

Lip cosmetics are valuable not only to accentuate the lips but also to provide lip lubrication and act as a sunscreen. Lip cosmetics can cover imperfections and redefine poorly formed lips due to congenital or surgical deformity. There are several types of lip cosmetics: lipsticks, lip crayons, lip creams, lip liners, lip sealers, and lip balms (Table 6-1).

LIPSTICK

Lipstick is an extruded rod of color dispersed in a blend of oils, waxes, and fats packaged in a roll-up tube. The perfect lipstick does not yet exist, since most women want a creamy, pleasant-tasting product that glides on easily, yet colors the lips for at least 8 hours.

History

Lip color has been used since the time of the Sumerians dating to 7000 bc. The practice has been handed down through many generations from the Egyptians to the Syrians to the Babylonians to the Persians to the Greeks to the Romans to present-day civilizations. Usually plant materials, such as hybrid saffron or brazilwood, were used to obtain a reddish color. The earliest true lipsticks consisted of beeswax, tallow, and pigment.[1]

Present-day lipstick was introduced around 1920, when the "push-up" holder, still used today, was invented. Other lipstick formulations, including liquids, pencils, and automatic applicators, have been introduced, but lipstick remains the product with the highest sales.[2]

Formulation

Lipsticks are mixtures of waxes, oils, and pigments in varying concentration to yield the characteristics of the final product. For example, a lipstick designed to remain on the lips for a prolonged period of time is composed of high wax,

Table 6-1. Lip Cosmetics

Lipsticks	Appearance	Coverage	Wearability	Main Ingredients
Lipsticks				
Pigmented	Matte	Full	Moderate	Wax, oil, pigment
Frosted	Pearlescent	Full	Moderate	Wax, oil, pigment
Transparent	Shiny	Very sheer	Short	High percentage of oil, soluble dyes
Indelible	Matte	Moderate	Very long	Wax, oil, bromo acid dyes
Lip crayons	Pearlescent or matte	Full	Moderate	Wax, less oil lipstick, pigment
Lip liners	Matte	Not applicable	Long	Wax, pigment
Lip creams and gloss pots	Shiny	Sheer	Very short	Petrolatum, oil, pigment
Lip sealants	Matte	Not applicable	Long	Water, glycerin, wax, oil, dimethicone
Lip balm	Matte	None	Long	Wax, mineral oil, chemical sunscreen

See glossary for definition of terms.

Coverage: very sheer = transparent, sheer = semitransparent, moderate = translucent, heavy = semiopaque, full = opaque.

Wearability: very short = 2 hours, short = 3 hours, moderate = 4 hours, long = 8 hours.

low oil, and high pigment concentrations. On the other hand, a product designed for a smooth creamy feel on the lips is composed of low wax and high oil concentrations.[2]

The waxes commonly incorporated into lipstick formulations are white beeswax, candelilla wax, carnauba wax, ozokerite wax, lanolin wax, ceresin wax, and other synthetic waxes. Usually, lipsticks contain a combination of these waxes carefully selected and blended to achieve the desired melting point. Oils are then selected, such as castor oil, white mineral oil, lanolin oil, hydrogenated vegetable oils, or oleyl alcohol, to form a film suitable for application to the lips. The oils are also necessary for dispersion of the pigments.

Several types of coloring agents are used in lipsticks.[3] Indelible coloring, or lip staining, is achieved through the use of bromo acids, consisting of fluoresceins, halogenated fluoresceins, and related water-insoluble dyes. Other pigments consist of insoluble dyestuffs and lake colors. Metallic lakes are insoluble dyes precipitated or ''laked'' on a metallic substrate such as aluminium. For example, FD&C Blue No. 1 is an azo dye precipitated on aluminium that transforms the insoluble dye to a pigment. Other lake colors are based on calcium or barium salts.

The safety of the coloring agents used in lipsticks has received a great deal of attention due to the inevitable entry of lipsticks into the mouth. The FDA divides certified colors into three groups: Food, Drug and Cosmetic (FD&C) colors, Drug & Cosmetic (D&C) colors, and External Drug & Cosmetic colors. Only the first two groups can be used in lipsticks. The External Drug & Cosmetic colors can only be used in locations where they are not likely to enter

Table 6-2. Lipstick Colorants Permitted in the United States

FD&C or D&C Blue No. 1, Al Lake	D&C Red No. 11, Ca
FD&C or D&C Blue No. 2, Al Lake	D&C Red No. 12, Ba
FD&C or D&C Red No. 2, Al Lake	D&C Red No. 13, Sr
FD&C or D&C Red No. 3, Al Lake	D&C Red No. 19, Al Lake
FD&C Yellow No. 5, Al Lake	D&C Red No. 21
D&C Yellow No. 5, Zr-Al Lake	R&C Red No. 27
D&C Yellow No. 6, Al Lake	D&C Red No. 27, Al Lake
FD&C or D&C Yellow, No. 6, Al Lake	D&C Red No. 30
	D&C Red No. 36
D&C Orange No. 5	D&C Blue No. 1, Al Lake
D&C Orange No. 5, Al Lake	Iron oxide—all shades
D&C Orange No. 10	Carmine
D&C Orange No. 10, Al Lake	Bronze powder
D&C Orange No. 17, Ba Lake	Carbon black
D&C Red No. 3, Al Lake	Guanine
D&C Red No. 6, Na or Ba	Manganese violet
D&C Red No. 7, Ca	Mica
D&C Red No. 8, Na	Aluminum powder
D&C Red No. 9, Ba	Bismuth oxychloride
D&C Red No. 10, Na	Carotene

Adapted from deNavarre,[1] with permission.

the mouth. The colorants listed in Table 6-2 are currently approved for use in lipsticks in the United States.[1]

Preservatives, antioxidants, perfumes, and surface characteristic additives complete the formulation.[4]

Manufacture

Lipstick manufacture consists of pigment grinding, mixing, molding, and flaming.[5] Pigment grinding involves forming small particles of color that are evenly suspended in an oily base ready for mixing with the remaining ingredients. The mixture is then heated until all the waxes are melted and stirred to ensure uniformity. The warm mixture is then poured into molds of desired shape. Flaming involves passing the finished lipstick rod through a gas flame to reheat the surface rapidly. This removes blemishes from handling and yields a high gloss on the product, which consumers consider desirable.[6]

Application

Lipstick is applied by stroking the pigmented rod across the lips. The product must be artistically applied to color the entire vermillion, yet create a smooth, even, pleasant lip outline. The outline of the lips can be drawn in any fashion desired, making lipstick a useful camouflage cosmetic in patients with lip deformity.

Adverse Reactions

Several ingredients unique to lipstick formulation can cause difficulty in the sensitized patient.[7] Castor oil, found in almost all lipsticks due to its excellent ability to dissolve bromo acid dyes, can rarely cause allergic contact dermatitis.[8–10] More common lipstick sensitizers in the mid-1920s were the bromo acid dyes, one of which is eosin (D&C Red No. 21).[11] Eosin was commonly used in the indelible red lipsticks popular at that time. These indelible lipsticks are now making a comeback as active professional women want a long-wearing lip product. Other causes of lipstick dermatitis include ricinoleic acid,[12] benzoic acid,[13] lithol rubine BCA (Pigment Red 57-1),[14] microcrystalline wax,[15] oxybenzone,[16] propyl gallate,[17] and C18 aliphatic compounds.[18]

Lip cosmetics can be open or closed patch tested ''as is'' since their irritating potential is low.

TYPES OF LIP COSMETICS

Lip cosmetics can be molded in a variety of shapes, depending on the wishes of the consumer. Subtle formulation changes can yield a remarkably different-appearing product.

Lip Crayons

Lip crayons are formed by encasing the extruded rod in wood. Sharpening with a pencil type sharpener is required to expose the product. Lip crayons generally contain more wax and have a higher melting point wax than lipsticks. This yields a firmer rod, but makes the product less creamy and more difficult to apply. Carnauba wax, with a melting point of 85°C, is used in higher concentration for firmer lip crayons, while candelilla wax or beeswax is used for softer products.

Lip Creams

Lip creams and gloss pots differ from lipsticks and lip crayons in that they are packaged in a small jar and are rolled on or applied with the finger. The cream formulation is obtained by lowering the wax content, increasing the oil content, and using waxes with a lower melting point. Lip creams usually contain both pigment and titanium dioxide, producing an opaque lip cosmetic. Gloss pots provide transparent color to the lips since no titanium dioxide is employed.

Products aimed at adolescents may also contain a strong perfume and/or flavor. The aim of both products is to provide high lip shine, but the weartime is short.

Problems can be encountered with lip creams or gloss pots. Their increased oil content allows running, or "bleeding," of the cosmetic into tiny fissures around the lips, making them unsuitable for the mature patient. Additionally, the oils incorporated may be comedogenic, making them unsuitable for the adolescent prone to perioral comedones.

Lip Liners

Lip liners are thin extruded rods encased in wood or placed in an automatic pencil type holder. Their formulation is similar to that of lipsticks, except that stiffer waxes with higher melting points are used with minimal oil. This creates an extremely hard rod that applies a thick layer of pigment to the lips. Lip liners are used to define the outer edge of the lips and are valuable in reconstructing a normal lip contour. The thick wax layer applied around the lips also prevents creamier lip products from bleeding. Lip liner is usually selected one to two shades darker than the lipstick.

Lip Sealants

Lip sealants are similar in function to eye shadow setting creams in that both products prepare the skin for increased cosmetic wearability. Lip sealants prevent movement of the product into the fine lines around the lips, encouraging the lip cosmetic to remain in place. They contain water, talc, glycerin, wax, mineral oil, and dimethicone. The cream is applied to the lips like lipstick or with the finger and allowed to dry before a pigmented lip cosmetic is applied. Facial foundation can also be applied to the lips as a sealant.

Lip Balms

Lip balms are not used for decoration of the lips, but rather to provide moisturization of the lips and protection from the sun and cold. These products form a moisture-resistant film over the lips, but contain no colorants. They contain mineral oil, wax, and possibly a chemical sunscreening agent.

SPECIALTY LIP COSMETICS

A variety of additives can be incorporated into lip cosmetics to alter their ability to remain on the lips or to provide fashionable surface characteristics.[19] Consumer desires dictate the specialty additives found in currently marketed formulations.[20]

Long-Wearing Lip Cosmetics

Lip cosmetics can be formulated to impart color to the lips for 8 hours or more. Obviously, the lipstick film will not stay on the lips this long, but the lips can be stained to impart long-lasting color. The most common stain employed is acid eosin, a tetrabromo derivative of fluorescein. Acid eosin, also known as bromo acid or D&C Red No. 21, is naturally colored orange but changes to a red salt at a pH of 4. Conditions present on the lip change the orange lipstick to a vivid red indelible stain that is long lasting. Acid eosin and other bromo acids (D&C Red No.2, D&C Red No. 27, D&C Orange No. 10, D&C Orange No. 5) have become unpopular due to their bitter taste and ability to cause allergic contact dermatitis or photosensitization resulting in cheilitis. For this reason, FDA has banned the use of D&C Red No. 2 and has placed restrictions on the use of D&C Orange No. 5.

Opaque Lip Cosmetics

An opaque lip cosmetic is preferred for patients who require lip camouflaging. The opaqueness is due to incorporation of high titanium dioxide concentrations into the lipstick. Titanium dioxide provides the best coverage of all the white pigments, including zinc oxide. It must be ground to a fine powder to enable smooth application of the lipstick. It also adds color brightness to lip cosmetics and is used to create pastel shades.

Frosted Lip Cosmetics

Frosted lipsticks obtain their pearlesence through the addition of guanine crystals from fish scale, titanium dioxide–coated mica, or bismuth oxychloride. Fish scales are now rarely used with bismuth oxychloride alone or coated onto mica as the preferred low cost pearlescent additive.

Transparent Lip Cosmetics

Transparent lipsticks do not use any opaque insoluble pigments or lakes. Instead, soluble dyes are used, which allow the underlying lips to be seen while providing a colored glaze. This lipstick provides a natural look but cannot cover lip defects.

LIP TATTOOING

Definition of the vermilion border can be enhanced through lip tattooing. Less conventional than the use of lip liners, this method is practiced by dermatologists and plastic surgeons. Lip tattooing is performed by inserting a red pigment such as cinnabar, a red dye containing mercuric sulfide, into the upper dermis along the vermilion border through punctures created by a specially designed needle. The normal lip contour can be followed, resulting in the appearance of permanent lipstick, or the pigment can be placed to reshape malformed lips. Lip tattooing can also be used to reconstruct the vermilion border in patients with treated actinic cheilitis or leukoplakia. It is possible to develop a tattoo granuloma since cinnabar is the most allergenic of the tattoo pigments.

This technique is not recommended for women, except in cases of extreme surgical deformity, since fashion dictates the desirable lip appearance and the patient will not be able to wear lighter lipstick shades in pink or peach. However, the permanence of lip color may be more desirable for male patients, who do not require fashion flexibility. Patients should recognize that there is some fading of the pigment color with time, and movement of the pigment within the dermis occurs due to macrophage phagocytosis.

LIP COSMETICS FOR ACNE PATIENTS

Acne patients should select lip cosmetics with low oil content to minimize the formation of comedones around the vermilion border and perioral acne. Lip creams and gloss pots contain the most oil and should be avoided in favor of lip crayons and lipsticks. Lip cosmetics with a higher oil content have a creamy feel and a glossy shine on application. Acne patients with oily complexions will also notice movement of the lip cosmetic away from the lips as sebum combines with the cosmetic. Lip crayons and the use of a lip liner will provide the longest wear in these patients. The use of a lip stain may also be considered.

LIP COSMETICS FOR MATURE PATIENTS

Color can be added to a pale face quickly with lip cosmetics. In addition, only minimal application skill is required, and the steady hand necessary for eye cosmetic application is not needed. These characteristics make lip cosmetics popular among mature patients. The most common complaint in this age group is the movement, or "bleeding," of lip cosmetics into the fine wrinkles that develop on the upper and lower lips from elastic tissue degeneration or gingival bone resorption. Often mature persons with dry lips select a moisturizing lipstick and subsequently experience lipstick bleeding. Lip cosmetic bleeding can be minimized by preparing the lips first with a lip sealant or facial foundation, using a stiff lip liner, and avoiding creamy lipsticks or lip creams in favor of lip crayons. All lipsticks are moisturizing to some extent. Stiff lip balms or sticks cannot be applied as moisturizers under lipsticks, since this will encourage lipstick bleeding.

Mature patients may wish to use a lip cosmetic to cover lentigines, venous lakes, or actinic cheilitis. Darker lipstick colors provide better coverage than lighter colors. Lipsticks that contain titanium dioxide are superior to lip crayons or lip creams. Application to the lips of a facial foundation containing titanium dioxide adds additional coverage. The selection of bluish-red lipstick will have the added advantage of seeming to whiten discolored teeth.

CORRECTIVE LIP COSMETICS

Abnormal lip shape due to congenital causes or surgery can be masked by effective application of lip cosmetics. A well proportioned mouth in a closed, relaxed state should be positioned between the medial aspect of the irises (Fig. 6-1).[21] Lips that do not extend this distance are perceived as small. Small lips

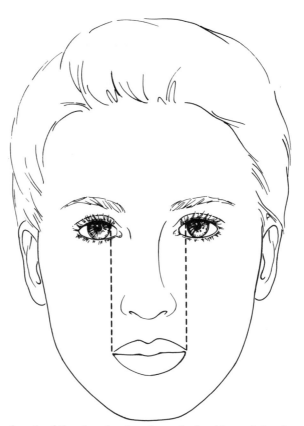

FIG. 6-1. The length of the closed, relaxed mouth should equal the distance between the medial aspect of the irises in the well-proportioned face.

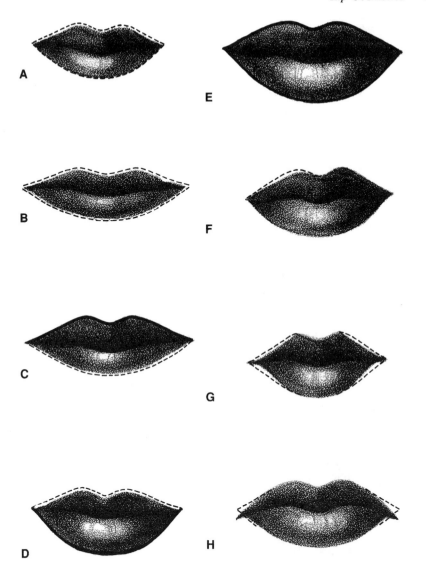

FIG. 6-2. Contouring of the lips (**A**) to enlarge small lips, (**B**) to thicken thin lips, (**C**) to thicken a thin lower lip, (**D**) to thicken a thin upper lip, (**E**) to decrease the size of thick lips, (**F**) to correct crooked lips, (**G**) to correct bow lips, and (**H**) to correct down-turned lips.

can be enlarged by using a lip liner to draw the lip boundary on the outer edge of the vermilion and then filling in with a deeply pigmented, matte finish lipstick (Fig. 6-2A). Uniformly thin lips (Fig. 6-2B), a thin lower lip possibly due to lip advancement surgery (Fig. 6-2C), or a thin upper lip (Fig. 6-2D) can be thickened by also lining outside the vermilion where required and selecting a lighter, frosted finish lipstick. Conversely, thick lips possibly due to a congenital hemangioma are lined inside the vermilion (Fig. 6-2E). Figure 6-2 also demonstrates the lip lining technique with a dashed line for crooked (Fig. 6-2F), bow (Fig. 6-2G), and down-turned lips (Fig. 6-2H). The lip liner should be one shade darker than the lipstick for optimal effect.

REFERENCES

1. deNavarre MG: Lipstick. p. 767. In The Chemistry and Manufacture of Cosmetics. Vol. IV. 2nd Ed. Allured Publishing Company, Wheaton, IL, 1975
2. Cunningham J: Color cosmetics. p. 143. In Williams DF, Schmitt WH (eds): Chemistry and Technology of the Cosmetics and Toiletries Industry. DF Williams and WH Schmitt eds, Blackie Academic & Professional, London, 1992
3. Boelcke U: Requirements for lipstick colors. J Soc Cosmet Chem 12:468, 1961
4. Poucher WA: Perfumes, Cosmetics and Soaps. Vol 3, 8th Ed. Chapman and Hall, London, 1984
5. Fishbach AL: Lipsticks: their formulation, manufacture, and analysis. J Soc Cosmet Chem 5:242
6. Torry LP: Lipstick, Rouge, Eye Make-up, Manicure Preparations. p. 304. In HW Hibbott (ed): Handbook of Cosmetic Science. Macmillan Company, New York, 1963
7. Sulzgerger MD, Boodman J, Byrne LA, Mallozzi ED: Acquired specific hypersensitivity to simple chemicals. Cheilitis with special reference to sensitivity to lipsticks. Arch Dermatol 37:597, 1938
8. Sai S: Lipstick dermatitis caused by castor oil. Contact Dermatitis 9:75, 1983
9. Brandle I, Boujnah-Khouadja A, Foussereau J: Allergy to castor oil. Contact Dermatitis 9:424, 1983
10. Andersen KE, Neilsen R: Lipstick dermatitis related to castor oil. Contact Dermatitis 11:253, 1984
11. Calan CD: Allergic sensitivity to eosin. Acta Allergol 13:493, 1959
12. Sai S: Lipstick dermatitis caused by ricinoleic acid. Contact Dermatitis 9:524, 1983
13. Calnan CD: Amyldimethylamino benzoic acid causing lipstick dermatitis. Contact Dermatitis 6:233, 1980
14. Hayakawa R, Fujimoto Y, Kaniwa M: Allergic pigmented lip dermatitis from lithol rubine BCA. Am J Contact Dermatitis 5:34, 1994
15. Darko E, Osmundsen PE: Allergic contact dermatitis to Lipcare lipstick. Contact Dermatitis 11:46, 1984
16. Aguirre A, Izu R, Gardeazabal J et al: Allergic contact cheilitis from a lipstick containing oxybenzone. Contact Dermatitis 27:267, 1992
17. Cronin E: Lipstick dermatitis due to propyl gallate. Contact Dermatitis 6:213, 1980
18. Hayakawa R, Matsunaga K, Suzuki M et al: Lipstick dermatitis due to C18 alipathic compounds. Contact Dermatitis 16:215, 1987
19. Lauffer PGI: Lipsticks. p. 367. In Balsam MS, Sagarin E (eds): Cosmetics Science and Technology. Vol 1. Wiley-Interscience, New York, 1972
20. Consumer Reports: Lipsticks, February, p. 75, 1988
21. Powell N, Humphreys B: Proportions of the Aesthetic Face. Thieme-Stratton Inc, New York, 1984

7

Camouflaging Cosmetics

Special color cosmetics are available for individuals with acquired or congenital contour and color defects of the face. These cosmetics are known as "camouflage cosmetics" since they attempt to recreate a more attractive appearance. They do not, however, duplicate the appearance of a freshly washed, unadorned face. It is obvious to all that the individual is wearing a cosmetic. Therefore, camouflage cosmetics are designed to minimize facial defects while accentuating attractive features of the face.[1]

Camouflaging cosmetics are used by paramedical camouflage artists, estheticians, dermatologists, plastic surgeons, and cosmetics consultants. Their successful use requires a well-formulated, quality product applied with the skill of a stage makeup technician and the artistic abilities of a painter.

FACIAL CAMOUFLAGING COSMETICS AND TECHNIQUES

Facial Defects

Key to understanding the use of camouflage cosmetics is a basic knowledge of the types of facial defects that can occur. There are defects of contour, pigmentation, and a combination of both.

Contour and Texture Defects

Defects of contour are defined as areas where the scar tissue is hypertrophied or atrophied. In addition, the scar tissue may also demonstrate a texture difference due to absence of follicular ostia and hair.

69

Table 7-1. Facial Pigmentation Defects

Facial Color	Disease Process	Foundation Color
Red	Psoriasis, lupus, rosacea	Green undercover foundation
Yellow	Solar elastosis, chemotherapy, dialysis	Purple undercover foundation
Brown hyperpigmentation	Chloasma, lentigenes, nevi	White undercover foundation
Hypopigmentation and depigmentation	Postinflammatory, congenital, vitiligo	Brown undercover foundation

Pigmentation Defects

Pigmentation defects are abnormalities solely in the color of the skin with no texture abnormalities. Some pigmentation abnormalities arise from tumors of the skin, while others are due to systemic abnormalities or extrinsic effects, such as sun exposure (Table 7-1).[2,3]

Camouflaging Principles

Camouflaging principles are adapted from stage makeup texts since many of the same techniques are employed.[4] Camouflaging is the art of illusion and demands that the cosmetics be applied with both skill and artistic ability. Fortunately, the cosmetics can be easily applied and removed, providing opportunity for experimentation and easy alteration of a bad result.

Facial Scar Contouring

The basic concept of facial scar recontouring is predicated on the fact that dark colors make surfaces recede while light colors make surfaces appear to project (Fig. 7-1).[5] Thus, lighter colors will minimize depressed areas of scarring while darker colors will minimize protuberant areas of the scar.

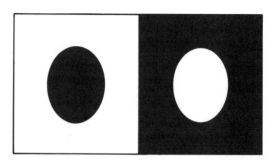

FIG. 7-1. The two fundamental rules of facial contouring: dark contours look smaller and appear to recede, light contours look larger and appear to come forward.

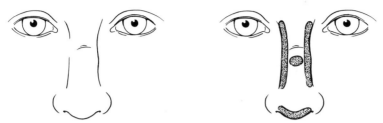

FIG. 7-2. Cosmetic camouflaging of depressed scar on nose.

Figure 7-2 demonstrates this technique on a patient who has sustained a depressed scar following surgical removal of a skin cancer on the nose. The scar itself is lightened to compensate for decreased light reflection while the sides and tip of the nose are darkened to draw attention away from the surgical defect.

Pigmentation Defect Camouflaging

Pigmentation defects can be camouflaged either by applying an opaque cosmetic that allows none of the abnormal underlying skin tones to be appreciated or by applying foundations of complementary colors (Table 7-1). For example, red pigmentation defects can be camouflaged by applying a green foundation, which is the complementary color to red. The blending of the red skin with the green foundation yields a brown tone, which can be readily covered by a more conventional facial foundation. Furthermore, yellow skin tones can be blended with a complementary colored purple foundation to also yield brown tones. Skin areas that are lighter or darker than desired can be camouflaged by applying facial foundations with the appropriate amount of brown pigment to hide the defect.[6]

Camouflage Cosmetics

There are many companies in the United States and Europe that manufacture cosmetics specifically designed for camouflaging purposes. Table 7-2 lists some of the more popular products presently available. A good camouflage artist will generally purchase a color palette from at least two different companies to provide the necessary mixture of cosmetic shades required to match a given patient's skin tone.[7]

Formulation

Different formulations of camouflaging cosmetics are designed to meet the needs of each defect to be concealed. The basic products required for camouflaging are makeup bases, lining colors, and rouges.

Table 7-2. Camouflage Cosmetic Manufacturers

Trade Name	Manufacturer/Distributor	Trade Name	Manufacturer/Distributor
Astarté	Astarté Cosmetics, Inc. 460 West 34th street New York NY 10001 USA	Hide and Sleek	RH Cosmetics 80 39th Street Brooklyn NY 11232 USA
Cinema Secrets	Cinema Secrets Inc. 4400 Riverside Drive Burbank CA 91505 USA	Keren Happuch	Keren Happuch, Ltd. PO Box 809 Oconomowoc WI 53066
Columbia Cosmetics	Columbia Cosmetics Manufacturing, Inc. 1661 Timothy Drive San Leandro CA 94577 USA	Keromask Cover Cream	USA Innoxa Ltd. 202 Terminus Road Eastbourne, Sussex BN21 3DF
Corrective Concepts	Pattee Products European Crossroads—Bordeaux Building 2829 West Northwest Highway Dallas TX 75220 USA	Laboratoire Dr. Renaud Lady Burd/private label	England Renaud Skin Care 1040 Rockland Road Montreal PQ H2V 3A1 Canada Lady Burd Exclusive Private Label Cosmetics
Coverette	Ben Nye Company, Inc. 5935 Bowcroft Street Los Angeles CA 90016 USA	Marvin Westmore	73 Powerhouse Road Roslyn Heights NY 11577 USA Westmore Academy of
Covermark	Lydia O'Leary 1 Anderson Avenue Moonachie NJ 07074 USA	Cosmetics	Cosmetic Arts 15445 Ventura Boulevard, #8
Cover Tone	Fashion Fair Cosmetics 820 South Michigan Avenue Chicago IL 60605 USA	Natural Cover	Sherman Oaks CA 91403 USA LS Cosmetics PO Box 32203
Cream Makiage	Il-Makiage PO box 1064 Long Island City NY 11101 USA	Naturalessa	Baltimore MD 21208 USA Naturalessa 5-02 Banta Place Fair Lawn NJ 07410 USA
Danielle Cosmetics	Danielle Cosmetics Division Teka Fine Line Brushes, Inc. 3307 Avenue N Brooklyn NY 11234 USA	Patricia Milton Rhetorique	C'est La Vie 3401 Dufferin Street Suite 306 Toronto ON M6A 2T9 Canada
Dermablend	Dermablend Corrective Cosmetics PO Box 3008 Lakewood NJ 08701 USA	Pevonia	Cosmopro, Inc. 320 Fentress Boulevard Daytona Beach FL 32114 USA
Dermaceal	Joe Blasco Cosmetics 1708 Hillhurst Avenue Hollywood CA 90027 USA	dVeil	Atelier Esthetique 386 Park Avenue South Suite 209 New York NY 10016 USA
Dermacolor	Kryolan Corporation 132 Ninth Street San Francisco CA 94103 USA	Your Name Cosmetics	Your Name div. of Mana Products 32-02 Queens Boulevard Long Island City NY 11101
Grafton Products	Grafton Products Corporation 25 Butler Street Norwalk CT 06850 USA		USA

From Draelos,[13] with permission.

Makeup Bases   Makeup bases or facial foundations are designed to create the desired skin color. They are available as hard grease paints, soft grease paints, pancakes, and liquids. Hard grease paints come in stick form and consist of pigments in an anhydrous, waxy base. Application requires great skill and is more time consuming than other makeup bases. This product is extremely long wearing, but is mainly reserved for theatrical uses.

Soft grease paints come in a jar or are squeezed from a tube and have a creamy texture due the incorporation of low viscosity oils in addition to waxes in the anhydrous preparation. They usually contain a high proportion of titanium dioxide to provide superior coverage.[8] These products tend to have a high shine and do not survive body heat; thus some type of setting preparation is required to prolong wear.

Pancake products are packaged in a flat, round container. The product is removed from the compact by stroking with a wet sponge. It is composed of talc, kaolin, zinc oxide, precipitated chalk, titanium dioxide, and iron oxide.[9] This product dries quickly and possesses a matte, or dull, finish. Unfortunately, it is easily removed with body warmth and perspiration, but is easy to retouch, if necessary.

Liquid makeups for camouflaging are similar to those marketed for general use; however, increased amounts of titanium dioxide provide superior coverage. These products also usually contain a higher concentration of oils to allow full color development and improved wearability.

Special liquid makeups are available for application under a traditional facial foundation. These products, discussed previously, are formulated with green and purple pigments to camouflage red and yellow color defects, respectively.

Lining Colors and Rouges   Special colors are required in localized facial areas to provide shading and highlighting for contour defects. Products used for this purpose are known as lining colors, also called moist rouges, and dry (or powdered) rouges.[4] Lining colors are available in all shades of gray, maroon, red, brow, green, blue, white, and black. They are packaged in both hard sticks and soft tins. These products can be mixed to obtain the desired final specialty color for use.

Dry rouges are compressed powder compacts and are available in shades of red. They do not wear as long as their oil-containing counterparts; however, they are easily used for quick touch-up and final shading purposes.

Application

The most popular camouflage facial foundations are the creamy products that are scooped from a jar or tin with a spatula and applied to the hand for warming. These products are the easiest to use since they have long playtime, good blending characteristics, minimal application skill requirements, excellent coverage, and adequate wearability for most individuals.[10]

Initially, a makeup base must be selected that is closest to the patient's natural skin color. Blending usually is necessary, but no more than three colors should be combined or a final muddy color quality can result. If the patient has an underlying pigmentation problem, this counts as one color. In this case, the pink color of the wound due to an increased vascular supply to promote healing counts as one color. Other color abnormalities may be due to increased melanin, producing a brown color; increased hemosiderin, producing a rust color; degenerated facial elastin, producing a yellow color; and so forth.

Depending on the situation, it may be desirable to camouflage the red hues by initially applying a green undercover cosmetic and then a traditional facial foundation, thus avoiding the surgical products. If, however, the color contrast is too great, a high coverage surgical foundation that covers all underlying skin tones may be a better camouflaging makeup selection.

Once the closest foundation color has been selected, it may be necessary to blend in yellow, if the individual has a sallow complexion, or reds, if the patient has a ruddy complexion, etc. All facial tones should be represented in the final foundation blend if a good color match is to be obtained. Blending is usually done by applying a small amount of the makeup to the back of the hand. This provides a good surface for blending that can be easily held up to the face to evaluate the color match; this also warms the product, allowing easier mixing and application.

The final foundation color mix is then dabbed, not rubbed, over the scarred area and then applied from the central face outward into the hairline for approximately 1/4 inch and blended over the ears and beneath the chin. It is necessary to feather the cosmetic where application ends to achieve a more natural appearance. The importance of dabbing cannot be overemphasized, since scars do not contain appendageal structures, such as follicular ostia, that are necessary for good cosmetic adherence. Rubbing will remove the makeup as it is applied. The cosmetic should actually be pressed into the skin and allowed to dry 5 minutes.

Following this brief drying period, the cosmetic must be set with an unpigmented finely ground talc-based powder to prevent smudging, improve wearability, provide waterproof characteristics, and impart a matte finish. Camouflaging makeups are designed to be worn with this powder and do not function properly without it. The powder should be pressed, not dusted, on top of the foundation.

Lastly, shading and highlighting principles, discussed above, are employed to minimize the scar contour abnormalities. Unfortunately, the camouflage foundation may actually accentuate the surface irregularities of the scar and normal skin structures, such as pores and wrinkles. Depressed scars usually appear darker than the surrounding skin, even though the same color foundation has been applied, due to presence of shadows. Figure 7-2 demonstrates areas to be highlighted in an atrophic scar. Thus, a lighter powdered rouge is applied over the scar. If the scar were elevated, a darker powdered rouge would be applied. Lastly, a reddish powdered rouge is dusted over the central face (central forehead, nose, and chin) and upper cheeks to mimic natural color variations of the face. Unfortunately, the high-coverage surgical makeup also covers these facial landmarks, resulting in a flat, mask-like face. Other colored facial cosmetics (eye shadow, eyeliner, mascara, etc.) are usually necessary to give an attractive final appearance.[11]

In general, removal of camouflaging cosmetics requires more than soap and water washing due to the waterproof nature of the product. Most companies provide an oily cleanser for cosmetic removal and then recommend soap and water cleansing of the skin. The cosmetic should only be worn when needed and definitely thoroughly removed at bedtime.[12]

Adverse Reactions

Camouflage cosmetics are generally used by patients without difficulty. Usually, a specially trained paramedical camouflage artist or esthetician will train the patient in blending and application of the makeup. Two to three hourly session are enough to solve most of the problems encountered with the cosmetic, but sometimes special difficulties arise.

Most camouflage foundations contain a high concentration of oils, which may rarely cause comedone formation in predisposed individuals. Evaluating ingredient lists for the absence or presence of comedogenic oils is not of much practical value; rather, the foundation should be use tested by the patient. This is accomplished by applying a small amount of the cosmetic to the upper lateral cheek for a 2 to 4 week period followed by dermatologic evaluation.

Acne can also arise in certain susceptible individuals who use camouflaging foundations. Camouflaging cosmetics are much more likely to be acnegenic than comedogenic, since they are worn for a prolonged period of time and must be occlusive to provide adequate coverage and waterproof properties. The occlusion may also lead to miliaria formation.

Allergic contact dermatitis to camouflage makeups is rare since the formulation is generally fragrance-free with a low preservative concentration. It is possible, however, for both allergic and irritant contact dermatitis to occur with camouflage cosmetics. These products can be open or closed patch tested "as is."

BODY CAMOUFLAGING COSMETICS AND TECHNIQUES

Camouflaging cosmetics appropriate for covering macular pigmentation defects on the legs, arms, and body are also available. The easiest products to apply are thinner creams squeezed from a tube that spread better over larger areas, but provide less coverage than the thicker facial products. Unfortunately, application is difficult and unsatisfactory in body areas densely covered with hair. Application with a sponge is recommended followed by loose powder to improve wearability and impart a better waterproof finish. A special removal product is required.

These products use either zinc oxide or titanium dioxide for coverage, iron pigments for color, methyl cellulose or other waxes for viscosity, and glycerin or other nonevaporating substances for increased adherence of the product to the skin. They are a rare cause of irritant or allergic contact dermatitis and can be open or closed patch tested "as is."

REFERENCES

1. Stewart TW, Savage D: Cosmetic camouflage in dermatology. Br J Dermatol 86: 530, 1972
2. Draelos ZK: Cosmetic camouflaging techniques. Cutis 52:362, 1993
3. Benmaman O, Sanchez JL: Treatment and camouflaging of pigmentary disorders. Clin Dermatol 6:50, 1988
4. Buchman J: Stage Makeup. Watson-Guptill Publications, New York
5. Helland JR, Schneider MF: Special Features. M Evans and Company, New York, 1985
6. Draelos ZD: Use of cover cosmetics for pigmentation abnormalities. Cosmet Dermatol 2:14, 1989
7. Rayner V: Clinical Cosmetology: A Medical Approach to Esthetics Procedures. Milady Publishing Company, Albany, NY, 1993
8. Schlossman ML, Feldman AJ: Fluid foundation and blush makeup. p. 748. In deNavarre MG (ed): The Chemistry and Manufacture of Cosmetics. Allured Publishing Company, Wheaton, IL, 1988
9. Wilkinson JB, Moore RJ: Harry's Cosmeticology. 7th Ed. Chemical Publishing, New York, 1982
10. Reisch M: Masking agents as adjunct therapy in cutaneous disorders. Clin Med 8: 5, 1961
11. Draelos ZD: Cosmetics have a positive effect on the postsurgical patient. Cosmet Dermatol 4:11, 1991
12. Thomas RJ, Bluestein JL: Cosmetics and hairstyling as adjuvants to scar camouflage. p. 349. In Thomas RJ, Richard G (eds): Facial Scars. CV Mosby, St. Louis, 1989
13. Draelos Z: Cosmetics and Toiletries: Camouflage Cosmet Techniques 109:75, 1994

8

Postsurgical Facial Care and Cosmetics

Careful skin care and cosmetic selection is important immediately following surgery to maximize, and not impede, wound healing. Furthermore, cosmetics assume medical importance when used by post-surgical patient to facilitate return to normal daily activities and improve emotional well-being.[1,2]

SKIN CARE AND COSMETIC USE

Cosmetic selection criteria for the post-surgical patient depend upon the type of wound involved. Incisional wounds, closed by sutures, expose only a small amount of unhealed skin to topical cosmetics, while large surface area wounds, such as those created by shave excisions, dermabrasions, and chemical peels, are allowed to heal by secondary intention, exposing large unhealed skin areas to topical cosmetics.

Wounds Healing by Primary Intention

Incisional wounds, closed by sutures that remain in place for 5 to 14 days, require a clean surgical site free of foreign bodies. Therefore, cosmetics should not be applied to the sutured area until the sutures are removed. Facial foundations especially should be avoided, as they contain finely ground titanium dioxide, which could act as a foreign body and impede wound healing through initiation of an inflammatory response or by inciting milia formation. Furthermore, facial foundation pigments, such as iron oxide, can become embedded within the dermis during healing, resulting in permanent tatooing of the skin.

Wounds Healing by Secondary Intention

Large surface area wounds healing by secondary intention are devoid of the protective stratum corneum, making post-surgical cosmetics selection important. No cosmetics should be applied to the wound until serous drainage has stopped. This is generally not a problem for patients since cosmetics will not adhere to the skin until an epithelial barrier has been reestablished. Premature application of cosmetics can create the same foreign body problem and pigment tattoos discussed above. Individuals who attempt to apply facial foundation too soon following chemical peeling or dermabrasion may also encourage milia formation, a common side effect of both procedures. Bland moisturizers to impede transepidermal water loss, such as purified petroleum jelly, are recommended, however, until reepithelialization has occurred.

COLORED COSMETIC SELECTION

The application of colored cosmetics to the face may be important for the patient to reestablish social and emotional well-being following surgery. New cosmetics may need to be selected on a temporary or permanent basis following surgery.

Facial Foundations

Facial foundation is the most important cosmetic used by the post-surgical patient. It can camouflage redness and scarring while providing physical and/ or chemical sun protection.[3] The foundation selected should be easy to apply and remove and contain a paucity of ingredients.

Cream or cream/powder formulations are recommended Cream foundations are dipped from a jar or squeezed from a tube, while cream/powder foundations are wiped from a compact with a dry sponge (powder) or a moistened sponge (cream).[4] Examples of appropriate foundations are listed in Table 8-1. These

Table 8-1. Post-Surgical Facial Foundations

Name/Company	Type	Cost	Color Selection	Availability
Continuous Coverage (Clinique)	Cream	+ + +	Fair to medium	Cosmetic counter
Pan-Cake Makeup (Max Factor)	Cream/powder	+	Fair to medium	Mass merchandise
Powdercreme Makeup (Revlon)	Cream/powder	+ +	Fair to medium	Mass merchandise
Dual Finish Creme/ Powder Makeup (Lancome)	Cream/powder	+ + + + +	Fair to dark	Cosmetic counter
Maximum Cover (Estee Lauder)	Cream	+ + + +	Fair to medium	Cosmetic counter
Creme Powder Makeup (Almay)	Cream/powder	+	Fair to medium	Mass merchandise
Ultimate Coverage Makeup (Ultima II)	Cream	+ + +	Fair to medium	Cosmetic counter

Cost: +, $4–5; + +, $5–10; + + +, $10–20; + + + +, $20–30; + + + + +, $30–40 foundations are more difficult to contaminate bacterially than liquid foundations due to their low water content. The cream also provides a good barrier to transepidermal water loss and smoothes easily around any remaining desquamating stratum corneum. They are less irritating, since a volatile vehicle is not required to suspend the pigment, as in most liquid foundations.

The patient may need to alter her color selection in the immediate postoperative period. The color of the foundation may need to contain more reddish hues; however, most patients can return to their pre-surgery foundation formulation after 4 to 6 weeks.

Undercover Foundations

Some patients with pronounced, long-lasting redness or bruising following surgery may wish to use a product known as an ''undercover'' foundation or a ''color corrector'' foundation. These products, as opposed to heavy-coverage, surgical facial foundations, are designed to mask undesirable tones present in the skin through complementary color combination.[5] Use of these color correctors allows the patient to wear a moderate-coverage foundation, which appears more natural and may be more acceptable to the patient. The products are discussed in detail in Chapter 7. For example, redness of the face common after dermabrasion and chemical peeling procedures can be minimized through the use of a green color corrector, since the complementary color to red is green. The yellow to rust tones present in the skin due to hemosiderin and melanin deposition as facial bruising resolves may be masked with a purple to mauve undercover foundation, since purple is the complementary color to yellow.[6]

Powders and Blushers

Facial powders and blushers are applied alone or on top of a facial foundation. Generally, their use should not be resumed until the face has healed to the point where facial foundations can be worn, as discussed previously Powders without ground particulate matter, such as nut shells or mica, should be selected to avoid damaging the follicular ostia, which can lead to milia and closed comedone formation. Thus, powders with a dull or matte finish are preferred.

Facial blushers are colored powders designed to add color to the cheeks and face. These products are extremely useful in the post-surgical patient to

1. Restore facial landmarks, such as cheekbones, in patients who are wearing high-coverage foundations
2. Camouflage facial redness by applying the blusher to the upper cheeks, central forehead, nasal tip, and central chin
3. Add color to impart the appearance of health

As with facial powders, blushers should be selected with a matte finish to avoid light-reflective particulate matter.

Eye Cosmetics

Most patients can resume wearing selected eye cosmetics immediately following surgery, unless the surgery involved the eye area (i.e., eyelid tumor, blepharoplasty, eyelid chemical peel). Mascara, applied to darken, lengthen, and thicken the eyelashes, may be immediately resumed. Water-soluble varieties are recommended, however, since the solvents required to remove waterproof varieties may cause cutaneous stinging. Water-soluble eyeliners may also be resumed to highlight and cosmetically enlarge the eye. Eye shadows, on the other hand, represent a pigmented powdered cosmetic and should not be worn until facial foundation use is resumed.

Lip Cosmetics

Lip cosmetics can also be resumed immediately following surgery unless the surgical site involves the lips (i.e., lip tumor removal, lip advancement flap, upper lip dermabrasion or chemical peel). Lip cosmetics are highly recommended as they represent a quick way to add color to the face and restore an acceptable cosmetic appearance.

Cosmetic Removal

Post-surgical patients should wear cosmetics only when necessary and thoroughly remove them as soon as possible. All cosmetics should definitely be removed prior to going, to bed. Ideally, the cosmetic should be removed with mild soap and water; however, the waterproof camouflaging foundations require a special removal product. Each surgical makeup company manufactures a special oily removal product that should be purchased with the foundation. Solvent makeup removers should be avoided until healing is complete.

REFERENCES

1. Theberge L, Kernaleguen A: Importance of cosmetics related to aspects of self. Precept Mot Skills 48:827, 1979
2. Cash TF, Cash DW: Women's use of cosmetics: psychosocial correlates and consequences. Int J Cosmet Sci 4:1, 1982
3. Brauer EW: Coloring and corrective make-up preparations. Clin Dermatol 6:62, 1988

4. Schlossman ML, Feldman AJ: Fluid foundation and blush make-up. p. 748. In deNavarre MG (ed): The Chemistry and Manufacture of Cosmetics. Wheaton IL: Allured Publishing Corp, 1988
5. Draelos ZK: Cosmetic camouflaging techniques. Cutis 52:362, 1993
6. Draelos ZK: Use of cover cosmetics for pigment abnormalities. Cosmet Dermatol 5:14, 1989

9

Moisturizers

Many terms are used by the cosmetics industry to describe the effects of creams and lotions: lubricants, moisturizers, repair or replenishing products, emollients, and so forth. These terms do not have scientific meaning since the mechanisms for rehydrating dry skin or rejuvenating damaged skin remain to be elucidated. In basic terms, "lubricants" refers to those products that increase skin slip in dry skin that is rough and flaky; "moisturizers" impart moisture to the skin, increasing skin flexibility; and "repair" or "replenishing" products are intended to reverse the appearance of aging skin. All three classes of products are based on emollients. An understanding of the function of moisturizers and their formulation is essential to the dermatologist who must maintain the health of xerotic skin once the dermatitis has resolved.[1]

PHYSIOLOGY OF XEROSIS

Xerosis is a result of decreased water content of the stratum corneum, which leads to abnormal desquamation of corneocytes. For the skin to appear and feel normal, the water content of this layer must be above 10%.[2] Water is lost through evaporation to the environment under low humidity conditions and must be replenished by water from the lower epidermal and dermal layers.[3] The stratum corneum must have the ability to maintain this moisture, or the skin will feel rough, scaly, and dry. However, this is indeed a simplistic view, as there are minimal differences between the amount of water present in the stratum corneum of dry and normal skin.[4] Xerotic skin is due to more than simply low water content.[5] Electron micrographic studies of dry skin demonstrate a stratum corneum that is thicker, fissured, and disorganized.

There are three intercellular lipids implicated in epidermal barrier function: sphingolipids, free sterols, and free fatty acids.[6] In addition, it is thought that the lamellar bodies (Odland bodies, membrane-coating granules, cementsomes), containing sphingolipids, free sterols, and phospholipids, play a key role in barrier function and are essential to trap water and prevent excessive water loss.[7,8] The lipids are necessary for barrier function since solvent extraction of these chemicals leads to xerosis directly proportional to the amount of lipid removed.[9] The major lipid by weight found in the stratum corneum is ceramide, which becomes sphingolipid if glycosylated via the primary alcohol of sphingosine.[10] Ceramides possess the majority of the long-chain fatty acids and linoleic acid in the skin. Perturbations within the barrier result in rapid lamellar body secretion and a cascade of cytokine changes associated with adhesion molecule expression and growth factor production.[11] If skin with barrier perturbations is occluded with a vapor-impermeable wrap, the expected burst in lipid synthesis is blocked. However, occlusion with a vapor-permeable wrap does not prevent barrier recovery.[12] Therefore, transepidermal water loss is necessary to initiate synthesis of lipids to allow barrier repair.[13,14]

Remoisturization of the skin must then occur in four steps: initiation of barrier repair, alteration of surface cutaneous moisture partition coefficient, onset of dermal–epidermal moisture diffusion, and synthesis of intercellular lipids.[15] It is generally thought in the cosmetics industry that a stratum corneum containing between 20% and 35% water will exhibit the softness and pliability or normal stratum corneum.[16]

Other disease states, such as psoriasis and atopic dermatitis, also demonstrate abnormal barrier function due to ceramide distribution.[17,18] Interestingly enough, xerosis tends to increase with age due to a lower inherent water content of the stratum corneum.[19] But this does not totally account for the scaliness and roughness of aged skin; probably an abnormal desquamatory process is also present.[20]

There are other lipids present in the stratum corneum, besides those previously discussed, that are worth mentioning: cholesterol sulfate, free sterols, free fatty acids, triglycerides, sterol wax/esters, squalene, and *n*-alkanes.[21] Cholesterol sulfate only comprises 2% to 3% of the total epidermal lipids, but is important in corneocyte desquamation.[22] It appears that corneocyte desquamation is mediated through the desulfation of cholesterol sulfate.[23] Fatty acids are also important since it has been demonstrated that barrier function can be restored by topical or systemic administration of linoleic acid–rich oils in essential fatty acid–deficient rats.[24]

MECHANISMS OF MOISTURIZATION

There are four mechanisms by which the stratum corneum can be rehydrated: occlusives, humectants, hydrophilic matrices, and sunscreens.[25]

Occlusives

There are 20 different generic classes of chemicals that can function as occlusives to retard transepidermal water loss. Each chemical imparts a different feel and thickness to the moisturizer. Some of the more widely used substances are[26]

Hydrocarbon oils and waxes: petrolatum, mineral oil, paraffin, squalene
Silicone oils
Vegetable and animal fats
Fatty acids: lanolin acid, stearic acid
Fatty alcohol: lanolin alcohol, cetyl alcohol
Polyhydric alcohols: propylene glycol
Wax esters: lanolin, beeswax, stearyl stearate
Vegetable waxes: carnauba, candelilla
Phospholipids: lecithin
Sterols: cholesterol

The most occlusive of the above chemicals is petrolatum.[27] It appears, however, that total occlusion of the stratum corneum is undesirable. While the transepidermal water loss can be completely halted, once the occlusive is removed, water loss resumes at its preapplication level. Thus, the occlusive moisturizer has not allowed the stratum corneum to repair its barrier function.[28] However, petrolatum does not appear to function as an impermeable barrier; rather, it permeates throughout the interstices of the stratum corneum, allowing barrier function to be reestablished.[29]

Humectants

Another concept in rehydrating the stratum corneum is the use of humectants. Humectants have been used in cosmetics for many years to increase shelf life by preventing product evaporation and subsequent thickening due to variations in temperature and humidity. For example, humectants are a necessary part of all oil-in-water creams to maintain their required water content. Substances that function as humectants are glycerin, honey, sodium lactate, urea, propylene glycol, sorbitol, pyrrolidone carboxylic acid, gelatin, hyaluronic acid, vitamins, and some proteins.[26,30]

Cosmetics chemists have theorized that humectants could be used to draw water from the environment, under conditions where the ambient humidity exceeds 70%, and more commonly from the deeper epidermal and dermal tissues to rehydrate the stratum corneum. Water that is applied to the skin in the absence of a humectant is rapidly lost to the atmosphere.[31] Humectants may also allow the skin to feel smoother by filling holes in the stratum corneum through swelling.[32] However, under low humidity conditions humectants, such as glycerin, will actually draw moisture from the skin and increase transepidermal water loss.[33] Therefore, a good moisturizer should combine both occlusive and humectant properties.

Hydrophilic Matrices

Hydrophilic matrices have also been available for many years in the form of colloidal oatmeal baths. The idea of the bath was to soothe, but also to provide a "blanket" against water evaporation. Hyaluronic acid is a high-molecular-weight substance that is one of the newer hydrophilic matrices found in some moisturizers.

Sunscreens

Many of the repair and replenishing moisturizing formulations have a sunscreen in addition to a more conventional emollient. The sunscreen agent is thought to prevent cellular damage and thus prevent dehydration. It may be a chemical sunscreen, a physical sunscreen, or a combination of both. A more detailed discussion of sunscreens is given in Chapter 23.

MECHANISMS OF EMOLLIENCY

Emolliency is important to consumer satisfaction with a moisturizing product, since smooth skin is expected following application, even though emolliency may not necessarily correlate with decreased transepidermal water loss. Emollients function by filling the spaces between the desquamating skin scale with oil droplets,[34] but their effect is only temporary.

Emollients can be divided into several categories: protective emollients, fatting emollients, dry emollients, and astringent emollients.[35] Protective emollients are substances such as diisopropyl dilinoleate and isopropyl isostearate that remain on the skin longer than average and allow the skin to feel smooth immediately upon application. Fatting emollients, such as castor oil, propylene glycol, jojoba oil, isostearyl isostearate, and octyl stearate, also leave a long-lasting film on the skin, but may feel greasy. Dry emollients, such as isopropyl palmitate, decyl oleate, and isostearyl alcohol, do not offer much skin protection but produce a dry feel. Lastly, astringent emollients, such as the dimethicones and cyclomethicones, isopropyl myristate, and octyl octanoate, have minimal greasy residue and can reduce the oily feel of other emollients.

FORMULATION

Most moisturizers consist of water, lipids, emulsifiers, preservatives, fragrance, color, and specialty additives. Interestingly, water accounts for 60% to 80% of any moisturizer; however, externally applied water does not remoisturize the skin. In fact, the rate of water passage through the skin increases with increased hydration.[36] The water functions as a diluent and evaporates, leaving the active agents behind. Emulsifiers are generally soaps in concentrations of 0.5% or less and function to keep the water and lipids in one continuous phase. Parabens are the most commonly used preservatives in moisturizers usually combined with one of the formaldehyde donor preservatives.[15] The variety of specialty additives incorporated into moisturizers is endless, limited only by the imagination of the cosmetics chemist.

A marketable moisturizer formulation must fulfill three criteria: it must increase the water content of the skin (moisturization), it must make the skin feel smooth and soft (emolliency), and it must protect injured or exposed skin from harmful or annoying stimuli (skin protectant).

Facial Moisturizers

Facial moisturizers and related products are the fastest growing product in the cosmetics market. There are two basic formulations: oil-in-water emulsions, in which water is the dominant phase, and water-in-oil emulsions, in which oil is the dominant phase. Oil-in-water formulations are used for the thinner daytime facial moisturizers, and water-in-oil formulations are used for night creams or facial replenishing creams. Oil-in-water emulsions can be identified by their cool feel and nonglossy appearance, while water-in-oil emulsions can be identified by their warm feel and glossy appearance.[37] Daytime moisturizers are generally composed of mineral oil, propylene glycol, and water in sufficient quantity to form a lotion. Night creams are composed of mineral oil, lanolin alcohol, petrolatum, and water to form a cream. Specialized eye creams are night creams with some of the more irritating ingredients removed to prevent eye stinging. The differences between products thus lie in the addition of fragrances, exotic oils, vitamins, protein or amino acid products, and other minor moisturizing aids.

The plethora of facial moisturizers has made categorization of the various products difficult; however, a brief look at the claims and composition of some key products is valuable. The cosmetics companies market facial moisturizers based on skin type. Naturally, products designed for oily complexions are oil-free or contain small amounts of light oils. Products for normal skin contain moderate amounts of light oils, and products for dry skin contain increased amounts of heavier oils. The lighter oil used is generally mineral oil, and the heavier oil is petrolatum. Thus, moisturizing products can be developed for all skin types based on varying water-to-oil ratios.

Oily complexion products that are oil-free are composed of water and silicone derivatives, such as cyclomethicone or dimethicone. This combination has been shown to be noncomedogenic in the rabbit ear assay. These products are nongreasy, since the bulk of the product evaporates from the face. Many oily complexion moisturizers also claim to provide oil control, which is accomplished through the use of oil-absorbing substances such as talc, clay, starch, or synthetic polymers.

Products designed for normal or combination skin contain predominantly water, mineral oil, and propylene glycol with very small amounts of petrolatum or lanolin. These products leave a greater oily residue on the face than oil-free formulations. Moisturizers in this line are also called "antiwrinkle lotions," "protective creams," or "sport creams" if they contain sunscreening agents.

Dry skin moisturizers contain water, mineral oil, propylene glycol, and larger amounts of petrolatum or lanolin in addition to low concentrations of numerous additives claiming to rebuild, renew, or replenish. The patient should realize that the perfect skin moisturizer does not exist. Creams and lotions that claim to restore or rebuild tissue in the dermis do not penetrate deeply to have any effect. The extremely high cost of some moisturizers is not justified by the value of the ingredients. Patients are buying a certain feel, fragrance, or image. If the patient achieves more self-confidence or an increased sense of well-being after using a certain facial cream, then the money has been well spent. The role of the physician should be to identify which cosmetics claims are unfounded so that patients have a medical perspective on the product they chooses to purchase.

It is important that patients select the appropriate facial moisturizer for their skin type. Most cosmetics companies clearly label which moisturizers are for oily, normal, and dry skin. Even though patients with oily skin may be hesitant to use a moisturizer, a product that contains oil-absorbing talc or kaolin can decrease facial shine. Patients with oily skin often use a soap containing benzoyl peroxide to remove unwanted oil and to aid in acne treatment. These soaps can leave the face scaly immediately following washing, interfering with foundation application. An oil-free moisturizer can help flatten scale, enabling smooth foundation application rather than preferentially adhering to skin scale. Patients selecting an oil-free foundation must use an oil-free moisturizer to ensure maximum foundation wear and minimize color drift.

Patients with dry skin will benefit from the selection of an appropriate moisturizer. Fine wrinkling due to cutaneous dehydration and roughness due to skin scale can be improved.

Body Moisturizers

Body moisturizers come in a variety of preparations, including lotion, cream, mousse, and ointment. Lotions are the most popular formulation. Creams and ointments can be used on the body, but are more difficult to spread, especially in hair-bearing areas. Female patients desire a nongreasy body lotion with a rich texture; however, a rich texture does not necessarily identify a superior moisturizer. Richness can be added to a thin lotion with water-soluble gums that impart a silky feel to the skin but do not provide improved moisture retention.

Body lotions are generally oil-in-water emulsions containing 10% to 15% oil phase, 5% to 10% humectant, and 75% to 85% water phase. More specifically, they are composed of water, mineral oil, propylene glycol, stearic acid, and petrolatum or lanolin. Most also contain an emulsifier such as triethanolamine stearate. Humectants such as glycerin or sorbitol may also be used. Other additives include vitamins, such as A, D. and E, and soothing agents, such as aloe and allantoin.

Hand Moisturizers

The simplest hand ointment is petroleum jelly, but most patients find this greasy. To improve cosmetic appeal, the petroleum jelly can be whipped with water, color, and fragrance to make a hand cream. Thus, hand creams are oil-in-water emulsions with 15% to 40% oil phase, 5% to 15% humectant, and 45% to 80% water phase.[38] The addition of silicone derivatives can also render the hand cream water-resistant through four to six washings. Some hand creams even include a sunscreen agent.

Liposome-Containing Moisturizers

Liposomes are not true moisturizers, but rather represent a novel method of delivering moisturizing substances to the epidermis. The reader is referred to page 256 for a complete discussion.

SPECIALTY ADDITIVES

Many substances can be added to moisturizers to enhance their marketing claims and possibly their efficacy. This section evaluates the scientific data published regarding the utility of the most popular moisturizer specialty additives.

Ceramides

Since ceramides play an important role in skin barrier formation, it has been postulated that topical application might enhance barrier repair. Chemically synthesized ceramides are available to the cosmetics chemist. More data are necessary before the value of topically applied ceramides can be assessed.

Essential Fatty Acids

Essential fatty acids, such as unsaturated linoleic, linolenic, and arachidonic acids, are referred to as "vitamin F" in the cosmetics industry. They are thought to become incorporated into the structural phospholipids of the epidermis, thus normalizing the cell lipid layers. Much of these data, however, are derived from topical application of sunflower oil on rodents who are essential fatty acid deficient.[24]

Vitamins

Vitamins are common moisturizer additives. Pantothenic acid, or vitamin B complex, is commonly used in many chemical forms: panthenol, pantethine, or pangamic acid. Some claim that bee pollen and jelly are useful for their high vitamin B content. However, there is no evidence that vitamin B penetrates the skin. Vitamin E is also a common additive and is said to enhance percutaneous absorption. Sometimes vitamins A, C, and D are added, but the usefulness of topical vitamins is dubious. Vitamins must be in a water-soluble form to have any chance of penetrating the stratum corneum, and thus oil-soluble preparations are of little value.[39] Oral administration of vitamins is far superior to cutaneous administration for the treatment of vitamin deficiencies. It is thought, however, that some vitamins can act as humectants, thus enhancing the efficacy of the moisturizing product. Another discussion of vitamins in cosmetic formulations is found in Chapter 24.

Natural Moisturizing Factor

There are a group of substances reported to regulate the moisture content of the stratum corneum, known as ''natural moisturizing factor'' (NMF). Natural moisturizing factor consists of a mixture of amino acids, derivatives of amino acids, and salts. More specifically, it contains amino acids, pyrrolidone carboxylic acid, lactate, urea, ammonia, uric acid, glucosamine, creatinine, citrate, sodium, potassium, calcium, magnesium, phosphate, chlorine, sugar, organic acids, and peptides.[34] Ten percent of the dry weight of the stratum corneum cells is composed of NMF. Skin that cannot produce NMF is dry and cracked.[44]

Sodium PCA

Sodium PCA has been termed one of the natural moisturizing factors, along with urea and lactic acid. It is a sodium salt of 2-pyrrolidone-5-carboxylic acid and experimentally has been shown to be a better moisturizer than glycerol.[39] Sodium PCA is used as a humectant in many cosmetics in concentrations of 2% or greater.

Urea

Urea is a penetrating moisturizer that possesses a high osmotic effect on the skin. It diffuses into the outer layers of the stratum corneum and disrupts hydrogen bonding, which exposes the water-binding sites on the corneocytes. Urea also promotes desquamation by dissolving the intercellular cementing substance between the corneocytes. In this manner it can promote the absorption of other topically applied drugs.[41] It must be kept at an acidic pH in formulation or it will decompose to ammonia. Problems with irritancy have been somewhat overcome by adsorbing the urea onto talc prior to dispersion into the emulsion.

Lactic Acid

Lactic acid, or sodium lactate, is also considered to be a natural moisturizing factor in that it enhances water uptake better than glycerin It is found in many therapeutic moisturizers, as it can increase the water-binding capacity of the stratum corneum. Additionally, it can increase stratum corneum pliability in direct proportion to the amount of lactic acid that is absorbed.[33]

Collagen, Elastin, Hyaluronic Acid

Collagen, elastin, and hyaluronic acid all are biologically derived substances included in the formulation of some moisturizers. The reader is referred to Chapter 24 for a complete discussion.

Aloe Vera and Other Botanicals

Aloe vera is a botanical additive to some moisturizers. The reader is referred to Chapter 24 for a complete discussion.

EFFICACY

The efficacy of moisturizers can be difficult to assess; however, several excellent noninvasive methods have been developed: regression analysis, profilometry, squametry, in vivo image analysis, twistometre, impedance measurement, and evaporimetry.[42]

Regression analysis is a method of evaluating moisturizer efficacy under clinical conditions. Patients are selected and treated by an objective observer with moisturizers at a predetermined test site for 2 weeks. The test site is evaluated on days 7 and 14. If improvement is noted, moisturizer application is discontinued and the test site evaluated daily for 2 weeks or until the baseline pathology has reappeared.[43] This method is particularly valuable since the efficacy of all moisturizers is excellent immediately following application, but the true effectiveness can only be assessed with the passage of time.[44]

Profilometry involves analysis of silicone rubber (Silflo) replicas of the skin surface. These silicone replicas are then cast into plastic positives, which are then measured with a computerized stylus instrument that provides a contour tracing of the surface. Thus a two- or three-dimensional topogram is created. Unfortunately, this method can be inaccurate since the silicone application to the skin surface tends to flatten and disturb the desquamating skin scale.[45]

Squametry involves analysis of skin squames harvested by pressing a sticky tape against the skin. The outermost, loosely adherent skin scale is then removed. The tape provides a specimen that retains the topographical relationships of the skin surface and the pattern of desquamation. Image processing is then used to evaluate the scaliness of the skin.[46]

In vivo image analysis is nothing more than feeding a video or 35 mm image into a computer image processing system to record and subsequently evaluate skin surface features.[47] Care needs to be taken to standardize lighting and camera angles to ensure accurate data for analysis.

Twistometre, impedance measurement, and evaporimetry, are mechanistic methods of evaluating skin dryness and moisturizer effectiveness. The twistometre uses torsion to measure in vivo the influence of stratum corneum hydration on skin extensibility. A weak torque is applied to a rotating disc that is placed in contact with the skin. It has been shown that dry skin is much less extensible than well-hydrated skin.[48]

Skin impedance can also be evaluated. A dry electrode consisting of two concentric brass cylinders separated by a phenolic insulator operating at 3.5 MHz is applied to the skin.[49] The impedance drops as the skin is better hydrated.[50] This technique can evaluate the efficacy and the duration of effect of moisturizers.[51]

Lastly, evaporimetry can be used to measure the cutaneous transepidermal water loss.[52] More occlusive substances would be expected to lower water loss, while some humectants, such as glycerin, actually increase water loss.[53,54]

Even though these sophisticated, noninvasive methods of cutaneous evaluation sound appealing, there is no substitute for the opinion of a trained, unbiased observer when evaluating moisturizer effectiveness. Mechanistic evaluation can be easily biased to produce data that serve the best interest of the manufacturer. Computers cannot yet accurately synthesize all the tactile and visual information that can be obtained with human evaluation. The noninvasive techniques simply present another tool for assessing moisturizer function.[55]

ADVERSE REACTIONS

Many patients with dry skin will claim that they are "allergic" to most moisturizers as a result of skin stinging experienced following application. This may represent an irritant contact dermatitis rather than a true allergic contact dermatitis.[56] These patients should avoid moisturizers containing propylene glycol, which may cause burning upon application to damaged skin. Other substances found in facial moisturizers that cause stinging include benzoic acid, cinnamic acid compounds, lactic acid, urea, emulsifiers, formaldehyde, and sorbic acid.

Moisturizing ointments, creams, lotions, and gels should be patch tested "as is." If an irritant reaction is experienced with closed patch testing, the product should be retested with open patch testing and provocative use testing.[57]

REFERENCES

1. Goldner R: Moisturizers: a dermatologist's perspective. J Toxicol-Cut & Ocular Toxicol 11:193, 1992
2. Boisits EK: The evaluation of moisturizing products. Cosmet Toilet 101 May 1986: 31, 1986

3. Wu MS, Yee DJ, Sullivan ME: Effect of a skin moisturizer on the water distribution in human stratum corneum. J Invest Dermatol 81:446, 1983

4. Wildnauer RH, Bothwell JW, Douglass AB: Stratum corneum biomechanical properties. J Invest Dermatol 56:72, 1971

5. Pierard GE: What does "dry skin" mean? Int J Dermatol 26:167, 1987

6. Elies PM: Lipids and the epidermal permeability barrier. Arch Dermatol Res 270: 95, 1981

7. Holleran WM, Man MQ, Wen NG et al: Sphingolipids are required for mammalian epidermal barrier function. J Clin Invest 88:1338, 1991

8. Downing DT: Lipids: their role in epidermal structure and function. Cosmet Toilet 106 December 1991:63, 1991

9. Grubauer G, Elias PM, Feingold KR: Transepidermal water loss: the signal for recovery of barrier structure and function. J Lipid Res 30:323, 1989

10. Petersen RD: Ceramides key components for skin protection. Cosmet Toilet 107 February 1992:45, 1992

11. Nickoloff BJ, Naidu Y: Perturbation of epidermal barrier function correlates with initiation of cytokine cascade in human skin. J Am Acad Dermatol 30:535, 1994

12. Elias PM: Epidermal lipids, barrier function, and desquamation. J Invest Dermatol 80:44s, 1983

13. Jass HE, Elias PM: The living stratum corneum: implications for cosmetic formulation. Cosmet Toilet 106 October 1991:47, 1991

14. Holleran W, Feingold K, Man MO et al: Regulation of epidermal sphingolipid synthesis by permeability barrier function. J Lipid Res 32:1151, 1991

15. Jackson EM: Moisturizers: What's in them? How do they work? Am J Contact Dermatitis 3:162, 1992

16. Reiger MM: Skin, water and moisturization. Cosmet Toilet 104 December 1989: 41, 1989

17. Motta S, Monti M, Sesana S et al: Abnormality of water barrier function in psoriasis. Arch Dermatol 130:452, 1994

18. Imokawa G, Abe A, Jin K et al: Decreased level of ceramides in stratum corneum of atopic dermatitis: an etiologic factor in atopic dry skin? J Invest Dermatol 96: 523, 1991

19. Potts RO, Buras EM, Chrisman DA: Changes with age in the moisture content of human skin. J Invest Dermatol 82:97, 1984

20. Wepierre J, Marty JP: Percutaneous absorption and lipids in elderly skin. J Appl Cosmetol 6:79, 1988

21. Brod J: Characterization and physiological role of epidermal lipids. Int J Dermatol 30:84, 1991

22. Lampe MA, Williams ML, Elias PM: Human epidermal lipids: characterization and modulation during differentiation. J Lipid Res 24:131, 1983

23. Long SA, Wertz PW, Strauss JS et al: Human stratum corneum polar lipids and desquamation. Arch Dermatol Res 277:284, 1985

24. Elias PM, Brown BE, Ziboh VA: The permeability barrier in essential fatty acid deficiency: evidence for a direct role for linoleic acid in barrier function. J Invest Dermatol 75:230, 1980

25. Baker CG: Moisturization: new methods to support time proven ingredients. Cosmet Toilet 102 April 1987:99, 1987

26. De Groot AC, Weyland JW, Nater JP: Unwanted Effects of Cosmetics and Drugs Used in Dermatology. 3rd Ed. Elsevier, Amsterdam, 1994

27. Friberg SE, Ma Z: Stratum corneum lipids, petrolatum and white oils. Cosmet Toilet 107 July 1993:55, 1993

28. Grubauer G, Feingold KR, Elias PM: Relationship of epidermal lipogenesis to cutaneous barrier function. J Lipid Res 28:746, 1987

29. Ghadially R, Halkier-Sorensen L, Elias PM: Effects of petrolatum on stratum corneum structure and function. J Am Acad Dermatol 26:387, 1992

30. Spencer TS: Dry skin and skin moisturizers. Clin Dermatol 6:24, 1988

31. Rieger MM, Deem DE: Skin moisturizers II. The effects of cosmetic ingredients on human stratum corneum. J Soc Cosmet Chem 25:253, 1974

32. Robbins CR, Fernee KM: Some observations on the swelling of human epidermal membrane. JSCC 37:21, 1983

33. Idson B: Dry skin: moisturizing and emolliency. Cosmet Toilet 107 July 1992:69, 1992

34. Wehr RF, Krochmal L: Considerations in selecting a moisturizer. Cutis 39:512, 1987

35. Brand HM, Brand-Garnys EE: Practical application of quantitative emolliency. Cosmet Toilet 107 July 1992:93, 1992

36. Warner RR, Myers MC, Taylor DA: Electron probe analysis of human skin: Determination of the water concentration profile. J Invest Dermatol 90:218, 1988

37. Idson B: Moisturizers, emollients, and bath oils. p. 37. In Frost P, Horwitz SN (eds): CV Mosby, St. Louis, 1982

38. Schmitt WH: Skin-care products. In Williams DF, Schmitt WH (eds): Chemistry and Technology of the Cosmetics and Toiletries Industry. Blackie Academic & Professional, London, 1992

39. Wilkinson JB, Moore RJ: Harry's Cosmeticology. 7th Ed. Chemical Publishing, New York, 1982

40. Rawlings AV, Scott IR, Harding CR, Bowser PA: Stratum corneum moisturization at the molecular level. Prog Dermatol 28:1, 1994

41. Raab WP: Uses of urea in cosmetology. Cosmet Toilet 105 May 1990:97, 1990

42. Grove GL: Noninvasive methods for assessing moisturizers. p. 121. In Waggoner WC (ed): Clinical Safety and Efficacy Testing of Cosmetics. Marcel Dekker, Inc, New York, 1990

43. Kligman AM: Regression method for assessing the efficacy of moisturizers. Cosmet Toilet 93:27, 1978

44. Lazar AP, Lazar P: Dry skin, water, and lubrication. Dermatol Clin 9:45, 1991

45. Grove GL, Grove MJ: Objective methods for assessing skin surface topography noninvasively p. 1. In Leveque JL (ed): Cutaneous Investigation in Health and Disease Marcel Dekker, New York, 1988

46. Grove GL: Dermatological applications of the Magiscan image analysing computer. p. 173. In Marks R, Payne PA (eds): Bioengineering and the Skin. MTP Press, Lancaster, England, 1981

47. Prall JK, Theiler RF, Bowser Pa, Walsh M: The effect of cosmetic products in alleviating a range of skin dryness conditions as determined by clinical and instrumental techniques. Int J Cosmet Sci 8:159, 1986

48. de Rigal J, Leveque JL: In vivo measurements of the stratum corneum elasticity. Bioeng Skin 1:13, 1985

49. Tagami H: Electrical measurement of the water content of the skin surface. Cosmet Toilet 97:39, 1982

50. Archer WI, Kohli R, Roberts JMC, Spencer TS: In Rietschel RL, Spencer TS (eds): Skin Impedance Measurement. Marcel Dekker, Inc, New York
51. Grove GL: The effect of moisturizers on skin surface hydration as measured in vivo by electrical conductivity. Curr Ther Res 50:712, 1991
52. Idson B: In vivo measurement of transdermal water loss. J Soc Cosmet Chem 29: 573, 1976
53. Rietschel RL: A method to evaluate skin moisturizers in vivo. J Invest Dermatol 70:152, 1978
54. Rietschel RL: A skin moisturization assay. J Soc Cosmet Chem 30:360, 1979
55. Grove GL: Design of studies to measure skin care product performance. Bioeng Skin 3:359, 1987
56. Lazar PM: The toxicology of moisturizers. J Toxicol-Cut & Ocular Toxicol 11: 185, 1992
57. Maibach HI, Engasser PG: Dermatitis due to cosmetics. In Fisher AA (ed): Contact Dermatitis. 3rd Ed. Lea & Febiger, Phildelphia, 1986

10

Nail Cosmetics

Nails function primarily to protect the tender fingertip and to facilitate manipulation of small items, but they are also an important area for cosmetic manipulation. Modern society assigns paramount importance to the appearance of the nails as a manner of determining social status. Persons who perform manual labor cannot maintain long nails, while individuals who work in managerial positions use longer nail length as one method of indicating success. It is mainly women who value long nails; however, some Mediterranean men allow the little fingernail to grow to indicate their white collar status.

The development of nail polishes, hardeners, bleaches, and moisturizers has provided increased access to nail cosmetics for both men and women (Table 10-1). This chapter discusses manicuring techniques and cosmetics available for adornment of the nails.

MANICURING TECHNIQUES

Manicuring of the nails is necessary for good grooming, but is also a source of dermatologic problems. Many techniques are employed.

The main goal of a manicure should be proper trimming of the nails to maintain a strong, healthy nail plate. The nail should be rounded at the tip for esthetics, but the corners should be left square to maximize strength. Too sharp an arc extending from the lateral to medial nail margin will weaken the nail structurally. Ideally, the nail plate should not be cut, but filed frequently with an orange stick to avoid cracking the nail plate through shearing forces generated by scissors or clippers. However, most patients groom their nails infrequently, necessitating cutting. Cutting should be done with a pair of curved nail clippers, since scissors may not cut the nail plate squarely. An angle on the distal nail plate can predispose to onychoschizia. Any remaining sharp edges should be filed with a diamond dust file.[1] Under no circumstances should the cuticle be removed or traumatized, as this may precipitate the formation of paronychia, onychomycosis, or onychodystrophy.

Table 10-1. Nail Cosmetics

Nail Cosmetic	Main Ingredients	Function	Adverse Reactions
Nail polish	Nitrocellulose, toluenesulfonamide resin, plasticizers, solvents, and colorants	Add color and shine to nail plates	Allergic contact dermatitis to toluene sulfonamide resin, nail plate staining
Nail hardener	Formaldehyde, acetates, acrylics, or other resins	Increase nail strength and prevent breakage	Allergic contact dermatitis to formaldehyde
Nail enamel remover	Acetone, alcohol, ethyl acetate, or butyl acetate	Remove nail polish	Irritant contact dermatitis
Cuticle remover	Sodium or potassium hydroxide	Destroy keratin that forms excess cuticular tissue on nail plate	Irritant contact dermatitis
Nail white	White pigments	Whiten free nail edge	Practically none
Nail bleach	Hydrogen peroxide	Remove nail plate stains	Irritant contact dermatitis
Nail polish drier	Vegetable oils, alcohols, or silicone derivatives	Speed drying time of nail polish	Practically none
Nail buffing cream	Pumice, talc, or kaolin	Smooth ridges in nails	Practically none
Nail moisturizer	Occlusives, humectants, lactic acid	Increase water content of nails	Practically none

NAIL POLISH

History

Nail enamel or polish is useful for nail adornment, covering nail discolorations, and providing strength to weak nails. This nail cosmetic was introduced in the 1920s when lacquer technology was developed. During Word War I, excellent sources of nitrocellulose were developed as a military explosive. The nitrocellulose was created by reacting cellulose fiber, from cotton linters or wood pulp, with nitric acid. It was discovered that boiled nitrocellulose could be dissolved in organic solvents. Following evaporation of the solvents, a hard, glossy film of nitrocellulose was produced, known as a "lacquer." Extensive research on nitrocellulose lacquer undertaken by the automobile industry found the product preferable to slow-drying oil-based paints previously used to paint cars. This technology was directly adapted to the cosmetics industry.[2]

Prior to 1920, nails were manicured and then "polished" with abrasive powder to achieve a shine. Color was then added through the use of stains. The first lacquer marketed was clear and labeled a "nail polish" as it imparted a high shine to the nail plate. In 1930, Charles Revson developed the idea of adding pigments to the clear lacquer to form an opaque, colored nail polish. Based upon the success of this poor-quality nail polish, Charles Revson formed Revlon in 1932. He hired a company to formulate a better product, which became known as ''nail enamel.''

Originally, Revson's nail enamel was only available in salons. But tremendous consumer demand created a new industry with tremendous sales that continue 60 years later.

Formulation

Nail polish consists basically of pigments suspended in a volatile solvent to which film-formers have been added. The ingredients can include[3]

1. Primary film-former (nitrocellulose, methacrylate polymers, vinyl polymers)
2. Secondary film-forming resin (formaldehyde, *p*-toluene sulfonamide, polyamide, acrylate, alkyd and vinyl resins)
3. Plasticizers (dibutyl phthalate, dioctyl phthalate, tricresyl phosphate, camphor)
4. Solvents and diluents (acetates, ketones, toluene, xylene, alcohols)
5. Colorants (organic D&C pigments, inorganic pigments)
6. Specialty fillers (guanine fish scale or titanium dioxide–coated mica flakes or bismuth oxychloride for iridescence)
7. Suspending agents

Nitrocellulose is the most commonly employed primary film-forming agent in nail lacquer. It produces a shiny, tough film that adheres well to the nail plate. The film is somewhat oxygen permeable, thus allowing gas exchange between the atmosphere and the nail plate. But the nontoxic nitrocellulose film is too hard and must be modified with resins and plasticizers.

The first resin used to enhance the nitrocellulose film was toluene-sulfonamide-formaldehyde. This resin is still widely used; however, some individuals are sensitive to this substance, which is found on the standard dermatology patch test tray. The resin has been eliminated in some hypoallergenic nail enamels. A polyester resin or cellulose acetate butyrate is employed instead, but sensitivity is still possible and the enamel is less resistant to wear.[4] The wear of a nail polish is determined by the film hardness, water resistance, adhesion to the nail, and ability to resist abrasion.

Nail lacquers also contain plasticizers such as dibutyl phthalate. These function to keep the product soft and pliable.

All of the nail lacquer ingredients must dissolve in a solvent that dries and leaves the colored film on the nail. Common solvents include *N*-butyl acetate and ethyl acetate. Other substances such as toluene and isopropyl alcohol may be added to act as diluents. Diluents keep the nail lacquer thin and lower its cost.

A variety of other substances can then be added to the basic nail lacquer to yield its final appearance. Coloring agents, such as organic colors, can be selected from an FDA-approved list of certified colors. Inorganic colors and pigments may also be used, but must conform to low heavy metal content standards.[5] These colors can be suspended within the lacquer with suspending agents, such as stearalkonium hectorite, to produce colors ranging from white to pink to purple to brown to orange to blue to green. If the pigments are dissolved rather than suspended in the polish, nail staining is more likely.

Specialty fillers, such as guanine fish scale, bismuth oxychloride, or titanium dioxide–coated mica, can be added to give a frosted appearance due to enhanced light reflection. Chopped aluminum, silver, and gold can be added for a metallic shine. Nylon fibers can be added for nail strengthening purposes. Proteins, gelatins, and vitamins are also added to attempt to "beautify" the nail plate.

Application

A professional nail enamel application requires three layers of polish: a base coat, a pigmented nail enamel, and a top coat. The base coat ensures good adhesion to the nail plate and prevents polish chipping. It contains no pigment, less primary film-former, and more secondary film-former resin and is of a lower viscosity since a thinner film is desirable. The second layer is the actual pigmented nail enamel. The top coat, or third layer, provides gloss and resistance to chipping. It contains increased amounts of primary film former, more plasticizer, and less secondary film-forming resins. Some top coats may contain sunscreens but do not contain pigment.

Adverse Reactions

Problems associated with nail enamels include nail plate discoloration and allergic contact dermatitis. The nail staining, as mentioned previously, is seen with dissolved rather than suspended pigments and is most common in deep red nail polishes containing D&C Reds No. 6, 7, 34, or 5 Lake.[6] The nail plate will be stained yellow after 7 days of continuous wear. The staining will fade without treatment in approximately 14 days, once the enamel has been removed. Scrapping of the nail plate with a scapel blade can be used to confirm that only the nail surface has been stained, an important distinction in nail pigmentation abnormalities.[7]

Allergic contact dermatitis is seen in sensitive individuals who may develop proximal nail fold erythema and edema, fingertip tenderness and swelling, and/or eyelid dermatitis.[8] The North American Contact Dermatitis Group determined that 4% of positive patch tests were due to toluenesulfonamide/formaldehyde resin.[9] Even though the allergic reaction is most commonly due to wet nail enamel, Tosti et al.[10] found that 11 out of 59 patients who were patch test positive to wet polish also reacted to the dried enamel. Allergic reactions can be severe, necessitating lost work time or, rarely, hospitalization.[11]

There is some concern that the use of nail polish can contribute to nail dryness and brittleness. This actually is not the case. Nail polish prevents contact of detergents with the nail, thus acting as a protectant. Furthermore, it decreases nail water vapor loss from 1.6 to 0.4 mg/cm^2/hour.[12]

Nail polish can be tested "as is," but should be allowed to dry thoroughly as the volatile solvent can cause an irritant reaction if not allowed to evaporate rapidly. The toluenesulfonamide/formaldehyde resin can be also tested alone in 10% petrolatum.[13] Patients who are allergic to this resin may experience no difficulty with hypoallergenic nail polishes, but allergic contact dermatitis is still a possibility.[14]

NAIL HARDENER

Nail hardeners are used to increase the strength of brittle nails, thus allowing the nails to reach longer lengths before traumatic breakage occurs. The cause of brittle nails is thought to be dehydration of nail plate, largely due to excessive contact with detergents and water.

Formulation

A variety of formulations exist for nail hardeners. Some products that cause concern are those containing high formaldehyde concentrations (greater than 10%), which are responsible for onycholysis, subungual hyperkeratosis, reversible subungual hemorrhage and bluish discoloration of the nail plate.[15–17] Furthermore, these products proved to be a cause of allergic contact dermatatis.[18,19]

Formaldehyde in concentrations greater than 5% is no longer used in nail hardener preparations manufactured for interstate sale, as mandated by the FDA. Products that are produced and sold within a given state, however, may contain any concentration of formaldehye desired since these are outside the jurisdiction of the FDA, falling under state control.

Free formaldehyde in concentrations of 1% to 2% is still permitted, but acetates, toluene, nitrocellulose, acrylic, and polyamide resins are now used to reinforce the nail plate structurally. Some products actually contain 1% nylon fibers and are known as "fibered nail hardeners." Other additives purported to strengthen the nail include hydrolyzed proteins, modified vegetable extracts, glycerin, propylene glycol, and metal salts.[3]

Application

Nail hardeners are essentially a modification of clear nail enamel with different solvent and resin concentrations. They are the first coat of enamel applied to the clean nail plate, functioning as a base coat to allow better adhesion of the colored nail enamel.

Adverse Reactions

Nail hardeners may contain the same toluenesulfonamide/formaldehyde resin as nail polish and can also be a source of allergic contact dermatitis, as discussed previously. These products can be open or closed patch tested ''as is,'' but should be allowed to dry thoroughly prior to occluding.

NAIL ENAMEL REMOVER

Formulation

Nail polish removers are liquids designed to strip nail polish from the nail plate. They may contain solvents such as acetone, alcohol, ethyl acetate, or butyl acetate. Conditioning nail enamel removers are available, containing fatty materials such as cetyl alcohol, cetyl palmitate, lanolin, castor oil, or other synthetic oils. It is thought that these oily substances act as occlusive nail moisturizers, retarding water evaporation.

Application

Nail enamel remover is applied to a tissue or cotton ball and then wiped across the nail plate to remove old or unwanted nail polish. Several applications and rubbing may be required to remove the polish if several coats have been applied. The polish can also be removed by chipping, but this can damage the smooth nail plate surface.

Patients who wear sculptured nails must use a special acetone-free product to remove polish. Failure to do so may result in removal of the nail sculpture from the natural nail plate.

Adverse Effects

Nail polish remover can irritate and dry the nail plate and paronychial tissues.[20] It also can contribute to nail dryness and resulting brittleness. These problems can be minimized by using the product once a week or less.

Only open patch testing should be attempted with nail polish remover due to its high solvent concentration.[21] It may be tested at a concentration of 10% dissolved in olive oil.

CUTICLE REMOVER

Formulation

Cuticle removers are formulated as liquids or creams and contain an alkaline substance to destroy the keratin that comprises the cuticle. The cuticle is considered unattractive by cosmetologists and is removed routinely as part of a professional manicure. This practice accounts for many of the dermatologic problems associated with manicuring.

Cuticle remover may contain sodium or potassium hydroxide, a primary irritant, in a 2% to 5% concentration, with propylene glycol or glycerin added as a humectant. Milder preparations can be made with trisodium phosphate or tetrasodium pyrophosphate, but they are also less effective.[22]

A subset of products within this category are known as "cuticle softeners." These are quaternary ammonium compounds in a 3% to 5% concentration, sometimes combined with urea, designed to soften the cuticular protein and facilitate mechanical removal.

Application

Cuticle removers dissolve excess cuticular tissue on the nail plate. They are not intended to remove the fibrous cuticular ridge; however, vigorous use can remove the entire cuticle. The product is applied with a cotton ball and left on the nail plate for 10 minutes followed by removal with wiping.[23]

Adverse Reactions

Removal or manipulation of the cuticle is not recommended; paronychial inflammation with secondary bacterial infection or yeast colonization can occur. Cuticle removers can also damage the nail plate through softening.

Due to the high alkali content of these products, irritant contact dermatitis is common if the product is left on too long. Thus these products should not be used in closed patch testing.[21] They may be open patch tested in a 2% aqueous concentration, if necessary.

NAIL WHITE

Nail white is a paste or pencil applied beneath the free nail edge to create an even margin and a white appearance. It is based on white pigments, such as zinc oxide, titanium dioxide, kaolin, talc, or colloidal silica. The pencil formulations have largely replaced the pastes.[22]

There are no reports of adverse reactions from these products. The products may be open or closed patch tested "as is."

NAIL BLEACH

Nail bleaches are designed to remove stains from the nails. Stains may result from handling foods, tobacco products, or industrial materials. The bleaches are based on hydrogen peroxide in high volumes and are a possible cause of irritant contact dermatitis.[22] Closed patch testing should not be performed. Open patch testing may be performed with a 3% aqueous solution.

NAIL POLISH DRIER

Nail polish drier is designed to speed the drying time of nail polish. It is brushed or sprayed over the completed nails and induces rapid hardening of the enamel by drawing off the solvent present in the nail polish. Formulations consist of vegetable oils, alcohols, and silicone derivatives.

No reports of adverse reactions to this product have been published, although it could be a mild irritant. It should be allowed to dry thoroughly prior to close patch testing. Patch testing may be performed ''as is.''

NAIL BUFFING CREAM

Nail buffing creams are used to smooth ridges in the nail plate. Longitudinal nail ridging is especially common in mature individuals and thought to be due to whorls of degenerative cells in the nail matrix.[24] These ridges can be sanded smooth with creams containing finely ground pumice, talc, kaolin, or precipitated chalk as abrasives. Waxes are also added to increase nail shine.[25]

Certainly, nail buffing removes part of the nail plate and can weaken the nail if done aggressively or frequently. Some mature individuals already have a defective nail plate at the site of the longitudinal ridge as manifested by frequent splitting of the nail along the ridge. These patients should be discouraged from nail buffing. Usually, these products are not patch tested due to their abrasive quality.

NAIL MOISTURIZER

Nail moisturizers are valuable for patients with dry, brittle, fissured, and/or splitting nails.[26] The normal nail contains about 16% water, becoming soft with saturation at 30%. The water content of nail keratin is proportional to relative humidity, being 7% at 20% relative humidity and 30% at 100% relative humidity.[12] The idea of applying a cream or lotion to the nails for purposes of increasing the nail water content is somewhat new.

Formulation

Nail moisturizers are usually creams or lotions containing occlusives, such as petrolatum, mineral oil, or lanolin. Humectants, such as glycerin, propylene glycol, and proteins, may also be added. Alpha-hydroxy acids, lactic acid, and urea are active ingredients used to increase the water-binding capacity of the nail plate. A well-formulated nail moisturizer should contain substances from all of the aforementioned groups to treat the dehydrated nail plate maximally.

Recent studies demonstrated that daily oral biotin supplementation may be helpful in the treatment of brittle nails.[27] However, there is no evidence that topical biotin added to nail moisturizers has a similar beneficial effect. Furthermore, there is no evidence that topical gelatin, calcium, iron, botanical extracts, biological extracts, and so forth are effective at treating nail dehydration.

Application

Nail moisturizers function best if the nails are first soaked for 10 to 20 minutes in lukewarm water, preferably at bedtime. The moisturizer should then be generously applied under occlusion with a light cotton glove or sock. This procedure should be repeated nightly for at least 3 months. Certainly, activities contributing to dry nails, such as frequent contact with water, detergents, solvents, and nail polish remover, should be discontinued.[30]

Adverse Reactions

Alpha-hydroxy acids, lactic acid, and urea can cause stinging and irritant contact dermatitis in susceptible individuals. Wounds on the hands or fissured cuticles can also experience burning if high concentrations of these substances are employed. Most over-the-counter preparations contain 5% or less of these active agents; however, prescription preparations of lactic acid are available in 12% and 30% strengths.

Both open and closed patch testing can be performed "as is" with nail moisturizers, as long as the patient does not report immediate stinging on contact. Lactic acid in a 5% to 10% concentration is used to detect individuals who are prone to experience stinging when cosmetics products are applied to the face.[31]

REFERENCES

1. Engasser PG, Matsunaga J: Nail cosmetics. p. 214. In Scher RK, Daniel CR (eds): Nails: Therapy, Diagnosis, Surgery. WB Saunders, Philadelphia, 1990
2. Wimmer EP, Scholssman ML: The History of Nail Polish. Cosmet Toilet September 1992 107:115, 1992
3. Wing HJ: Nail preparations. p. 983. In deNavarre MG (ed): The Chemistry and Manufacture of Cosmetics. Wheaton, IL: Allured Publishing Corporation, 1988
4. Schlossman ML: Nail-enamel resins. Cosmet Technol 1:53, 1979
5. Schlossman ML: Nail polish colorants. Cosmet Toilet 95:31, 1980

6. Samman PD: Nail disorders caused by external influences. J Soc Cosmet Chem 28:351, 1977
7. Daniel DR, Osmet LS: Nail pigmentation abnormalities. Cutis 25:595, 1980
8. Scher RK: Cosmetics and ancillary preparations for the care of the nails. J Am Acad Dermatol 6:523, 1982
9. Adams RM, Maibach HI: A five-year study of cosmetic reactions. J Am Acad Dermatol 13:1062, 1985
10. Tosti A, Buerra L, Vincenzi C et al: Contact sensitization caused by toluene sulfonamide-formaldehyde resin in women who use nail cosmetics. Am J of Contact Dermatitis 4:150, 1993
11. Liden C, Berg M, Farm G et al: Nail varnish allergy with far-reaching consequences. Br J Dermatol 128:57, 1993
12. Mast R: Nail products. p. 265. In Whittam JH (ed): Cosmetic Safety A Primer for Cosmetic Scientists. Marcel Dekker, Inc, New York, 1987
13. deGroot AC, Weyland JW, Nater JP: Unwanted Effects of Cosmetics and Drugs Used in Dermatology. 3rd Ed. Elsevier, New York, 1994
14. Shaw S: A case of contact dermatitis from hypoallergenic nail varnish. Contact Dermatitis 20:385, 1989
15. Jawny L, Spada FJ: Contact dermatitis to a new nail hardener. Arch Dermatol 95:199, 1967
16. Paltzik RL, Enscoe I: Onycholysis secondary to toluene sulfonamide formaldehyde resin used in a nail hardener mimicking onychomycosis. Cutis 25:647, 1980
17. Donsky HJ: Onycholysis due to nail hardener. Canad Med Assoc J 96:1375, 1967
18. Lazar P: Reactions to nail hardeners. Arch Dermatol 94:446, 1966
19. Huldin DH: Hemorrhages of the lips secondary to nail hardeners. Cutis 4:709, 1968
20. Wallis MS, Bowen WR, Guin JD: Pathogenesis of onychoschizia (lamellar dystrophy). J Am Acad Dermatol 24:44, 1991
21. Maibach HI, Engasser PG: Dermatitis due to cosmetics. p. 384. In Fisher AA (ed): Contact Dermatits. 3rd Ed. Lea & Febiger, Philadelphia, 1986
22. Wilkinson JB, Moore RJ: Harry's Cosmeticology. 7th Ed. Chemical Publishing, New York, 1982
23. Brauer E: Cosmetics: the care and adornment of the nail. p. 289. In Baran R, Dawber RPR (eds): Diseases of the Nail and their Management. Blackwell, Oxford, 1984
24. Lewis BL, Montgomery H: The senile nail. J Invest Dermatol 24:11, 1955
25. Cohen PR, Scher RK: Nail changes in the elderly. J Geriatr Dermatol 1:45, 1993
26. Scher RK: Brittle nails. Int J Dermatol 28:515, 1989
27. Hochman LG, Scher RK, Meyerson MS: Brittle nails: response to daily biotin supplementation. Cutis 51:303, 1993
28. Cohen PR, Scher RK: Geriatic nail disorders: diagnosis and treatment. J Am Acad Dermatol 26:521, 1992
29. Fisher AA: Paresthesia due to contactants. p. 483. In Contact Dermatitis. 3rd ed. Lea & Febiger, Philadelphia, 1986

11

Cosmetic Nail Techniques

Cosmetic nail techniques can be applied solely for the elongation or beautification of the nail plate, but can also function as effective camouflaging for discolored, dystrophic, or malformed fingernails. Unfortunately, this group of cosmetics is responsible for both allergic contact dermatitis and nail damage. This chapter discusses the use of cosmetics designed to elongate the nail plate artificially: preformed artificial nails, nail sculptures, nail tips, nail wraps, and nail mending kits.

PREFORMED ARTIFICIAL NAILS

The most popular type of artificial nail is a preformed plastic nail. These nails are available in a variety of styles: precolored, uncolored, pre-cut, and uncut. The nails also come in a variety of sizes and shapes to match the patient's natural nail plate.[1] Even with the variety available, most patients do not find a suitable preformed nail, accounting for the increasing popularity of custom-made sculptured nails.

Preformed nails come in press-on, preglued forms and in forms requiring glue application. The acrylic glue used for adhesion is typically methacrylate-based and a possible cause of allergic contact dermatitis. A stronger nail adhesive made from ethyl 2-cyanoacrylate provides better adhesion, but can cause onycholysis.[2] Traumatic removal of artificial nails may result in onychoschizia and nail pitting.[3]

Preformed nails cannot be used effectively by patients with nail dystrophy, congenital nail deformity, or nail plate irregularities, since a smooth nail surface is required for adhesion.

SCULPTURED NAILS

An increasingly popular method of obtaining long, hard nails is the application of sculptured nails. The word ''sculptured'' is used since the custom-made artificial nail is sculpted on a template attached to the natural nail plate. The sculpted nail fits perfectly and, if well done, can be hard to differentiate from a natural nail.

Application

Nail sculpture application is an involved process requiring approximately 2 hours to sculpt 10 fingernails. The basic process is as follows:

1. All nail polish and oils are removed from the nail.
2. The nail is roughened with a coarse emery board, pumice stone, or grinding drill to create an optimal surface for sculpted nail adhesion.
3. An antifungal, antibacterial liquid, such as decolorized iodine, is applied to the entire nail plate to minimize onychomycosis and paronychia.
4. The loose edges of the cuticle are trimmed, removed, or pushed back, depending on the operator.
5. A flexible template is fit beneath the natural nail plate upon which the elongated sculpted nail will be built.
6. The acrylic is mixed and applied with a paint brush to cover the entire natural nail plate and extended onto the template to the desired nail length. A clear acrylic is used over the natural nail plate attached to the nail bed so that the natural pink color shows through. A white acrylic is used from the nail plate's free edge distally. This combination perfectly simulates a natural nail, so enamel need not be worn. This allows both men and women to use nail sculptures.
7. The final sculpture is sanded to a high shine.
8. Nail polish, jewels, decals, and decorative metal strips may be added, depending on the fashion tastes of the patient.

Originally, methyl methacrylate was the monomer used to fashion the nail, but it has been removed from the market due to its sensitizing potential. Currently, liquid ethyl or isobutyl methacrylate is utilized as the monomer and mixed with powdered polymethyl methacrylate polymer. The product is allowed to polymerize in the presence of a benzoyl peroxide accelerator, and a formable acrylic is made that hardens in 7 to 9 minutes.[4] Usually, hydroquinone, monomethyl ether of hydroquinone, or pyrogallol is added to slow down polymerization.[5] As mentioned previously, this acrylic is shaped in accord with the patient's wishes.

Many patients are not aware that the finished nail sculptures require more care than natural fingernails. With continued wear of the sculpture, the acrylic loosens from the natural nail, especially around the edges. These loose edges must be clipped and new acrylic applied approximately every 3 weeks to prevent development of an environment for infection. The sculpture grows out with the natural nail plate and more polymer must be added proximally, depending on the nail growth rate. This procedure is known as ''filling.'' Failure to undergo filling every 2 to 3 weeks will result in creation of a lever arm that predisposes to traumatic onycholysis or damage to the natural nail plate. If necessary, the sculptured nails can be removed by soaking in acetone.

Damage to the natural nail plate can still occur with nail sculpture use even if the patient is conscientious. After 2 to 4 months of wear, the natural nail plate becomes yellowed, dry, and thin. Most operators prefer to allow the patient's natural nail to grow and act as a support for the sculpture. However, the nails become thin, bendable, and weak. For this reason, it is not advisable to wear sculptured nails for more than 3 months consecutively. One month should be allowed between applications.

Sculptured nails can be used to cover unsightly nails on both men and women. Dystrophic nails, psoriatic nails, discolored nails, and damaged nail plates can be cosmetically improved with sculptured nails. It takes more operator skill to apply nails to these patients, however. The entire nail bed must be covered with some type of nail plate for the plain sculptures to be used. For example, patients with median canal dystrophy cannot wear plain nail sculptures.

Adverse Reactions

There are many problems associated with the application and wearing of nail sculptures. An important issue is the failure of states to license operator training, application techniques, and facility cleanliness uniformly. Poorly trained operators may allow liquid acrylic to enter the proximal nail fold, resulting in nail matrix damage. Furthermore, failure to sterilize equipment or apply antifungal, antibacterial solutions to the nail plate may result in fungal, viral, and bacterial infections.

Allergic contact dermatitis remains as issue even though methyl methacrylate is no longer used; isobutyl, ethyl, and tetrahydrofurfuryl methacrylates are still strong sensitizers.[6,7] But it should be emphasized that the polymerized, cured acrylic is not sensitizing, only the liquid monomer.[8] Therefore, a careful operator who avoids skin contact with the uncured acrylic can avoid sensitizing the patient. Patch testing should be performed in suspected sensitized individuals with methyl methacrylate monomer, 10% in olive oil, and methacrylate acid esters, 1% and 5% in olive oil and petrolatum.[9]

Onycholysis is a common problem, since the bond between the sculpture and the natural nail plate is stronger than the adhesion between the natural nail and nail bed. Additionally, sensitivity to the acrylic can cause onycholysis[10,11] or, rarely, permanent loss of the fingernails.[12] Many patients are appalled at the broken, thinned, yellowed appearance of their nails following sculpture removal. This is due to interference with the nail's normal vapor exchange, nail plate trauma during the removal process, and damage to the underlying nail bed.[13]

Modified Sculptures

Sculptures With Artificial Tips

Another technique of elongating nails is to combine custom-made nail sculptures with preformed artificial tips. This involves applying the liquid acrylic to the natural nail and embedding an artificial tip at the distal end. This method is used for patients who wish to have extremely long nails or nails embedded with numerous jewels. The possibility of developing traumatic onycholysis is enhanced with this variation due to the extreme length of the nails.

Sculptures With Cloth Wraps

Silk or linen cloth may be combined with nail sculptures to add additional strength to the artificial nail or to aid in covering nail defects. This technique involves applying a layer of liquid acrylic to the natural nail plate and embedding a fitted piece of cloth prior to complete polymerization. Several layers of liquid acrylic are then applied to seal the cloth. The cloth texture appears through the clear nail sculpture, so these nails are generally polished. Linen wraps provide more nail strength than silk wraps. Cloth wraps can be used for patients with mild median canal dystrophy to bridge the dystrophic nail edges. Brittle psoriatic nails can also be strengthened.

Photobonded Nails

One variation of nail sculptures is known as "photobonded nails." These nails are also formed from a cured acrylic sculpted on the natural nail, but, instead of allowing the acrylic to cure with room temperature drying, the nails are placed under a magnesium light for 1 to 2 minutes. This technique is similar to restorative dental bonding. Photoonycholysis and paresthesias have been reported as a result of this procedure.[14]

COSMETIC TECHNIQUES FOR DAMAGED NAILS

External trauma and cosmetic trauma both may result in nail plate damage (see Table 11-1).[15,16] External trauma includes nail biting, habit tic picking, occupational damage, and exposure to harsh chemicals or solvents.[17] Nail biting and habit tic picking are difficult to treat in the unmotivated patient; however, nail enamel can act as a deterrent to manipulation, since picking damages the enamel, which is time-consuming to apply.

Occupational damage requires that the patient protect the nails with gloves or refrain from the damaging activity. In most situations, neither of these suggestions is practical. A common occupational problem is breakage of the nail plate proximal to the free edge. This may cause pain that cannot be remedied until

Table 11-1. Cosmetic Techniques for Damaged Nails

Damage	Possible Cosmetic Cause	Possible Cosmetic Solution
Nail color		
Yellowish stain	Nail polish containing D & C Reds No. 6, 7, 34, 5 Lake	Discontinue nail polish
Poor nail color	Numerous medical conditions	French manicure technique
Nail Structure		
Onychoschizia lamellina	Nail plate dehydration	Application of lactic acid- or urea-containing cream
Mild median canal dystrophy	Trauma	Sculptured nail with linen wrap
Uneven nail surface contour	Trauma to nail matrix	Artificial or sculptured nails
Nail fragility	Numerous medical conditions, idiopathic	Fibered nail polish
Nail thinning	Nail sculptures worn too long	Remove nail sculptures
Nail dystrophy	Numerous medical conditions, idiopathic	Sculptured nails
Broken nail	Trauma	"Tea bag repair" technique

See glossary for definition of terms.

the nail grows. A temporary, effective, inexpensive solution is to use the "tea-bag repair" method. This technique is so named because it requires a tea bag and fibered clear nail polish. The broken edges of the nail are reapproximated and the entire nail painted with fibered clear nail polish. A piece of tea bag paper, or other fibered paper, is then cut and shaped to fit over the nail surface and embedded in the wet polish. Several more nail polish coats are subsequently applied. This repair covers the rough broken nail edge and provides strength. Nail repair kits to accomplish the same end are available commercially,[18] but some use powdered acrylic that is mixed with ethyl cyanoacrylate prior to application. These products may cause difficulty in the methacrylate-sensitive patient.

Chemical and solvent nail damage generally results in nail dehydration,[19,20] brittleness,[21–23] and onychoschizia. Avoiding water and chemical contact is the logical solution, but this too is not always practical. A reasonable alternative is to have the patient briefly moisten the nails by soaking followed by application of a lactic acid cream. Evidence also suggests that biotin supplementation (2,500 μg per day) may aid in the treatment of brittle nails.[24]

COSMETIC TECHNIQUES FOR
MEDICAL NAIL CONDITIONS

Medical nail conditions create three correctable cosmetic problems: abnormal nail color,[25] abnormal nail surface contour, and longitudinal nail splitting (see Table 11-1).

Nail discoloration may be due to a variety of conditions, including onychomycosis and yellow nail syndrome.[26–29] The cosmetic appearance of the nail can be improved with a technique known as a "French manicure." A French manicure utilizes a number of colored nail enamels to simulate the natural appearance of unpainted nail. Initially, the nail is painted with an unpigmented opaque base coat to cover the discoloration. A light pink enamel is then added to the entire nail plate, followed by white enamel to the tip, simulating the nail free edge. Lastly, a clear top coat is applied to prevent enamel chipping. French manicures can be performed professionally by a manicurist or with kits available for home use.

Nail surface contour abnormalities result from a variety of medical conditions and may be temporary or permanent. Temporary abnormalities may be seen following treatment of a paronychia or hand dermatitis involving the proximal nail fold. Longer lasting ones can also occur, as with psoriasis. For patients who are bothered by poor nail appearance, only sculptured nails can offer a solution. The use of sculptured nails in these patients requires a skilled operator and a motivated patient. Poorly applied or poorly maintained nail sculptures could result in worsening of the nail abnormality. The physician should personally visit a number of nail sculpturing salons and select an operator for patient referral who upholds the highest standards of hygiene. It is also important that the artist work with the physician and accept suggestions for nail grooming. In these patients, the cuticle should never be removed, and meticulous care should be taken to avoid contact of liquid acrylic with skin. If a suitable salon cannot be found in the community, patients should not be offered this alternative.

The last cosmetically correctable medical nail abnormality to be discussed is splitting of the nail plate. This condition is seen in median canal dystrophy and trauma leading to onychorrhexis. If there is a small gap between the two edges of the longitudinally split nail, a sculptured nail with a linen wrap can be applied. The linen holds the two nail edges together and provides strength. This can be especially helpful for the patient who repeatedly traumatizes the nail edges.

None of the aforementioned techniques should be suggested to patients who are sensitized to those products required for the cosmetic repair.

REFERENCES

1. Brauer EW: Selected prostheses primarily of cosmetic interest. Cutis 6:521, 1970
2. Baran R: Pathology induced by the application of cosmetics to the nails. In Frost P, Horwitz SN (eds): Cosmetics for the Dermatologist. CV Mosby, St. Louis, 1982

3. Lazar P: Reactions to nail hardeners. Arch Dermatol 94:446, 1966
4. Barnett JM, Scher RK, Taylor SC: Nail cosmetics. Dermatol Clin 9:9, 1991
5. Viola LJ: Fingernail elongators and accessory nail preparations. p. 543. In Balsam MS, Sagarin E (eds): Cosmetics, Science and Technology. 2nd Ed. Wiley-Interscience, New York, 1972
6. Marks JG, Bishop ME, Willis WF: Allergic contact dermatitis to sculptured nails. Arch Dermatol 115:100, 1979
7. Fisher AA: Cross reactions between methyl methacrylate monomer and acrylic monomers presently used in acrylic nail preparations. Contact Dermatitis 6:345, 1980
8. Fisher AA, Franks A, Glick H: Allergic sensitization of the skin and nails to acrylic plastic nails. J Allergy 28:84, 1957
9. Baran R, Dawber RPR: The nail and cosmetics. In Samman PD, Fenton DA (eds): The Nails in Disease. 4th Ed. Yearbook Publishers, Chicago, 1986
10. Goodwin P: Onycholysis due to acrylic nail applications. J Exp Dermatol 1:191, 1976
11. Lane CW, Kost LB: Sensitivity to artificial nails. Arch Dermatol 74:671, 1956
12. Fisher AA: Permanent loss of fingernails from sensitization and reaction to acrylic in a preparation designed to make artificial nails. J Dermatol Surg Oncol 6:70, 1980
13. Baden H: Cosmetics and the nail. p. 99. In Diseases of the Hair and Nails. Yearbook Publishers, Chicago, 1987
14. Fisher AA: Adverse nail reactions and paresthesia from photobonded acrylate sculptured nails. Cutis 45:293, 1990
15. Baden HP: The physical properties of nail. J Invest Dermatol 55:115, 1970
16. Scott DA, Scher RK: Exogenous factors affecting the nails. Dermatol Clin 3:409, 1985
17. Samman PD: Nail disorders caused by external influences. J Soc Cosmet Chem 28:351, 1977
18. Scher RK: Cosmetics and ancillary preparations for the care of the nails. J Am Acad Dermatol 523, 1982
19. Finlay AY, Frost P, Keith AD, Snipes W: Effects of phospholipids and water on brittleness of nails. p. 175. In Frost P, Horwitz SN (eds): Cosmetics for the Dermatologist. CV Mosby, St. Louis, 1982
20. Finlay AY, Frost P, Keith AD, Snipes W: An assessment of factors influencing flexibility of human fingernails. Br J Dermatol 103:357, 1980
21. Scher RK: Brittle nails. Int J Dermatol 28:515, 1989
22. Kechijian P: Brittle fingernails. Dermatol Clin 3:412, 1985
23. Silver H, Chiego B: Nail and nail changes. III. Brittleness of nails (fragilitas unguium). J Invest Dermatol 3:357, 1940
24. Hochman LG, Scher RK, Meyerson MS: Brittle nails: response to daily biotin supplementation. Cutis 51:303, 1993
25. Daniel CR, Osment LS: Nail pigmentation abnormalities. Cutis 25:595, 1980
26. Mautner G, Scher RK: Yellow nail syndrome. J Geriatr Dermatol 1:106, 1993
27. Nelson LM: Yellow nail syndrome. Arch Dermatol 100:499, 1969
28. Venencie PY, Dicken GH: Yellow nail syndrome. J Am Acad Dermatol 10:187, 1984
29. Samman PD, White WF: The "yellow nail" syndrome. Br J Dermatol 76:153, 1964

12

Hair Shampoos

The purpose of shampoo is to cleanse hair. While this sounds like a simple task, the average woman has 4 to 8 m^2 of hair surface area to clean.[1] Shampoos are intended to remove sebum, sweat components, desquamated stratum corneum, styling products, and environmental dirt that is deposited on the hair.[2] It is very easy to formulate a shampoo that will remove dirt, but studies have shown that consumers do not favor a shampoo that only cleans efficiently. Hair that has had all the sebum removed is dull in appearance, coarse to the touch, subject to static electricity, and more difficult to style. Therefore, consumers want a shampoo that will not only clean but also beautify. This demand has led to the tremendous variety of shampoo formulations on the market.

HISTORY

Until the middle 1930s, bar soap was used to cleanse the hair. This was somewhat unsatisfactory since hard water in combination with bar soap left behind a scum that dulled the hair appearance. Early shampoo formulations were liquid coconut oil soaps that lathered and rinsed better than bar soap. Surfactant shampoos were introduced in the late 1930s and represented a significant advance, since they performed well even with the hardest water.[3]

FORMULATION

Shampoos contain detergents, foaming agents, conditioners, thickeners, opacifiers, softeners, sequestering agents, fragrances, preservatives, and specialty additives.[4] Detergents are the primary sebum and dirt removal components; however, excessive removal of sebum leaves the hair dull, susceptible to static electricity, and difficult to comb. Furthermore, consumers equate cleansing ability with foaming ability, thus demanding shampoos that produce an abundant, long-lasting foam. Excessive bubbles are not a technical requirement

115

for good hair cleansing and bacteria removal, but shampoo manufacturers add increased amounts of detergents, in addition to foam boosters, to obtain the foam that consumers desire. This increased concentration of detergent creates the need for conditioners and other additives in shampoos to improve their cosmetic acceptability.

Detergents

Shampoos function by employing detergents, also known as surfactants, that are both lipophilic (oil-loving) and hydrophilic (water-loving). The lipophilic component adheres to sebum, and the hydrophilic component allows water to rinse away the sebum.[5] A tremendous variety of detergents is available to the cosmetics chemist formulating a shampoo, including[6]

Alkyl sulfates
Alkyl ether sulfates
Alpha-olefin sulfonates
Paraffin sulfonates
Isethionates
Sarconsinates
Taurides
Acyl lactylates
Sulfosuccinates
Carboxylates
Protein condensates
Betaines
Glycinates
Amine oxides

Nevertheless, the most common detergents used in shampoos are[7]

Sodium laureth sulfate
Sodium lauryl sulfate
TEA lauryl sulfate
Ammonium laureth sulfate
Ammonium lauryl sulfate
DEA lauryl sulfate
Sodium olefin sulfonate

Shampoo detergents can be chemically classified as anionics, cationics, amphoterics, nonionics, and natural surfactants (Table 12-1). Anionic detergents are named for their negatively charged hydrophilic polar group. The commonly used anionics are fatty alcohols that clean well, but may leave the hair harsh.[8] There are several detergents contained within the anionic group:

Table 12-1. Shampoo Detergents

Surfactant Type	Chemical Class	Characteristics
Anionics	Lauryl sulfates, laureth sulfates, sarcosines, sulfosuccinates	Deep cleansing, may leave hair harsh
Cationics	Long-chain amino esters, ammoniosters	Poor cleansing, poor lather, impart softness and manageability
Nonionics	Polyoxyethylene fatty alcohols, polyoxyethylene sorbitol esters, alkanolamides	Mildest cleansing, impart manageability
Amphoterics	Betaines, sultaines, imidazolinium derivatives	Nonirritating to eyes, mild cleansing, impart manageability
Natural surfactants	Sarsaparilla, soapwort, soap bark, ivy, agave	Poor cleansing, excellent lather

1. Lauryl sulfates (sodium lauryl sulfate, triethanolamine lauryl sulfate, ammonium lauryl sulfate) are used in most shampoos as the main surfactant since they work well in both hard and soft water, produce rich foam, and are easy to remove. This group produces good cleansing but is hard on the hair.
2. Laureth sulfates (sodium laureth sulfate, triethanolamine laureth sulfate, ammonium laureth sulfate) produce rich foam, provide good cleansing, and leave hair in good condition. They also are a common main surfactant.
3. Sarcosines (lauryl sarcosine, sodium lauryl sarcosinate) are poor cleansers but are excellent conditioners. This group is commonly used as a secondary surfactant.
4. Sulfosuccinates (disodium oleamine sulfosuccinate, sodium dioctyl sulfosuccinate) are strong degreasers and commonly are used as a secondary surfactant in oily hair shampoos.

The cationic detergents are named for their positively charged polar group. They are relatively poor detergents and do not lather well, but their unpopularity is largely due to their incompatibility with other anionic surfactants. Some shampoos designed for dyed or bleached hair use cationic detergents, as they are excellent at imparting softness and manageability.[1]

The nonionic detergents are the second most popular and have no polar group. These are the mildest of all surfactants and are used in combination with ionic surfactants as a secondary cleanser.[9] Examples include polyoxyethylene fatty alcohols, polyoxyethylene sorbitol esters, and alkanolamides.

The amphoteric detergents contain both an anionic and a cationic group such that they behave as cationics at lower pH values and anionics at higher pH values. The detergents that fall within this group are the betaines, sultaines, and imidazolinium derivatives. Ingredients such as cocamidopropyl betaine and sodium lauraminopropionate can be found in baby shampoos, since they are nonirritating to the eyes. These surfactants foam moderately well and leave the hair manageable, making them a good choice for chemically treated and fine hair.

The last group of detergents are the natural surfactants, such as sarsaparilla, soapwort, soap bark, and ivy agave. These natural saponins have excellent lathering capabilities, but are poor cleansers and thus must be present at high concentration. Usually, they are combined with the other synthetic detergents outlined above.[5]

Foaming Agents

Foaming agents in shampoos introduce gas bubbles into the water. Many consumers believe that shampoos that generate copious foam are better cleansers than poorly foaming shampoos. This is not true. As the shampoo removes sebum from the hair, the amount of foam will decrease because sebum inhibits bubble formation. This accounts for the increased foam seen on the second shampooing, when the majority of the sebum has been removed.

Thickeners and Opacifiers

Thickeners and opacifiers have no part in hair cleansing. They simply make the product more appealing to the consumer. Many people incorrectly believe that a thick shampoo is more concentrated than a thin shampoo; others want a shampoo that appears opaque or pearlescent.

Conditioners

Conditioners impart manageability, gloss, and antistatic properties to the hair. They are found in most shampoos for dry, damaged, or treated hair. These are usually fatty alcohols, fatty esters, vegetable oils, mineral oils, or humectants. Many conditioners are used in dry-hair shampoos, including hydrolyzed animal protein, glycerin, dimethicone, simethicone, polyvinylpyrrolidone, propylene glycol, and stearalkonium chloride.[10] Other protein sources such as lanolin, beer, and egg yolk, which contain lecithin and cholesterol, are also used in dry-hair shampoos that claim to be "natural." Of all these conditioners, hydrolyzed animal protein is probably the best for extremely dry hair, since it has some substantivity for keratin and can mend split ends (trichoptilosis).[11] A more complete discussion of hair conditioners is given in Chapter 13.

Sequestering Agents

Sequestering agents make shampoos function better than bar soaps in cleansing the hair. They chelate magnesium and calcium ions so that other salts or insoluble particles known as "scum" are not formed. Without sequestering agents, shampoos would leave a film on the hair, rendering it dull. For this reason, patients should be encouraged to use shampoo and not bar soap when cleansing the hair. In areas of extremely hard water, the film that remains may contribute to scalp pruritus.

pH Adjusters

Some shampoos contain ingredients designed to alter pH, allowing the marketing claim of ''pH balanced.'' Most shampoos are alkaline, which can swell the hair shaft and render it more susceptible to damage. This is not a problem for patients with healthy, nonporous hair containing an intact cuticle. Patients with damaged or chemically treated hair with a fragmented cuticle may wish to avoid hair swelling by selecting a shampoo that has an acid added to balance the pH.

Specialty Additives

The key differences between similar purpose shampoos manufactured by various personal care product companies are the fragrance and special care additives. Additives such as wheat germ oil (containing vitamin E) and panthenol (a form of vitamin B) are added mainly for marketing reasons but are thought to leave hair more silky and manageable. Other producers add fatty substances such as plant extracts or mink oil. Proteins such as ribonucleic acid, collagen, and placenta may be added to act somewhat as conditioners. Some shampoos now include a chemical sunscreen.

TYPES OF SHAMPOO

Shampoos have been formulated in liquids, gels, creams, aerosols, and powders. Only the liquids are discussed here, as they are the most popular. A number of different types of shampoos are also available: basic shampoos (for normal, dry, oily, and chemically treated hair), baby shampoos, conditioning shampoos, medicated shampoos, and professional shampoos.

Basic Shampoos

Basic shampoos may be selected from several formulations, depending on the amount of scalp sebum production, hair shaft diameter, and hair shaft condition. The label usually indicates the intended consumer by stating the type of hair—normal hair, oily hair, dry hair, or damaged, colored-treated hair—for which it was designed. Some companies alter the concentrations of detergents and conditioners to make the different formulations, so the ingredients lists may be identical for all formulations. Other product lines have different formulations for each type.

Normal-hair shampoos use lauryl sulfate detergents, giving them good cleansing and minimal conditioning characteristics. These products work well for adults with moderate sebum production and coarse hair; however, they do not work well for persons with fine, unmanageable hair.

Oily-hair shampoos have excellent cleansing and minimal conditioning properties. They may use lauryl sulfate or sulfosuccinate detergents and are intended for adolescents with oily hair or persons who have extremely dirty hair. They can be drying to the hair shaft if used daily. Following an oily-hair shampoo with use of a heavy conditioner is self-defeating.

Dry-hair shampoos provide mild cleansing and good conditioning. Some companies recommend the same product for dry hair and damaged hair. These products are excellent for mature persons and those who wish to shampoo daily. They reduce static electricity and increase manageability in fine hair; however, some products provide too much conditioning, which may result in limp hair. Dry-hair shampoos may also cleanse so poorly that conditioner can build up on the hair shaft. This condition has been labeled as the ''greasies'' in popular advertising and may account for the observation that hair sometimes has more body after using a different shampoo.

Damaged-hair shampoos are intended for hair that has been chemically treated with permanent hair colors, hair bleaching agents, permanent waving solutions, or hair straighteners. Hair can also be damaged physically by over cleansing, excessive use of heated styling devices, and vigorous brushing or combing. Longer hair is more likely to be damaged than shorter hair, since it undergoes a natural process known as ''weathering'' whereby the cuticular scales are decreased in number from the proximal to distal hair shaft. As mentioned previously, damaged-hair shampoos may be identical to dry-hair shampoos or may contain mild detergents and increased conditioners. Hydrolyzed animal protein is the superior conditioner for damaged hair, since it can minimally penetrate the shaft and temporarily repair surface defects, resulting in hair with a smoother feel and more shine. It is important that the protein is hydrolyzed: larger protein molecules cannot penetrate the hair shaft.

Baby Shampoos

Baby shampoos are nonirritating to the eyes and are designed as mild cleansing agents since babies produce limited sebum. These shampoos use detergents from the amphoteric group.[12] Baby shampoos are also appropriate for mature hair and for individuals who wish to shampoo daily.

Conditioning Shampoos

Conditioning shampoos may be labeled as such or may be labeled as shampoos for dry or damaged hair. These products may actually be self-defeating since the shampoo is intended to remove sebum, the body's natural conditioner, and replace it with a synthetic conditioner, which consumers somehow interpret as cleaner. As a consequence, conditioning shampoos neither clean nor condition well.[13] Detergents used in conditioning shampoos are generally amphoterics and anionics of the sulfosuccinate type. These products are sometimes known as one-step shampoos, since a conditioner need not be applied following shampooing. Patients should not use a conditioning shampoo prior to permanent dyeing or permanent waving, because maximum color uptake or curling can be inhibited.

Medicated Shampoos

Medicated shampoos, also known as dandruff shampoos, contain additives such as tar derivatives, salicylic acid, sulfur, selenium disulfide, polyvinylpyrrolidone–iodine complex, chlorinated phenols, or zinc pyrithione.[14] Medicated shampoos have several functions: to remove sebum efficiently, to remove scalp scale, to decrease scalp scale production, and to act as an antibacterial/antifungal agent. The shampoo base removes sebum, while mechanical scrubbing removes scalp scale. Tar derivatives are commonly used as anti-inflammatory agents. Sulfur and zinc pyrithione are used for their antibacterial/antifungal qualities. Menthol is added to some shampoos to produce a tingling sensation, which some patients find esthetically pleasing.

Professional Shampoos

There are two types of professional shampoos: those intended for hair washing prior to cutting or styling and those intended to precede or follow a chemical process. Professional shampoos for hair washing are the same formulation as the over-the-counter varieties except that they are more concentrated and must be diluted eight to ten times before to use. Special anionic, acidic professional shampoos are used after bleaching to neutralize residual alkalinity and prepare the hair for subsequent dyeing. Acidic, cationic shampoos are used after dyeing to act as a neutralizing rinse. A subset of these shampoos includes those designed to maintain the color of bleached or dyed hair. These shampoos are only available to licensed cosmetologists.

ADVERSE REACTIONS

Shampoos do not represent a common cause of cutaneous irritant or allergic contact dermatitis due to their relatively brief contact with the skin prior to rinsing. Eye irritation, however, can be a problem that some shampoos overcome with the addition of imidazoline-type amphoteric surfactants, succinic ester sulfonates, silicone glycols, and fatty acid–peptide condensates.[3] Ingredients in shampoos that are possible sensitizers include formalin, parabens, hexa-chlorophene, and miranols.[15]

Shampoos should be diluted to form a 1% to 2% aqueous solution for closed patch testing and a 5% aqueous solution for open patch testing. However, it should be recognized that false-positive reactions due to irritation may still occur. A better assessment may be obtained by patch testing individual ingredients separately.[16]

REFERENCES

1. Bouillon C: Shampoos and hair conditioners. Clin Dermatol 6:83, 1988
2. Robbins CR: Interaction of shampoo and creme rinse ingredients with human hair. p. 122. In Chemical and Physical Behavior of Human Hair. 2nd Ed. Springer-Verlag, New York, 1988
3. Markland WR: Shampoos. p. 1283. In deNavarre MG (ed): The Chemistry and Manufacture of Cosmetics. Vol. IV. 2nd Ed. Allured Publishing Corporation, Wheaton IL, 1988
4. Fox C: An introduction to the formulation of shampoos. Cosmet Toilet 103:25, 1988
5. Zviak C, Vanlerberghe G: Scalp and hair hygiene. p. 49. In Zviak C (ed): The Science of Hair Care. Marcel Dekker, New York, 1986.
6. Shipp JJ: Hair-care products. p. 32. In Williams DF, Schmitt WH (eds): Chemistry and Technology of the Cosmetics and Toiletries Industry. Blackie Academic & Professional, London, 1992
7. Rieger M: Surfactants in shampoos. Cosmet Toilet 103:59, 1988
8. Tokiwa F, Hayashi S, Okumura T: Hair and surfactants. p. 631. In Kobori T, Montagna W (eds): Biology and Disease of the Hair. University Park Press, Baltimore, 1975
9. Powers DH: Shampoos. p. 73. In Balsem MS, Gershon SD, Reiger MM et al (eds): Cosmetics Science and Technology. 2nd Ed. Wiley-Interscience, New York, 1972
10. Harusawa F, Nakama Y, Tanaka M: Anionic–cationic ion-pairs as conditioning agents in shampoos. Cosmet Toilet 106:35, 1991
11. Karjala SA, Williamson JE, Karler A: Studies on the substantivity of collagen-derived peptides to human hair. J Soc Cosmet Chem 17:513, 1966
12. Wilkinson JB, Moore RJ: Harry's Cosmeticology. Chemical Publishing, New York, 1982
13. Hunting ALL: Can there be cleaning and conditioning in the same product? Cosmet Toilet 103:73, 1988
14. Spoor HJ: Shampoos. Cutis 12:671, 1973
15. Bergfeld WF: The side effects of hair products on the scalp and hair. p. 507. In Orfanos CE, Montagna W, Stuttgen G (eds): Hair Research. Springer-Verlag, New York, 1981
16. De Groot AC, Weyland JW, Nater JP: Unwanted Effects of Cosmetics and Drugs Used in Dermatology. Elsevier, Amsterdam, 1994

13

Hair Conditioners

The need for hair conditioners arose following the development of shampoos with extremely good detergent action.[1] These new shampoos cleaned too well: they so thoroughly removed sebum from the hair shaft that the hair became unmanageable, dull, and harsh to the touch. The role of a conditioner is to mimic sebum in making the hair manageable, glossy, and soft. Conditioners also attempt to recondition hair that has been damaged by chemical or mechanical trauma.[2] Common sources of trauma include excessive brushing, hot blow-drying, detergent shampoos, alkaline permanent waves, and bleaching. Obviously, since hair is nonliving tissue, any reconditioning that occurs is minimal and temporary until the next shampooing.

HISTORY

Hair conditioners were developed during the early 1930s when self-emulsifying waxes became available. These waxes were combined with protein hydrolysates, polyunsaturates, and silicones to give the hair improved feel and texture. Early sources of the proteins included gelatin, milk, and eggs.[3]

MECHANISM OF ACTION

Healthy, undamaged hair is soft, resilient, and easy to disentangle.[4] Unfortunately, shampooing, drying, combing, brushing, styling, dyeing, and permanent waving damage the hair, making it harsh, brittle, and difficult to disentangle.[5] Hair conditioners are designed to reverse this hair damage by improving sheen, decreasing brittleness, decreasing porosity, increasing strength, and restoring degradation in the polypeptide chain. Damage to the hair shaft can also occur through environmental exposures to sunlight, air pollution, wind, seawater, and chlorinated swimming pool water.[6] This type of hair damage is technically known as ''weathering.''[7]

Hair conditioners improve manageability by decreasing static electricity. Following combing or brushing, the hair shaft becomes negatively charged, thus repelling one another to prevent the hair from lying smoothly in a given style. Conditioners deposit positively charged ions onto the hair shaft, neutralizing the electrical charge. Improved manageability also derives from cuticle alterations and reduction of friction between hair shafts by as much as 50%.[8] This leads to enhanced disentangling of the hair, as well.

Hair gloss results from light reflected by individual hair shafts. The smoother the hair surface, the more light reflected.[9] Conditioners increase hair gloss primarily by Increasing adherence of cuticular scale to the hair shaft. Gloss is also related to the hair structure. Maximum gloss is produced by large-diameter, elliptical hair shafts with a sizeable medulla and intact, overlapping cuticle scales. Hair softness too results from an even overlap of cuticlar scales.[10]

Conditioners attempt to mend the split ends resulting from missing cortex, the structural component responsible for hair shaft strength. The resulting exposure of the soft keratin medulla results in a condition known as "trichoptilosis," or split ends. Conditioners temporarily reapproximate the frayed remnants of remaining medulla and cortex.

All the problems associated with damaged hair are magnified if the hair is fine in texture. There are more fine hair fibers per weight than coarse hair fibers, so the net surface area of fine hair is greater. Proportionally more irregular cuticle scales can develop, and more of these fine hair fibers are subject to static electricity. Thus, there are special conditioner formulations designed to meet the grooming needs of fine hair.

FORMULATION

Hair conditioners can contain as many as nine different conditioning agents from the following chemical classes:[11]

Alkanolamides
Glycols
Lipids
Protein derivatives
Quaternaries
Surface active agents
Specialty ingredients

Of these, the quaternaries, protein derivatives, and alkanolamides are the most frequently used. These chemical classes are discussed in detail and summarized in Table 13-1.[12]

Table 13-1. Hair Conditioner Formulations

Type	Ingredient	Advantage	Hair Type
Cationic detergent	Quaternary ammonium compounds	Smooth cuticle, decrease static	Chemically processed hair
Film former	Polymers	Fill shaft defects, decrease static, add shine	Dry hair, not fine hair
Protein-containing	Hydrolyzed proteins	Penetrate shaft	Split ends

Quaternary Conditioning Agents

The cationic detergents, also known as ''quaternaries'' or ''quaternary ammonium compounds'' (or quats), are conditioning agents found in both shampoos and hair conditioners.[13] They are excellent at increasing adherence of the cuticular scales to the hair shaft, which increases the light-reflective abilities of the hair, adding shine and luster. Additionally, they are able to neutralize static electricity based on the negative (anionic) charge of processed or damaged hair, which attracts the positively (cationic) charged quaternary compound to adhere to the hair shaft, thus improving manageability.[14] These qualities make them an excellent conditioner choice for patients with permanently dyed or permanently waved hair.

Film-Forming Conditioning Agents

Film-forming conditioners apply a thin layer of polymer, such as polyvinylpyrrolidone (PVP), over the hair shaft.[15] The polymer fills hair shaft defects, creating a smooth surface to increase shine and luster while eliminating static electricity due to its cationic nature. The polymer also coats each individual hair shaft, thus ''thickening'' the hair shaft. Film-former conditioners should not be used on fine hair, as the added weight of the polymer decreases the ability of the hair to hold a style. They are excellent, however, on normal to dry hair.

Protein Conditioning Agents

Protein-containing conditioners are the only product that can actually penetrate and alter the damaged hair shaft. These proteins, derived from animal collagen, keratin, placenta, and so forth, are hydrolyzed to a particle size (molecular weight 1,000 to 10,000) able to enter the hair shaft.[16] Hydrolyzed protein conditioners can temporarily strengthen the hair shaft and mend split ends until the subsequent shampooing, when the product must be reapplied. The source of the protein is not as important as the protein particle size.[17]

Table 13-2. Hair Conditioner Products

Type	Use	Indication
Instant	Apply following shampoo, rinse	Minimally damaged hair, aids wet combing
Deep	Apply 20–30 minutes, shampoo, rinse	Chemically damaged hair
Leave-in	Apply to towel dried hair, style	Prevent hair dryer damage, aid in combing and styling
Rinse	Apply following shampoo, rinse	Aid in disentangling if creamy rinse, remove soap residue if clear rinse

APPLICATION

Hair conditioners are available in three forms: instant conditioners, deep conditioners, leave-in conditioners, and rinses (Table 13-2). Consideration must also be given to the development of sunscreen products for hair application.

Instant Conditioners

Instant conditioners are so named as they are applied following shampooing, left on the hair for 5 minutes, and subsequently rinsed. These products provide minimal conditioning due to their short contact time with the hair and are basically useful to aid in wet combing and manageability. Their ability to repair damaged hair is somewhat limited. Nevertheless, they are the most popular type of conditioner for both home and salon use. Instant conditioners contain water, conditioning agents, lipids, and thickeners. The conditioning agents consist of combinations of cationic detergents, film formers, and proteins.

Deep Conditioners

Deep conditioners are creams, compared with instant conditioners, which are liquids. They contain the same conditioning agents as instant conditioners, but are more concentrated.[18] They remain on the hair for 20 to 30 minutes and may include the application of heat from a hair dryer or warm towel. The extended application time allows more conditioner to coat the hair shaft, while heat causes hair shaft swelling and allows increased conditioner penetration. These products are intended for extremely dry hair. Deep conditioners used prior to some permanent coloring or permanent waving procedures are called "fillers." Fillers are designed to condition the distal hair shaft and reverse some of the effects of weathering, allowing even application of the subsequent coloring or waving procedure.

Some salons offer a deep conditioning treatment known as "trichotherapy" or "aromatherapy." Aromatherapy involves several steps, the first of which is to condition the hair and scalp with rare oils and herbal extracts. The scalp is then vigorously brushed. A scalp and facial massage are also performed with fragrant oils to release tension and soothe the senses. The hair is then shampooed and conditioned. The value of this treatment is primarily esthetic.

Leave-In Conditioners

Leave-in conditioners are applied following towel drying of the hair and designed to remain on the hair shaft through styling. They are removed with the next shampooing. Products designed for straight hair are known as blow-drying lotions or hair thickeners. Blow-drying lotions are massaged through the scalp after towel drying and prior to heat drying. Since they contain no oils, they are not rinsed from the hair. They contain the same conditioning agents previously described for instant conditioners. The thin coating of conditioner on the hair only minimally prevents heat damage.

Hair thickeners are another form of leave-in conditioner. They do not thicken hair by increasing the number of hair shafts, but rather provide a coating on each shaft that increases its diameter minutely. These products are protein-containing, conditioning liquids that are massaged through a towel-dried scalp before styling to increase shine, improve manageability, and impart softness. A hair thickener is thicker than a blow-drying lotion and intended for persons with dry, damaged hair.

Special leave-in conditioners are used by Black and Asian individuals with tightly kinked hair to aid in combing, provide additional shine, improve manageability, and enhance styling options. These products are discussed more fully in Chapter 19.

Rinses

Rinses are applied immediately following shampooing and removed prior to drying the hair. There are two types: clear rinses and cream rinses. Clear rinses, formed from lemon juice and vinegar, were used prior to the development of pH-balanced shampoos with sequestering agents designed to prevent soap scum formation on the hair. These acidic chemicals removed calcium and magnesium soap residue and returned the hair to a neutral pH following use of an alkaline shampoo. Residue removal restores hair shine, while pH neutralization restores hair manageability. Clear rinses work well for patients with oily hair, but are not recommended for patients with normal to dry hair.

Cream rinses utilize cationic quaternary ammonium compounds, such as stearalkonium chloride and benzalkonium chloride. Cream rinses are thinner than conditioners, but the differences in formulation are small. Some companies even label their products as "cream rinse/conditioners." As a general rule, cream rinses provide less conditioning than conditioners and are intended for oily to normal hair.

Hair Sunscreens

A relatively new concern is photoprotection of the hair. While the hair is made up of nonliving material and cannot develop cancerous changes, its cosmetic value can be diminished through excessive exposure to the sun. Dryness, reduced strength, rough surface texture, loss of color, decreased luster, stiffness, and brittleness of the hair are all precipitated by sun exposure. Hair protein degradation is induced by light wavelengths from 254 to 400 nm.[19] Chemically, these changes are thought to be due to ultraviolet light–induced oxidation of the sulfur molecules within in the hair shaft.[20] Oxidation of the amide carbon of polypeptide chains also occurs, producing carbonyl groups in the hair shaft.[21] This process has been studied extensively in wool, where it is known as "photoyellowing."[22,23] Only recently have studies been undertaken by the cosmetics research community to document these effects. The OTC-FDA Advisory Review Panel in their 1978 monograph makes no mention of the effects of sunscreens on hair protein.[24]

Bleaching, or lightening of the hair color, is common with both brunette and blonde individuals who expose their hair to ultraviolet radiation.[25] Brunette hair tends to develop reddish hues due to photooxidation of melanin pigments, while blonde hair develops photoyellowing. The yellow discoloration is due to photodegradation of cystine, tyrosine, and tryptophan residues within the blonde hair shaft.[26] Furthermore, hair treated with permanent or semipermanent hair dyes may also shift color when exposed to sunlight.[27]

Sunscreen-containing conditioners are available; however, there is some debate as to their effectiveness in protecting the hair and the scalp. To develop a standardized rating system for hair products, the concept of HPF, or hair protection factor, has been proposed.[28] This is similar to the concept of SPF, or skin protection factor, except that tensile strength assessments of the hair shaft are used for grading instead of sunburn assessment. HPF ratings follow a logarithmic scale from 2 to 15. At present, shampoo formulations containing octyl-dimethyl PABA, and hair spray formulations containing benzophenones have been proposed. Both of these products seem to decrease ultraviolet light–induced melanin and keratin damage, thus preserving the color and structure of the hair shaft. In general, products that remain in contact with the hair and scalp for a short period of time prior to rinsing, such as shampoos and conditioners, may not leave much sunscreen residue as products that stay on the hair, such as hair sprays and styling aids.

ADVERSE REACTIONS

Since hair conditioners are applied to the hair and eventually rinsed, they must be nonirritating to the eyes as well as to the skin.[29] The most popular instant conditioners only remain in contact with the skin for a brief period of time and are therefore infrequent causes of allergic and/or irritant contact dermatitis. These products can be patch tested "as is" in an open or closed manner.

The leave-in conditioners based on film-forming polymers too are infrequent causes of contact dermatitis; however, contamination with monomeric impurities, such as acrylamide, ethyleneimine, or acrylic acid, can cause problems. Acrylamide is highly toxic, ethyleneimine is carcinogenic, and acrylic acid is highly irritating to the skin. The safety and performance of polymers used in hair conditioners is related to their purity.[30]

REFERENCES

1. Goldemberg RL: Hair conditioners: the rationale for modern formulations. p. 157. In Frost P, Horwitz SN (eds): Principles of Cosmetics for the Dermatologist. CV Mosby, St. Louis, 1982
2. Swift JA, Brown AC: The critical determination of fine change in the surface architecture of human hair due to cosmetic treatment. J Soc Cosmet Chem 23:675, 1972
3. deNavarre MG: Hair conditioners and rinses. p. 1097. In deNavarre MG (ed): The Chemistry and Manufacture of Cosmetics. Vol IV. 2nd Ed. Allured Publishing Corporation, Wheaton, IL, 1988
4. Garcia ML, Epps JA, Yare RS, Hunter LD: Normal cuticle-wear patterns in human hair. J Soc Cosmet Chem 29:155, 1978
5. Corbett JE: Hair conditioning. Cutis 23:405, 1979
6. Zviak C, Bouillon C: Hair treatment and hair care products. p. 115. Zviak C (ed): The Science of Hair Care. Marcel Dekker, Inc, New York, 1986
7. Rook A: The clinical importance of "weathering" in human hair. Br J Dermatol 95:111, 1976
8. Price VH: The role of hair care products. p. 501. In Orfanos CE, Montagna W, Stuttgen G (eds): Hair Research. Springer-Verlag, Berlin, 1981
9. Robinson VNE: A study of damaged hair. J Soc Cosmet Chem 27:155, 1976
10. Zviak C, Bouillon C: Hair treatment and hair care products. p. 134. In Zviak C (ed): The Science of Hair Care. Marcel Dekker, Inc, New York, 1986
11. Rieger M: Surfactants in shampoos. Cosmet Toilet 103:59, 1988
12. Corbett JF: The chemistry of hair-care products. J Soc Dyers Colour 92:285, 1976
13. Allardice A, Gummo G: Hair conditioning. Cosmet Toilet 108:107, 1993
14. Idson B, Lee W: Update on hair conditioner ingredients. Cosmet Toliet 98:41, 1983
15. Finkelstein P: Hair conditioners. Cutis 6:543, 1970
16. Fox C: An introduction to the formulation of shampoos. Cosmet Toilet 103:25, 1988
17. Spoor HJ, Lindo SD: Hair processing and conditioning. Cutis 14:689, 1974
18. Bouillon C: Shampoos and hair conditioners. Clin Dermatol 6:83, 1988
19. Arnoud R, Perbet G, Deflandre A, Lang G: ESR study of hair and melanin–keratin mixtures: the effects of temperature and light. Int J Cosmet Sci 6:71, 1984
20. Jachowicz J: Hair damage and attempts to its repair. J Soc Cosmet Chem 38:263, 1987

21. Holt LA, Milligan B: The formation of carbonyl groups during irradiation of wool and its releance to photoyellowing. Textile Res J 47:620, 1977
22. Launer HF: Effect of light upon wool. IV. Bleaching and yellowing by sunlight. Textile Res J 35:395, 1965
23. Inglis AS, Lennox FG: Wool yellowing. IV. Changes in amino acid composition due to irradiation. Textile Res J 33:431, 1963
24. Proposed Rules, Part II, Federal Register 38206, 1978
25. Tolgyesi E: Weathering of the hair. Cosmet Toilet 98:29, 1983
26. Milligan B, Tucker DJ: Studies on wool yellowing. Part III. Sunlight yellowing. Textile Res J 32:634, 1962
27. Berth P, Reese G: Alteration of hair keratin by cosmetic processing and natural environmental influences. J Soc Cosmet Chem 15:659, 1964
28. Nacht S: Sunscreens and hair. Cosmet Toilet 105:55, 1990
29. Whittam JH: Hair care safety. p. 335. In Whittam JH (ed): Cosmetic Safety. Marcel Dekker, Inc., New York, 1987
30. Robbins CR: Polymers and polymer chemistry in hair products. p. 196. In Chemical and Physical Behavior of Human Hair. 2nd Ed. Springer-Verlag, New York, 1988

14

Hair-Styling Cosmetics and Devices

Both men and women take pride in arranging their hair in currently fashionable styles. However, preparations for hair adornment are some of the oldest cosmetic products known. The Assyrians invented hair styling with elaborate layered cuts combined with oiling, perfuming, and hot iron curling. The complexity of the hair style indicated the societal status of the individual.[1] Modern hair styling can be divided into those manipulations involving styling aids and those involving nonelectric and electric devices.

STYLING AIDS

All hair-styling aids aim to maintain the hair in a groomed position. Styling aids also provide conditioning, shine, body, and increased manageability. The availability of styling aids keeps pace with popular hair fashions. Hair styles in the 1960s were long, straight, and ungroomed, so styling aids were minimal and consisted of hair spray alone. Hair styles in the 1970s were curly and short, so styling aids were destined to condition damage induced by permanent waving. Hair styles of the 1980s were gravity defying and demanded styling aids that provided maximum hold. The 1990s are marked by hair styles with emphasis on smoothness and shine, requiring styling products that impart gloss.

These products are applied following shampooing and are intended to be completely removed with the subsequent shampooing. There are three categories of modern styling products: sprays, mousses, and gels (Table 14-1). Pomades and brilliantines are discussed in Chapter. Older hair dressings such as gum-based dressings, alcohol-based lotions, oil-in-water emulsions, and water-in-oil emulsions are not discussed because of their lack of popularity.

Table 14-1. Hair Styling Aids

Styling Aid	Type	Main Ingredients	Purpose
Hair spray	Aerosol	Solution of film-forming resin	Hold finished hair style
Styling fix	Aerosol	Solution of film-forming resin	Add strong hold to finished hair style
Spritz	Aerosol	Solution of film-forming resin	Add strong hold to finished hair style
Styling gel	Gel	Gel of film-forming resin	Add moderate hold before styling
Sculpturing gel	Gel	Gel of film-forming resin	Add extreme hold before styling
Mousse	Foam	Aerosolized foam of film-forming resin	Add mild hold before styling

Hair Sprays

Formulation

Early hair sprays were aerosolized shellac, a natural resin composed of polyhydroxy acids and esters. Shellacs are no longer used, since they form insoluble films that are not easily removed. In addition, chlorinated propellants have not been used since their ban in 1979 by the Food and Drug Administration, and states are now imposing limits on volatile organic compound emissions from hair sprays and other personal care products.[2] Copolymers such as polyvinylpyrrolidone (PVP) are the main ingredient in hair sprays, now widely available in aerosol pumps. PVP is a resin that is soluble in water and easily removed by shampooing. However, it also is hydroscopic: the film becomes sticky upon water contact from rain, humidity, or perspiration. Once wet, the film loses its holding ability. Vinyl acetate (VA) was added to PVP to make the product less hydroscopic, but this also made removal difficult. Most hair sprays now combine PVP/VA and utilize anywhere from 30% to 70% PVP.[3] Other newer polymer combinations are constantly being developed, such as copolymer resins of vinylmethylether and maleic acid hemiesters (PVP/MA) or copolymer resins of vinyl acetate and crotonic acid or dimethylhydantoin–formaldehyde resins, with a few products now containing methacrylate copolymer (polyvinylpyrrolidone dimethylaminoethylmetharylate or PVP/DMAEMA).[4,5]

Besides polymer resins, hair sprays also contain plasticizers (mineral oil, lanolin, castor oil, butyl palmitate), humectants (sorbitol, glycerol), solvents (SD alcohol 40, isopropyl alcohol), and conditioners (panthenol, plant proteins, hydrolyzed animal proteins, quaternium-19). More expensive hair sprays contain panthenol and quaternium-19, which are more costly conditioning ingredients, while lower priced conditioning hair sprays use hydrolyzed animal protein.[6] Higher priced hair sprays may also include a more costly fragrance than the lower-priced brands.

Application

Hair sprays are usually applied following hair styling, but may also function as a setting lotion, although this is not recommended. Hair sprays are available in several formulations that provide varying degrees of hold. Regular-hold hair sprays are designed simply to keep the hair in place. Super- or extra-hold hair sprays, hair-styling fixes, and hair spritzes contain more copolymer than regular-hold products and afford tremendous gravity-defying hold. These products also contain a less volatile vehicle than standard hair sprays, thus prolonging the drying time and allowing complex hair styling.

Adverse Reactions

There was some concern in the 1960s regarding inhalation of PVP/VA aerosolized particles. These copolymers were originally developed in the medical industry for use as plasma diluents and were subsequently adopted by the cosmetics industry. Some reports indicated that thesaurosis was due to hair sprays and that inhalation of PVP solid particles could induce foreign body granuloma formation in the lung. After extensive animal testing, it was concluded that PVP resin did not provoke pulmonary lesions.[4,7] Nevertheless, persons who are predisposed to lung conditions or those with allergic tendencies should use hair spray products with care.[8]

Hair sprays may produce dermatologic problems, such as nail damage.[9] Patients who have their hair done weekly in a salon and styled with an excessive amount of hair spray may develop hair spray build up, resulting in hair shaft dullness. If applied as a coarse mist, the hair spray can bead on the hair shaft, which resembles pediculosis capitis or trichorrhexis nodosa. The hair spray will also attract dirt, causing scalp irritation. Finally, once weekly shampooing may not be adequate to control seborrheic dermatitis in predisposed patients. There is some debate in cosmetics circles as to whether alcohol, an inexpensive evaporating solvent, also contributes to hair shaft dryness.

Hair sprays may be open or closed patch tested "as is," but the volatile vehicle should be allowed to evaporate prior to occlusion.

Hair Gels

Formulation

Hair gels contain the same PVP-type copolymers as hair sprays except that they are formulated into a gel and packaged in soft plastic squeeze tubes. They are available in alcohol-containing and alcohol-free forms and have glossening agents that coat the hair shaft and restore shine. Conditioners (hydrolyzed animal proteins, panthenol, keratin polypeptides, amino acids) are also incorporated into some hair gels. Two formulations are available: styling gels and sculpturing gels. As the names suggest, sculpturing gels afford more hold than styling gels.

Hair gels may contain synthetic color, usually in unnatural shades, such as blue, red, or purple. The colored gel coats the hair shaft, imparting tones of the color that is selected. The color molecules are too large to penetrate the undamaged hair shaft, so the colored coating can be removed with one shampooing. However, persons with chemically dyed or waved hair have a porous shaft that could semipermanently absorb color molecules, requiring four to six shampooings for removal. Glitter may also be added to hair gels for effect.

Application

This product is applied to towel-dried, damp hair and distributed on the hair shafts by combing to form a thin film. If a small amount of gel is applied, the hair will have a natural look and feel. If a large amount is applied, the hair will have a wet, "spiky" look and a stiff feel. The product can also be applied to completely dry hair to achieve a wet, "spiky" look. Hair gels afford maximum hold and are used in conjunction with styling fixes to create gravity-defying hair styles.

Hair gels can be useful by persons with thinning, dull hair. The eye interprets hair thickness by the hair elevation over the crown, lateral displacement at the sides, and the extent of the visible scalp.[10] Hair gels can hold the hair away from the scalp, creating the illusion of fullness.[11]

Adverse Reactions

These products adhere well to the hair shaft since PVP/VA has some substantivity for keratin. The films are flexible and colorless on the hair shaft, but can be removed by combing and brushing. This results in white polymer flakes in the hair that may resemble seborrheic dermatitis. The high concentration of PVP/VA also makes these products sticky with water contact. Persons who are exposed to moisture, such as athletes who perspire, should not use these styling products, since the PVP/VA will fix the hair upon redrying, possibly in an undesirable position.

Hair gels can be both open and closed patch tested "as is," but they should be allowed to dry prior to occlusion. They are of low irritant potential, but could cause allergic contact dermatitis in those methacrylate-sensitive patients who choose a product containing a methacrylate-based polymer.

Hair-Styling Mousses

Formulation

Hair-styling mousses are a foam released under pressure from an aerosolized can of the same copolymer-containing hair styling aid, as discussed for hair gels.

Hair-styling mousses may contain glossening and conditioning agents and can be colored to provide either natural or unnatural highlights. For example, persons with less than 15% gray hair can use a colored mousse with brown or auburn hues to blend gray hair. Unnatural colors such as yellow, green, red, orange, purple, and blue are also available. The color is temporary and removed with one shampooing unless applied to chemically treated hair.

Application

The mousse is applied in the same manner as a hair gel to towel-dried hair. It can also be applied to dry hair to create a wet, "spiky" look. Hair mousse yields a lighter copolymer application and does not provide as strong a hold as gel formulations. It also produces less flaking and less stickiness under moist conditions. Men generally prefer this product.

Hair-styling mousses can be used to create natural-appearing fullness more easily than hair gels due to their lower moisture content. A half-dollar-sized mound of mousse is placed in the palm. Small amounts are then dabbed onto the fingers and massaged into the proximal hair shaft. Drying occurs almost immediately. The mousse adds stiffness to the hair shaft, creating the illusion of fullness. This technique can be used by both men and women with thinning hair. A small amount of mousse applied to the palms and lightly touched to a finished style can smooth unmanageable hairs. Mature persons would probably find hair mousse more satisfactory than hair gel as a styling aid.

STYLING DEVICES

Two types of modern hair-styling devices are available: nonelectric and electric. Nonelectric styling devices include dry rollers, combs, brushes, and a variety of hair clasps. Electric styling devices include hair dryers, curling irons, electric curlers, and crimping irons.

Nonelectric

Nonelectric rollers function to impart curl and add body to create a desirable hair style. A variety of sizes and styles are available, with larger rollers forming looser curls while smaller rollers form tighter curls. Toothed rollers are designed to hold the hair without the aid of a hair pin, but may fracture the hair shaft on removal. Hair breakage can be minimized by using toothless smooth rollers held in place with hair pins and a hair net.

Wet hair is required to produce optimal curls with nonelectric rollers. Physically, wet hair is more elastic than dry hair, allowing partial transformation of the normal alpha-keratin structure to a beta-keratin structure under tension. This transformation shifts the relative position of the polypeptide chains and brings about a disruption of ionic and hydrogen bonds. During the drying process, new ionic and hydrogen bonds are formed, blocking return to the natural alpha-keratin configuration and allowing the hair to remain in its newly curled position. Wetting the hair, however, returns hair bonds immediately to the natural alpha configuration.[12] Hair must be rolled under tension to provide the load required for bond breakage, but hair should not be stretched beyond the point at which more than one-third of the alpha-keratin bonds have been unfolded to beta-keratin bonds. Excessive stretching will result in permanent deformation causing the inelastic hair to fracture.

Since wet hair is more elastic than dry hair, vigorous combing of the moist fibers can stretch the shaft to the point of fracture. Wet hair should be combed gently, if at all. The comb should possess smooth, rounded, coarse teeth to slip easily through the hair. Soft plastic combs are recommended since they bend when caught in tangled hair.

Extensive hair brushing should also be avoided while hair is wet. A good brush should have smooth, ball-tipped, coarse, bendable bristles. The brush should not tear the hair, but rather gently glide through it. Brushes used while blow drying hair should be vented to prevent increased heat along the brush, which could damage hair. Patients should be encouraged to brush and manipulate their hair as little as possible to minimize breakage. Older teachings that the hair should be brushed 100 strokes a day and the scalp vigorously massaged with the brush should be dispelled.

Common sense applies to the selection of appropriate hair pins and clasps. Rubber bands should never be used; hair pins should have a smooth, ball-tipped surface; and hair clasps should have spongy rubber padding where they contact the hair. Loose-fitting clasps also minimize breakage. The fact remains, however, that all hair pins or clasps break some hair since they must hold the hair tightly to stay in place. To minimize this problem, the patient should be encouraged to vary the clasp placement so that hair breakage is not localized to one scalp area. This problem is particularly apparent in women who wear a ponytail. These women frequently state that their hair is no longer growing when in actuality it is repeatedly broken at the same distance from the scalp due to hair clasp trauma. Pulling the hair tightly with clasps or braids can also remove hair shafts from the scalp, a condition known as traction alopecia.

Electric

Heat can also re-form hair shaft bonds, allowing development of numerous electric hair-styling appliances. The most popular appliance is the hair dryer, which can be hooded or hand-held. Hooded hair dryers are mainly used in professional salons. The patient, with wet hair on rollers, is placed inside the hood to dry the hair in its newly curled position. Hooded dryers are more efficient at drying the hair than blow dryers, but can cause more hair and scalp damage, especially if excess heat is present between the hood and scalp. Hand-held blow dryers avoid heat build up but must be held a sufficient distance from the scalp to avoid burns. Overheating can damage hair protein through denaturation. A vented styling brush is generally used to shape hair while blow drying.

The next most popular hair appliance is the curling iron, which is a modern version of the oven-heated metal rods that were wrapped with hair in the pre-electric era. Modern curling irons are thermostatically controlled to prevent overheating, but temperatures capable of producing first- and second-degree burns are still attainable. Some irons come with variable temperature settings, but most patients prefer the hottest setting since the curls produced are tighter and longer lasting. It is recommended that patients remove excess heat from the curling iron before use by placing it in a moist towel. This lowers the rod temperature, preventing burns of the hair and scalp.

Removal of hair from the curling iron without damage is another frequently encountered problem. Most curling irons have a spring-loaded clip to hold the hair to the rod. Failure to release the clip completely can cause hair breakage. Newer rods are now coated with nonstick materials to facilitate hair release; however, certain styling products, such as hair spray, can melt and glue hair to the rod. Thus, patients should curl their hair first and then add hair spray or other styling products.

Electric curlers are individually heated, plastic-coated rods of varying sizes. A curler set is more expensive than a curling iron, but the chance of burning is lessened since hot metal does not come in contact with the hair or scalp. Many patients prefer curling irons, since they have a shorter heating period, but fast, 60-second heating curlers are available. A variation on the firm, molded electric roller is a smaller diameter, rubber-coated, bendable rod or disk. The shape and type of curlers available are fashion dictated.

The last major type of electric hair-styling appliance is a variation on the old-fashioned hair iron. Two hinged metal plates are heated with hair placed between them. If the plates are corrugated, the device is known as a "crimping iron" and produces tight bends in the hair shaft. If the plates are smooth, the device is known as a hair straightener for those with kinky hair. Cautions and recommendations for its use are the same as for the curling iron.

It is important for the physician to consider electric styling device burns in the patient with scarring alopecia, especially of the frontal and vertex areas. In these locations, it is not only easier for the heated device to rest on the head, but also most women curl this area more frequently than the sides of the head, increasing the opportunity for burns.

REFERENCES

1. Henkin H: Hair grooming. p. 1111. In The Chemistry and Manufacture of Cosmetics. 2nd Ed. Allured Publishing Corporation, Wheaton, IL, 1988
2. Oteri R, Tazi M, Walls E, Kosiek JC: Formulating hairsprays for new air quality regulations. Cosmet Toilet July 106:29, 1991

3. Wells FV, Lubowe II: Hair grooming aids, part III. Cutis 22:407, 1978
4. Zviak C: The Science of Hair Care. Marcel Dekker, New York, 1986
5. Stutsman MJ: Analysis of hair fixatives. In Senzel AJ (ed): Newburger's Manual of Cosmetic Analysis. 2nd Ed. Published by the Association of Official Analytical Chemists, Inc, Washington, DC, 1977
6. Lochhead RY, Hemker WJ, Castaneda JY: Hair care gels. Cosmet Toilet October 102:89, 1987
7. Wells FV, Lubowe II: Hair grooming aids, part IV. Cutis 22:557, 1978
8. Wilkinson JB, Moore RJ: Harry's Cosmeticology. Chemical Publishing, New York, 1982
9. Daniel DR, Scher RK: Nail damage secondary to a hair spray. Cutis 47:165, 1991
10. Clarke J, Robbins CR, Reich C: Influence of hair volume and texture on hair body of tresses. J Soc Cosmet Chem 42:341, 1991
11. Rushton DH, Kingsley P, Berry NL, Black S: Treating reduced hair volume in women. Cosmet Toilet 108:59, 1993
12. Robbins CR: Chemical and Physical Behavior of Human Hair. 2nd Ed. Springer-Verlag, New York, 1988

15

Hair Removal

No single method of hair removal is appropriate for all body locations. The following discussion provides information on methods of hair removal and their appropriateness for a given patient (Table 15-1). Methods discussed include shaving, plucking, epilating, waxing, hair removing gloves, abrasives, threading, chemical depilatories, and electrolysis.

SHAVING

Shaving is the most widespread method of hair removal due to its rapid speed, effectiveness, and low expense. Shaving is the preferred removal technique for facial hair in men and underarm or leg hair in women. A major limitation of this technique is rapid, bristly regrowth due to a hair shaft now devoid of a naturally tapered tip.[1,2]

Many factors influence the closeness of a shave, mainly achieved by the optimum interaction between the blade and the skin. Contributing skin factors to shave closeness include abundant facial subcutaneous fat (resulting in improved resiliency), the absence of deep pits around hair ostia, and ostia containing only one hair.[3] Factors that lead to increased shaving irritation are old razor blades, large shaving angle, thin lathers, high skin tension, shaving against the direction of hair growth, repeat shaving over a given facial area, and increased shaving pressure.[4]

There are two methods of shaving: wet shaving with a razor blade and dry shaving with an electric razor.

Wet Shaving

Wet shaving employs a manual razor blade and shaving cream applied to moistened hair. Shaving cream functions to soften the beard, through hair shaft swelling, and lubricate the skin, thereby reducing razor drag.[5] Shaving creams with the highest viscosity seem to prevent surface trauma most effeciently.

Table 15-1. Methods of Hair Removal

Technique	Equipment	Cost	Regrowth Period	Body Sites for Use	Advantages	Disadvantages
Shaving	Razor or shaver	+	Days	Face, arms, legs, axilla	Fast, easy	Irritating, rapid regrowth
Plucking	Tweezers	+	Weeks	Eyebrows, facial hair	Longer regrowth period	Painful, slow
Epilating	Epilator	+	Weeks	Arms, legs	Longer regrowth period, fast	Painful, irritating
Waxing	Wax and melting pot	+ +	Weeks	Face, eyebrows, groin	Longer regrowth period	Painful, slow
Hair removing glove	Sandpaper gloves	+ +	Days	Legs, male face	None	Irritating, slow
Abrasives	Pumice stone	+ +	Days	Legs, male face	None	Irritating, slow
Threading	Thread	+	Days	Legs, arms	None	Painful, slow
Depilatories	Depilatory	+ +	Days	Legs, groin	Quick	Irritating
Electrolysis	Trained professional	+ + + +	May be permanent	All	May be permanent	Painful, time-consuming, expensive
Bleaching	Peroxide bleach	+ +	Does not remove hair	Female facial and arm hair	Quick	Irritating

Cost: + = $2–4, + + = $4–5, + + + = $5–10, + + + + = $10–20. This cost represents the average cost per hair removal session.

However, shaving cream must be left in contact with the hair and skin for at least 4 minutes to diminish razor burn and prolong razor blade life. (A more detailed discussion of shaving creams is given below.) Research has also determined that an angle of 28 to 32 degrees between the blade and the skin produces the closest shave with the least amount of irritation.[3]

The main advantage of wet shaving is that it allows the hair to be cut closely at the skin surface. It is an excellent hair removal technique for large, well-keratinized body surfaces, such as the legs in women and the face in men, where rapid regrowth and a coarse skin texture are not a problem. Women who have keratosis pilaris on the upper outer thighs should use wet shaving instead of dry shaving as shaving cream can soften the perifollicular keratotic material, thus minimizing skin trauma.

Problems with wet shaving include skin irritation, skin trauma, and the chance of spreading skin infections (such as impetigo or viral verruca) through microscopic tears in the stratum corneum. The regrown hair shafts also have a sharp tip that may reenter the skin, resulting in pseudofolliculitis barbae, commonly seen in the neck area of Black patients.[6,7]

Patients who experience undue irritation from wet shaving may not be using shaving cream, allowing insufficient time for hair softening to occur, shaving against the direction of hair growth, or stretching the skin tightly while shaving.

Dry Shaving

Dry shaving uses an electric shaver with no moisture or shaving cream. The electric shaver contains blades that rotate or vibrate, thereby cutting the hair shaft. In general, an electric shaver cannot cut the hairs as closely to the skin surface as a razor, but skin abrasion is not as great a problem. Skin irritation and the spread of cutaneous infections may still occur.[8]

Advantages of this hair removal method include the rapidity and the ease with which the hair can be removed. Large surface areas can be shaved with minimal effort, as long as the hair shafts are short. Clippers, a variant of the electric razor, can be used to shave longer hairs more easily.

In areas where rapid hair regrowth or bristly hair is a problem, such as the face of women, dry shaving should not be used. Furthermore, the sharp regrowing hair shafts may cause irritation in intertrigenous areas such as the underarms or inguinal folds. Dry shaving may also cause irritation of the follicular ostia, resulting in perifollicular pustules, a problem seen especially in the female pubic area. In these instances, other methods of hair removal are recommended.

PLUCKING

Plucking of the hair is a method of removing the entire hair shaft, including the bulb, with a pair of tweezers.[9] It is an easy, inexpensive method of hair removal, requiring minimal equipment, but is tedious and mildly uncomfortable.

Plucking does not encourage rapid regrowth. Removal of hair from large areas is not feasible, but plucking is effective for removal of stray eyebrow hairs or isolated coarse hairs on the chin of postmenopausal women. Only terminal hairs can be efficiently plucked, as vellus hairs usually break close to the skin surface.

Plucking produces little skin damage and provides a longer regrowth period due to complete hair shaft removal. It should be remembered, however, that repeated plucking of a given hair may result in ingrown hairs or failure of the hair to regrow, due to follicular damage.[10] For this reason, overplucking of the eyebrow area should be avoided.

EPILATING

"Epilating" has now come to refer to a mechanized method of plucking hair.[11] Most electric hand-held epilating devices are stroked over the skin much like an electric shaver. They consist of a rotating, tightly coiled spring that traps the hair and pulls it out at the level of the hair bulb. Retail cost for the device is $30 to $50. This efficient plucking of the hair provides a long regrowth period, but is somewhat painful. Additionally, the device functions poorly on curved surfaces, such as the underarms, and can do considerable damage to body areas with thin skin, such as the face.

Epilating is best used on large flat surfaces such as the arms and legs, but the hair must be of sufficient length for entrapment in the coiled spring. Follicular disruption is a problem that can result in ingrown or coiled hairs beneath the skin surface.[12,13] Infection may also be a problem, so use of an antibacterial agent prior to and following hair removal is recommended. If the epilator is pressed too firmly against the skin, purpura may result.

WAXING

Waxing is another variation on plucking of the hair. Two waxing techniques are available: hot waxing and cold waxing. Hot wax is composed of rosin, beeswax, paraffin wax, petrolatum, and mineral or vegetable oil. Some products are mentholated. The wax is melted in a double boiler or professional wax pot and applied to the hairs with a wooden spatula. Hair becomes embedded within the wax, which is allowed to cool and harden. The hair is then pulled out at the level of the hair bulb as the wax is ripped from the skin. Care must be taken not to burn the skin.

Cold waxing, a newer method, employs a wax-like substance that is squeezed as a liquid from a pouch, thus eliminating the need for melting. Sometimes cold waxing uses a cloth piece that is initially placed on the hair removal area followed by liquid application. The cloth is then ripped from the skin with the hair and the wax. The advantage of the cloth is that it provides strength so the wax can theoretically be removed in one piece rather than numerous smaller pieces.

Waxing has the advantage of adequate removal of both terminal and vellus hairs. This is important on the upper lip, chin, eyebrows, cheeks and groin of women where removal of all hair is desirable. Men generally do not find waxing of facial hair acceptable as the hair has to grow to at least 1/16 inch before it can be reliably removed by waxing. Excess hair present in Becker's nevi, congenital hairy nevi, and benign hairy nevi can be removed in both males and females with this technique.

The major disadvantages of waxing are discomfort and poor removal of hairs shorter than $\frac{1}{16}$ inch. Patients may also need to tweeze a few hairs that were not removed, and thick hair growth may require two treatments for complete removal.

The results of waxing are identical to hair plucking. The 2 week regrowth period is longer than that for shaving, since the hair is removed by the root. When regrowth occurs, the hair has a tapered tip rather than the sharp, blunt tip produced by shaving. No damage to the surrounding skin occurs, but patients must test the heated wax prior to application to avoid a burn. Waxing can be done professionally in a salon or at home. Professional fees vary depending on the size of the removal area. For example, it costs about $20 to have the eyebrows professionally waxed. Home waxing is much less expensive: $4 will purchase sufficient wax to remove excess eyebrow hair for 30 treatments.

HAIR REMOVING GLOVES

Hair removing gloves consist of a mitten of fine sandpaper that is rubbed over the hair-bearing skin in a circular fashion.[14] This mechanically fractures the hair shaft, but is also irritating to the skin. This is a method used to remove female leg hair and male facial hair in some countries, but is not popular in the United States.

ABRASIVES

Pumice stone or other abrasives can also be rubbed over the skin to remove hair through mechanical friction.[14] Again, this is very irritating to skin and not a popular hair removal technique in the United States.

THREADING

Threading is a hair removal technique popular in India. It is performed by looping a cotton thread around the neck of the operator and twisting the other end into a loop held in one hand. Then the ends are twisted and the loop pulled across the skin. The thread catches the hair and removes some at the level of the follicle while other hair breaks above the skin surface.[9]

DEPILATORIES

Chemical depilatories function by sufficiently softening the hair shaft above the skin surface so it can be gently wiped away with a soft cloth. Presently marketed chemical depilatories are available in pastes, powders, creams, and lotions with formulations specially adapted for use on the legs, groin area, and face. All formulations function by softening the cysteine-rich hair disulfide bonds to the point of dissolution. This is accomplished by combining five different classes of ingredients.

The agents combined to produce a chemical depilatory are detergents, hair shaft swelling agents, adhesives, pH adjusters, and bond-breaking agents.[15] Together they function to prepare the hair for and facilitate removal. Detergents such as sodium lauryl sulfate, laureth-23, or laureth-4 remove protective hair sebum and allow penetration of the bond-breaking agent. Further penetration is accomplished with swelling agents such as urea or thiourea. Adhesives such as paraffin allow the mixture to adhere to the hairs, while adjustment of pH, to between 9.0 and 12.5, is important to minimize cutaneous irritation. Lastly, the bond-breaking agent is able to destroy the hair shaft successfully.

Several bond-breaking agents are available: thioglycolic acid, calcium thioglycolate, strontium sulfide, calcium sulfide, sodium hydroxide, and potassium hydroxide. The most popular commercial bond-breaking agents are the thioglycolates, as they minimize cutaneous irritation while effectively breaking disulfide bonds; however, they are less effective at dissolving coarse hair such as in the male beard. Sulfide bond-breaking agents are faster acting, but are more irritating and sometimes produce an undesirable sulfur odor. Sodium hydroxide, also known as "lye," is the best bond-breaking agent, but is extremely damaging to the skin.

It is interesting to note that the consumer pays from $2 to $7 for a package of chemical depilatory, a profit of approximately 1,000% to 5,000% over the cost of the ingredients.

Chemical depilatories are designed to be left in contact with the skin for 5 to 10 minutes, shorter for fine hair and longer for coarse hair. The products are somewhat selective for hair shaft damage, since the hair shafts contain more cysteine than the surrounding skin, but are still irritating to skin, especially if contact is prolonged. The hairs are wiped away once they assume a corkscrew appearance. Under no circumstances should chemical depilatories be applied to abraded or dermatitic skin.

The main advantage of chemical depilatory hair removal is slower regrowth than with shaving, and, if used properly, the technique is painless and without scarring. The major disadvantage is the skin irritancy. A study by Richards et al.[9] found that fewer than 1% of their female study population could tolerate facial depilatories.

Chemical depilatories are best used for removal of hair on the legs to include the upper thigh. Darkly pigmented hair seems somewhat more resistant to removal than lighter hair, and coarse hair is more resistant than fine hair. This explains why these products are difficult to use on the male beard. However, a variety of powder depilatories, containing barium sulfide, are available for the Black male who has difficulty with pseudofolliculitis barbae.[16,17] These powdered products are mixed with water to form a paste and applied to the beard with a wooden applicator for 3 to 7 minutes. The hair and depilatory are then removed with the same applicator and the skin rinsed with cool water. This procedure should be performed no more frequently than every other day.

Both allergic and irritant contact dermatitis can occur with the use of chemical depilatories. Allergic contact dermatitis is less common but may be seen due to fragrances, lanolin derivatives, or other cosmetic additives. Irritant contact dermatitis is common, especially in individuals who use the product more than once weekly or apply it close to mucous membranes. Generally, the product is not appropriate for any patient with dermatologic problems. Most cutaneous problems can be remedied by discontinuing use and applying a topical corticosteroid. Depilatories also can damage fabrics and furniture.

ELECTROLYSIS

Electrolysis is the only permanent method of hair removal presently available to patients. Physicians are well aware of the complications of electrolysis, which include scarring, failure to destroy the germinative follicular cells, and transmission of viral and bacterial diseases. Yet electrolysis is a tremendously popular hair removal technique among women for unwanted hairs on the face, chin, neck, and bikini areas.[18] There are three electrolysis techniques: galvanic electrolysis, thermolysis, and the blend.

History

The first individual to use electrolysis for hair removal was a Missouri ophthalmologist named Dr. Charles E. Michel, who in 1875 used the technique in the treatment of trichiasis. The technique became well known during the later part of the 19th century. In 1924, the technique of thermolysis was developed by Dr. Henri Bordier of Lyon, France. The combination of electrolysis and thermolysis, known as "the blend," was developed by Arthur Hinkel and Henri St. Pierre in 1945, and a patent was granted for the technique in 1948.[19]

General Principles

All electrolysis techniques involve the insertion of a needle into the follicular ostia down to the follicular germinative cells. The dermal papillae must be destroyed to prevent hair growth permanently. There are several important considerations in determining the effectiveness of electrolysis techniques.

Telogen vs. Anagen

Only hairs that are visible can be removed by electrolysis, and only anagen hairs can be adequately treated. Follicles in the telogen phase, without a visible hair shaft, cannot be treated. If there is a high telogen to anagen ratio, a substantial amount of hair growth will be seen in the treated area. This ratio varies depending on body area.[9]

Many electrologists advise that their clients shave the hair in the area to be treated several days prior and refrain from other temporary hair removal techniques. This ensures that only anagen hair follicles are treated. Prior waxing or plucking of the hairs may delay regrowth, thus decreasing the thoroughness of electrolysis.

Moisture Content

Moisture content of the hair follicle is also important in determining the success of electrolysis. The lower part of the hair follicle is wetter than the more superficial follicle. Water is necessary for transmitting electrical energy between the needle and dermal papillae. For this reason, the electrolysis needle must be inserted to the depth of the hair follicle.

Depth

The depth of needle insertion is determined by the hair shaft diameter. As is readily demonstrated in Table 15-2, larger diameter hairs require deeper needle insertion for adequate destruction. Knowledge of follicular depth is necessary to ensure adequate follicular destruction without scarring.

Table 15-2. Hair Shaft Diameter and Hair Follicle Depth

Hair Shaft Diameter (inches)	Description of Hair	Hair Follicle Depth (mm)
<0.001	Very fine	>1
0.001–0.002	Fine	1–2
0.002–0.003	Medium	2–3
0.003–0.004	Coarse	3–4
0.004–0.005	Very coarse	4–5
0.005–0.006	Extra coarse	5
>0.006	Super coarse	5

(Adapted from Richards and Meharg,[19] with permission.)

Intensity and Duration

Dermal papillae damage depends on both the intensity and duration of the current administered. High intensity energy may be used for a short duration, or lower intensity energy may be used for a longer duration. The decision of how much energy to use depends upon both the technique used by the electrologist and the pain tolerance of the client. As might be expected, pain increases with higher intensity energy. Low intensity energy, however, is not able to destroy some hairs. In general, coarse hairs require a longer treatment duration than fine hairs.[20]

Follicular Shape

Electrolysis is much more difficult to perform on individuals with curly, wavy, or kinky hair. This is due to difficulty in placing the needle accurately into the hair follicle.

Theory

Electrolysis, thermolysis and the blend represent the three techniques that can be used to remove unwanted hair permanently.[21] Other advertised methods, such as electronic tweezers, do not work.

Electrolysis

This technique is properly known as ''galvanic electrolysis'' and utilizes direct current (DC), which is passed through a stainless steel needle into sodium chloride and water in the tissue surrounding the hair follicle. The DC current causes ionization of the salt (NaCl) and water (H_2O) into free sodium (Na^+), chloride (Cl^-), hydrogen (H^+), and hydroxide (OH^-) ions. These free ions then recombine into sodium hydroxide (NaOH), known as ''lye,'' and hydrogen gas (H_2). The caustic sodium hydroxide destroys the hair follicle while the hydrogen gas escapes into the atmosphere. The amount of sodium hydroxide produced is greater at the base of the hair follicle due to increased moisture content and minimal at the skin surface. Less lye production near the skin surface accompanied by the protective effect of sebum decrease the skin irritancy potential of this technique. The amount of follicular destruction induced is measured in units of lye, defined by Arthur Hinkel as the amount of lye produced 0.1 milliamp of current flows for 1 second.[22]

Galvanic electrolysis is the most effective method of producing permanent hair removal, but is tedious and slow. This has led to the development of multiple needle techniques.

Thermolysis

Thermolysis, also known as ''short-wave radio frequency diathermy,'' differs from galvanic electrolysis in that alternating high frequency (AC) current is passed down the needle. This current causes vibration of the water molecules around the hair follicle and produces heat. Thus, heating occurs in the same manner as in a microwave oven.[23]

The needle begins to heat at the tip first and spreads toward the skin surface. This means that the heat remains longer around the hair follicle than at the skin surface, minimizing discomfort and cutaneous damage. If too much AC current is administered, steam is produced that exits through the follicular ostia, resulting in a burn and possible scarring.

Thermolysis is much faster than galvanic electrolysis, but does not destroy the hair follicle as reliably. Additionally, thermolysis does not work well on distorted or curved hair follicles. An extremely rapid method of thermolysis, known as the "flash" method, was introduced several years ago, but unfortunately yields high regrowth.

Blend

The blend is a combination of both galvanic electrolysis and thermolysis.[20] Both direct and high-frequency alternating current are passed down the needle at the same time to produce sodium hydroxide and heat. The hot lye is extremely effective in destroying the dermal papillae, allowing superior results with less regrowth. Furthermore, the tissue damage induced by the thermolysis allows the lye to spread through the hair follicle more rapidly. The blend requires only one-fourth the time of galvanic electrolysis alone.

Needle Selection

Needle selection is important to the success of electrolysis. Needles are available in a variety of shapes: straight, tapered, bulbous, and insulated.[24] Most electrologists prefer to use a straight needle with a gently rounded tip. Tapered needles (narrower at the tip than at the base) are sometimes selected for the removal of deep terminal hairs. Electrolysis of these hairs requires more energy, which can be delivered at the tip without exposing the more superficial tissues to excessive damage.

A variety of sizes are also available since the needle diameter should match the diameter of the hair shaft to be treated. Smaller needles generally get hotter than larger needles. Client pain can be reduced by selecting the largest needle possible.

Stainless steel is the standard material from which needles are made. However, one company markets a gold-plated needle that is termed "hypoallergenic."

Sometimes the electrologist may use multiple needles at one time to speed the treatment. A computerized electrolysis machine is used to administer sequentially energy to the needles in the proper order and for the specified length of time.

Needle Insertion Techniques

The needle must be properly inserted into the follicular ostia to ensure destruction of the hair follicle without cutaneous scarring. The most popular technique for needle insertion is known as the "forehand" technique. The needle holder is held much like a pencil between the thumb and forefinger. The removal forceps are then placed between the needle holder and thumb of the same hand. This allows the free hand to be used for stretching the skin. Skin stretching is important to open the follicular ostia for needle insertion.

The needle is always inserted parallel to the hair shaft opposite to the direction of hair growth. Hairs may exit the skin at angles varying between 10 and 90 degrees. The needle must be inserted at the same angle as hair growth. If the hair is long and lays on the skin surface, it should be clipped to gain a better appreciation of its exit angle. The needle should also always be inserted below the hair shaft. These steps are necessary to destroy the follicle without scarring the surrounding skin.

It is important that needle insertion occur to the proper depth. A general rule is that coarse hairs have deeper follicles than fine hairs. A slight dimpling of the overlying skin and resistance means that the bottom of the follicle has been reached and the needle should be withdrawn slightly until the dimpling disappears. A proper needle insertion should be painless and bloodless for the client. Shallow needle insertions may result in pain and scarring for the client.

Hair Removal Techniques

Once the hair has been treated, the needle should be withdrawn at exactly the same angle as it was inserted. The forceps held between the thumb and needle holder are now positioned 90 degrees to the hair shaft for epilation. The hair should be grasped firmly and gently slide out of the follicle, if the treatment has been properly performed. Resistance in removing the hair means that the hair has been epilated and not treated with electrolysis; thus regrowth may occur.

Adverse Reactions

Electrolysis must be properly performed to minimize client scarring. Table 15-3 summarizes the pointers that must be followed for successful electrolysis.[19] Care must also be taken to perform the procedure under sanitary conditions to prevent the spread of bacterial and viral infections.[25] The real concern regarding electrolysis is the lack of regulation, as 23 states do not require licensing of electrologists. This lack of licensing means that training and health standards are apt to vary tremendously between salons. Improper techniques can result in permanent scarring, and failure to sterilize equipment adequately can result in the transmission of bacterial and viral infections. If a good operator with

Table 15-3. Recommendations for Electrolysis Scar Prevention

The treated hair should be pulled effortlessly from the follicular ostia.
The needle size should be the same as the hair diameter.
The skin should be dry.
The skin should not be blanched following treatment.
The current should only flow when the needle has been completely inserted into the follicular ostia to the level of the follicle.
The needle should only be removed when the current has stopped.
The same follicular ostia should not be re-entered or treated twice.

superior health standards can be found, electrolysis may be useful for the female with a few unwanted facial hairs on the upper lip or chin. This technique is not suitable for removal of large hairy areas, such as the male beard, as only 25 to 100 hairs can be removed per sitting.

BLEACHING

Bleaching is not a method of hair removal, but is included in this section because it can make unwanted hair less apparent. Commercial products are available for bleaching hair; however, a home bleach can be made by mixing 40 ml hydrogen peroxide with 7 ml 20% ammonia. The bleach is left in contact with the hair until the color is removed, about 5 to 10 minutes. This product is irritating to the skin and should not be used around the eyes or mucous membranes.

Hair bleaching is most appropriate for the female patient who notes excess pigmented hair on the arms, upper lip, or jawline. The hair may be pigmented due to a Hispanic, Mediterranean, or Middle Eastern genetic background. Bleaching may be the most acceptable alternative when shaving produces an unacceptable regrowth appearance and the area is too large for waxing.

REFERENCES

1. Bhaktaviziam C, Mescon H, Matolsky AG: Shaving. Arch Dermatol 88:242, 1963
2. Lynfield YL, MacWilliams P: Shaving and hair growth. J Invest Dermatol 55:170, 1970
3. Hollander J, Casselman EJ: Factors involved in satisfactory shaving. JAMA 109: 95, 1937
4. Elden HR: Advances in understanding mechanisms of shaving. Cosmet Toilet 100: 51, 1985
5. Bogaty H: Shaving with razor and blade. Cutis 21:609, 1978
6. Strauss J, Kligman AM: Pseudofolliculitis of the beard. Arch Dermatol 74:533, 1956

7. Spencer TS: Pseudofolliculitis barbae or razor bumps and shaving. Cosmet Toilet 100:47, 1985
8. Brooks GJ, Burmeister F: Preshave and aftershave products. Cosmet Toilet 105: 67, 1990
9. Richards RN, Uy M, Meharg G: Temporary hair removal in patients with hirsuitism: A clinical study. Cutis 45:199, 1990
10. Blackwell G: Ingrown hairs, shaving, and electrolysis. Cutis 19:172, 1977
11. Scott JJ, Scott MJ, Scott AM: Epilation. Cutis 46:216, 1990
12. Wright RC: Traumatic folliculitis of the legs: a persistent case associated with use of a home epilating device. J Am Acad Dermatol 27:771, 1992
13. Dilaimy M: Pseduofolliculitis of the legs. Arch Dermatol 112:507, 1976
14. Wagner RF: Physical methods for the management of hirsutism. Cutis 45:319, 1990
15. Breuer H: Depilatories. Cosmet Toilet 105:61, 1990
16. de la Guardia M: Facial depilatories on black skin. Cosmet Toilet 91:37, 1976
17. Halder RM: Pseudofolliculitis barbae and realted disorders. Dermatol Clin 6:407, 1988
18. Goldberg HC, Hanfling SL: Hirsutism and electrolysis. J Med Soc NJ 62:9, 1965
19. Richards RN, Meharg GE: Cosmetic and Medical Electrolysis and Temporary Hair Removal. Medric Ltd., Ontario, 1991
20. Hinkel AR, Lind RW: Electrolysis, Thermolysis and the Blend. Arroway Publishers, California, 1968
21. Fino G: Modern Electrology. Milady Publishing Corp., New York, 1987
22. Cipollaro AD: Electrolysis: discussion of equipment, method of operation, indications, contraindications, and warnings concerning its use. JAMA 110:2488, 1938
23. Wagner RF, Tomich JM, Grande DJ: Electrolysis and thermolysis for permanent hair removal. J Am Acad Dermatol 12:441, 1985
24. Gior F: Modern Electrology. Milady Publishing Corporation, New York, 1987
25. Petrozzi JW: Verrucae planae spread by electrolysis. Cutis 26:85, 1980

16

Hair-Coloring Agents

Hair dyes represent a major hair cosmetic used by both men and women. It is estimated that 40% of women regularly use hair dyes to blend gray tones, cover gray hair, add colored highlights, produce unnatural temporary colors, and either lighten or darken the original hair color. A number of different hair dye cosmetics have been developed to fulfill all of these needs: gradual, temporary, semipermanent, and permanent. Approximately 65% of the hair dye market is for permanent hair colorings, 20% for semipermanent colorings, and 15% for the remaining types.

HISTORY

Hair coloring is an ancient tradition that was common among the Persians, Hebrews, Greeks, and Romans. The use of henna, a naturally occurring plant dye, dates to the third dynasty of Egypt 4,000 years ago. The Egyptians mixed the *Lawsonia* plant (henna) with hot water and placed the material on the head to produce an orange-red hair color. Metallic dyes containing lead acetate, obtained by dipping lead combs in sour wine, were used by Roman men to cover gray hair.[1] Roman women, on the other hand, attempted to lighten their hair by applying lye followed by sun exposure.

The modern concept of permanent hair dyeing dates to 1883, when Monnet patented a process for coloring fur using *p*-phenylenediamine and hydrogen peroxide. Feathers and hair were later dyed in 1888, and the first human applications were in Paris in 1890 and in St. Louis, Missouri, in 1892.[2] Temporary and semipermanent dyes were not developed until the 1950s, when they were incorporated from the textile industry into the cosmetics industry. Bleaching of the hair with hydrogen peroxide was first demonstrated at the Paris Exposition of 1867 by Thillary and Hugo.[3] All of these products form the basis for modern hair coloring.

HAIR COLOR PHYSIOLOGY

Pigment comprises less than 3% of the fiber mass of hair, yet is one of the most important hair cosmetics aspects.[4] Three pigment types produce the tremendous variety of color seen in human hair: eumelanins, pheomelanins, and oxymelanins. Eumelanins are insoluble polymers accounting for the brown and black hues consisting mainly of 5,6-dihydroxyindole, with lesser amounts of 5,6-dihydroxyindole-2-carboxylic acid. Pheomelanins are soluble polymers accounting for the yellow to red hues containing 10% to 12% sulfur and 1,4-benzothiazinylalanine. Eumelanin contains less sulfur than pheomelanin.[5] A lesser pigment, known as "oxymelanin," is yellow or reddish in color and probably represents bleached eumelanin pigment arising from partial oxidative cleavage of 5,6-dihydroxyindole units. Oxymelanin is distinct in that it contains no sulfur.[6] Hair dyes attempt to mimic these pigments in reproducing a natural-appearing hair color.

The principle use for hair dyeing is to cover gray hair. The mechansim of graying is not totally understood, however. It is thought that the death of some melanocytes within the hair–melanocyte unit triggers a chain reaction resulting in the death of the rest of the unit melanocytes in a relatively short period.[7] A possible mechanism of death is the accumulation of a toxic intermediate metabolite, such as dopaquinone.[8]

TYPES OF HAIR DYES

Hair dyes can be divided into several types based on their formulation and permanency: gradual, temporary, semipermanent, and permanent (Table 16-1).

Gradual

Gradual hair dyes, also known as "metallic" or "progressive" hair dyes, require repeated application to result in gradual darkening of the hair shaft. This product will change the hair color from gray to yellow-brown to black over a period of weeks.[9] There is no control over the final color of the hair, only the depth of color, and lightening is not possible. Gradual dyes employ water-soluble metal salts that are deposited on the hair shaft in the form of oxides, suboxides, and sulfides. The most common metal used is lead, but silver, copper, bismuth, nickel, iron, manganese, and cobalt have also been used. In the United States, 2% to 3% solutions of lead acetate or nitrate are used to dye the hair, while 1% to 2% solutions of silver nitrate are used to dye eyelashes and eyebrows.[10]

Metallic hair dyes are inexpensive and do not require a professional operator for application. Their disadvantages include poor color quality and resulting stiff, brittle, or dull hair that may not withstand further chemical processing.

Table 16-1. Hair Coloring

Type	Main Ingredient	Duration of Effect	Effect on Hair	Advantages/ Disadvantages
Gradual	Aqueous solution of lead or silver oxides, suboxides, and sulfides	Color persists with continued use	Darkens gradually by "plating" hair shaft	Cannot be combined with permanent dye or permanent wave
Temporary	High-molecular-weight, textile dyes	Removal with one shampooing	Large color molecules deposited on hair shaft	Can blend or tone undesirable hair color
Semipermanent	Low-molecular-weight, natural or synthetic textile-type dye	Removal with four to six shampooings	Small color molecules penetrate hair cortex	Tone-on-tone coloring. Will cover less than 30% gray. May be allergenic
Permanent	Oxidation coloring employing primary intermediates, couplers, and an oxidant	Permanent	New color molecules formed within hair shaft	Lighten (two-step processing) or darken (one-step processing). Will cover gray 100%. Need to cover new growth with monthly dyeing. May be allergenic

In addition, the trace metals left on the hair will cause permanent dyes or permanent waving solutions to perform poorly. The metal can cause breakdown of the hydrogen peroxide in bleaching or permanent waving products, resulting in rupture of the hair shaft. The hair that has been treated with the gradual hair colorant must therefore grow out before other dyeing or waving procedures are used, to guarantee an optimal result.[11]

The gradual color change induced by metallic dyes requires continued use if the color is to be maintained; however, the hair shaft damage induced by the product is permanent. Therefore, metallic dyes are not appropriate for female patients who desire more color darkening than the product can provide and who are likely to undergo permanent waving. These products are most appropriate for male patients who cut their hair frequently, only need minimal darkening, and are unlikely to process their hair further.[12]

Temporary

Temporary hair-coloring agents are designed to be removed in one shampooing.[13] They are used to add a slight tint, brighten a natural shade, or improve an existing dyed shade. Their particle size is too large to penetrate through the cuticle, accounting for their temporary nature.[1] Temporary dyes can be easily rubbed off the hair shaft, however, and will run onto clothing if the hair gets wet from rain or perspiration. They can be formulated as a liquid, mousse, gel, or spray.

Liquid temporary hair colorants are also referred to as "hair rinses," since they are frequently applied in the shower following shampooing, with the excess dyestuff removed by rinsing. They contain acid dyes of the same type used to dye wool fabrics and belong to the following chemical classes: azo, anthraquinone, triphenylmethane, phenzainic, xanthenic, or benzoquinoneimine.[14] These dyes are known as FDC and DC blues, greens, reds, oranges, yellows, and violets. No damage is imparted to the hair shaft by these dyes because they are composed of large molecules that are deposited on the surface of the hair and are unable to penetrate due to size.

The liquid rinse formulation is most popular, especially among mature patients with gray hair who wish to remove undesirable yellow tones and achieve a purer platinum color. A sample product for this purpose may contain a 0.001% concentration of methylene blue, acid violet 6B, and water-soluble nigrosine in an aqueous preparation. Temporary hair colorants are recommended for mature patients since the hair shaft will not be damaged and many patients only require weekly shampooing. The liquid rinse can also be used by patients who have achieved an undesirable permanent dye color and wish to tone the bad result until the poorly colored hair grows out and is cut.

Mousse formulations of temporary hair colorants are available in both natural and party colors. They are applied following shampooing to towel-dried hair and are not removed. Because the coloring agent is dispersed in a styling polymer, such as polyvinylpyrrolidone/vinyl acetate (PVP/VA), the mousse serves as both styling agent and temporary colorant. This product may be used to add highlights or blend gray hair in brunette patients with less than 15% gray hair. Mousse temporary coloring agents are ideal for the female patient with minimal bitemporal graying. These products are also available in party colors such as yellow, orange, blue, green, purple, and red, which can be used to create special multicolored effects.

Gel formulations of temporary hair colorants are identical to mousse formulations, except that they are packaged as a gel in a tube rather than as a foam released from an aerosol can. Gel temporary hair colorants also combine a styling aid with coloring; however, the hold provided by the gel is generally superior to that provided by the mousse. These products are only available in party colors, with some lines including a hair glitter. Gel temporary hair colorants are only appropriate for creating unusual hair styles.

Spray formulations of temporary hair colorants are also available to professional cosmetologists. A pressurized aerosol spray is used to apply the temporary liquid dyestuff to the hair.[15]

Temporary hair coloring agents should be used with care in patients with damaged or chemically treated hair because the hair shaft has increased porosity due to loss of the cuticular scale. The porous hair shafts allow entrance of the color molecules into the hair shaft, rendering them more permanent. Under these conditions, it may take more than one shampooing to remove the color.

Semipermanent

Textile Dyes

Semipermanent hair coloring is popular with both men and women. Formulated for use on natural, unbleached hair, it can cover gray, add highlight, or rid hair of unwanted tones. Semipermanent hair dyes are removed in four to six shampooings due to their intermediate-sized particles that can both enter and exit the hair shaft.[16] Recently, longer lasting products within this category incorporating hydrogen peroxide have become available. The dyes are retained in the hair shaft by weak polar and Van der Waals attractive forces; thus dyestuffs with increased molecular size will remain longer. The formulation of a typical semipermanent hair dye is dyes (nitroanilines, nitrophenylenediamines, nitroaminophenols, azos, anthraquinones), alkalizing agent, solvent, surfactant, thickener, fragrance and water.[17] Usually, 10 to 12 dyes are mixed to obtain the desired shade.[18]

Semipermanent dyes are available as lotions, shampoos, and mousses. The shampoo-in process is most popular for home use. The dyestuff is combined with an alkaline detergent shampoo to promote hair shaft swelling so that the dye can penetrate, a thickener so that the product will remain on the scalp, and a foam stabilizer so that the product will not run and stain facial skin. The mousse formula incorporates the dyestuff in an aerosolized foam. Both products are applied to wet, freshly shampooed hair and then rinsed after 20 to 40 minutes. Semipermanent dyes can become more permanent if applied to porous, chemically treated hair.

Semipermanent dyes produce tone-on-tone coloring rather than effecting drastic color changes, so their role is actually in toning rather than dyeing hair. The less color change required by the patient, the more satisfied he or she will be with the semipermanent dye result. Semipermanent dyes are best suited for patients with less than 30% gray hair who want to restore their natural color.[19] This is done by selecting a dye color that is lighter than the natural hair color since the dye will penetrate both the gray and the nongray hairs, resulting in an increased darkening of the nongray hairs. It is not possible to lighten hair with semipermanent dyes, since they do not contain hydrogen peroxide, nor is it possible to darken hair more than three shades beyond the patient's natural hair color. Thus, in the cosmetics industry, semipermanent dyes are known as suitable only for staying ''on shade.''

Stains

A newer type of semipermanent hair coloring is hair stain. Hair stain is a synthetic polymer, usually in unnatural shades such as reds, blues, purples, or yellows, that imparts a hue or highlight to the hair. For example, brunette hair with a red stain will have a reddish glow or blond hair with a yellow stain will have a yellow glow. The stain appears transparent so that it blends with the underlying hair color. The stain does not cover, but only tones. If heat is added to the staining process, the stain is more resistant to shampoo removal, and, if both heat and hydrogen peroxide are added to the staining process, the stain can penetrate the hair shaft deeply and become permanent.

Rarely, individuals with multiple dye sensitivities may wish to stain hair with natural agents, such as walnut stain (Cosmetochem USA, Herbasol extract of walnut leaves). This extract of black walnut leaves produces a deep brownish-black color when applied to the hair.

Vegetable Dyes

Vegetable dyes, the first form of hair coloring developed, fall under the semipermanent category because they minimally penetrate the cuticle, although four to six shampooings are required for removal. The only vegetable dye remaining today is henna, derived from the *Lawsonia alba* plant. As originally used, the dried plant leaves were ground to form a powder that was activated with water to form an acidic naphthoquinone dye that was then applied as a paste to the hair for 40 to 60 minutes. The henna imparted a reddish hue to the hair. Metallic salts were combined with henna to produce what was termed a ''compound henna'' to provide a wider range of colors. Today, natural henna dyes have been replaced by synthetic henna-type products with dye shades ranging from auburn to blonde to gray. These synthetic henna products combine a conditioning agent with the dye, but they are still powders mixed with water to form a paste that remains in contact with the hair for 40 minutes. Hennas can be used for darkening, but not lightening, of the original hair color. Natural hennas are inferior to synthetic hennas because they leave the hair stiff and brittle after repeated applications. Henna has not been reported to cause allergic contact dermatitis when used as a hair dye.[20]

Permanent

Permanent hair coloring accounts for $3 of every $4 spent on hair dyeing in the United States. It is more popular with women than men since women are more likely to effect a complete hair color change than men. Permanent hair coloring is so named because the dyestuff penetrates the hair shaft to the cortex and forms large color molecules that cannot be removed by shampooing.[20] It can be used both to cover gray hair and to produce a completely new hair color. Redyeing is necessary every 4 to 6 weeks, as new growth, known in the cosmetics industry as ''roots,'' appears at the scalp.

This type of hair coloring does not contain dyes, but rather colorless dye precursors that chemically react with hydrogen peroxide inside the hair shaft to produce colored molecules.[21] The process entails the use of primary intermediates (*p*-phenylenediames, *p*-toluenediamine, *p*-aminophenols) that undergo oxidation with hydrogen peroxide. These reactive intermediates are then exposed to couplers (resorcinol, 1-naphthol, *m*-aminophenol, and so forth) to result in a wide variety of indo dyes. These indo dyes can produce shades from blonde to brown to black with highlights of gold to red to orange. Variations in the concentration of hydrogen peroxide and the chemicals selected for the primary intermediates and couplers produce this color selection.[22] Red is produced by using nitroparaphenylenediamine alone or in combination with mixtures of para-aminophenol with metaphenylenediamine, alphanaphthol, or 1,5-dihydroxynaphthalene. Yellow is produced by mixtures of orthoaminophenol, orthophenylenediamine, and nitro-orthophenylenediamine. Blue has no single oxidation dye intermediate and is produced by combinations of paraphenylenediamine, phenylenediamine, methyltoluylenediamine, or 2,4-diaminoanisol.[23]

Permanent dyeing allows shades to be obtained both lighter and darker that the patient's original hair color. Higher concentrations of hydrogen peroxide can bleach melanin; thus the oxidizing step functions in both color production and bleaching. Due to the use of hydrogen peroxide in the formation of the new color molecules, hair dyes must be adjusted so that hair lightening is not produced with routine dyeing.[24] However, hydrogen peroxide cannot remove sufficient melanin alone to lighten dark brown or black hair to blonde hair. Boosters, such as ammonium persulfate or potassium sulfate, must be added to achieve great degrees of color lightening. The boosters must be left in contact with the hair for 1 to 2 hours for an optimal result. Nevertheless, individuals with dark hair who choose to dye their hair a light blonde color will notice the appearance of reddish hues with time. This is due to the inability of the peroxide/booster system to remove reddish pheomelanin pigments completely, which are more resistant to removal than brownish eumelanin pigments.

Permanent hair dyes are sold as two bottles containing colorless liquid within a kit. One bottle contains the dye precursors in an alkaline soap or synthetic detergent base, and the other contains a stabilized solution of hydrogen peroxide. The two bottles are mixed immediately prior to use and applied to the hair. The dye precursors and hydrogen peroxide diffuse into the hair where the new color is created.

Permanent hair dyes are the most damaging to the hair. This type of hair dye alters the internal hair shaft structure and therefore decreases its strength. Several key points should be remembered to minimize hair shaft damage:

1. If both permanent waving and permanent dyeing are to be performed, the hair should be permanently waved first and permanently dyed second. Ten days should be allowed between the procedures.
2. Lightening, or bleaching, the hair is more damaging than dyeing the hair to a darker color.
3. Each redyeing procedure further damages the hair shaft; thus the period between redyeing should be as long as possible, and the dye should be concentrated on the new proximal hair growth, not the previously dyed distal hair shaft.

Permanent hair coloring agents are available for both home and professional salon use. The chemistry is identical for both home and salon products, except that more drastic color changes require a salon product. Permanent hair coloring agents for home use are available in several different formulations: liquid, cream, and gel. The liquid shampoo-in formulas are most popular. All formulations come with a hair color tint and developer that must be mixed immediately before application on dry hair. The product must saturate the hair with thicker cream formulations requiring parting and sectioning of the hair to ensure even application. The excess dye is then rinsed, and frequently a conditioner is applied. Home permanent dye products can be purchased to lighten or darken the hair by three shades. Products that lighten the hair contain ammonia and more hydrogen peroxide, thus bleaching as well as dyeing the hair. Most home products are designed to achieve a 35% coverage of gray hair. More dramatic color changes require professional products.

Even though oxidation dyes are termed "permanent," some color drift or "off-shade fading" does occur. This is due to slow chemical changes in the indo dyes, which produce a reddish to yellowish cast. Thus, permanent hair colors may become "brassy" with age. Semipermanent hair colorings may be used to cover the brassy tones until redyeing occurs. Sometimes, undesirable reddish and yellowish tones develop immediately following dyeing. In this case "drabbers" are used to remove the harshness from a color. Examples of drabbers are resorcinol to yield dark green to brown colors, pyrocatechol to yield deep gray, pyrogallol to yield gold, alphanaphthol to yield bright violet, betanaphthol to yield red brown, and hydroquinone to yield yellow brown.[23]

Professional permanent hair dyeing techniques can be classified into one- and two-step processing. One-step processing permanently darkens the hair color, whereas two-step processing permanently lightens the hair color.

One-Step Processing

In one-step processing, a cream tint is used in a shampoo formulation. Often a conditioner or filler must be used prior to processing to ensure even uptake of the dye by the entire hair shaft. Damaged distal hair shafts or previously treated hair will absorb or "grab" color more quickly. The filler prevents the distal hair shaft from dyeing darker than the proximal hair shaft. However, in extremely damaged hair, a filler cannot ensure even dye uptake. In these cases the dyestuff is applied to the scalp first and the ends last so that the distal hair shafts have a shorter dyeing time. The cream tint is then rinsed, and a postdyeing conditioner may be applied. Sometimes the hydrogen peroxide used in the oxidation dyeing process can lighten the existing hair color, a phenomenon known as "lift." Hair cosmetic companies formulate one-step permanent oxidation dyes to avoid lift.

Two-Step Processing

Two-step hair processing involves bleaching or lifting the natural hair color, with subsequent redyeing to the desired lighter shade. This technique is used when patients wish to dye their hair much lighter than their natural color.

The bleaching is achieved with an alkaline mixture of hydrogen peroxide and ammonia, which causes swelling of the hair shaft to allow easier penetration of the dye, known as a toner.[25] A toner must be used since the hair, when completely stripped of color, has an undesirable appearance. The toner can be either a permanent or semipermanent dye.

The hair must be lightened to the desired color group and then dyed to the desired shade. There are seven levels of lightening:

Black
Brown
Red
Red gold
Gold
Yellow
Pale yellow

A patient with black natural hair color would have to go through all seven stages of lightening to become a pale yellow blonde, whereas a patient with natural gold hair color would have to go through three stages of lightening to become a pale yellow blonde. The more stages of lightening required to achieve the end result, the stronger the bleaching agent used and the more damaging the process to the hair.[26] A ''booster'' such as ammonium persulfate or potassium persulfate may be added to the hydrogen peroxide and ammonia solution for patients who desire extreme hair color lightening.[17] Allergic reactions to ammonium persulfate have been reported.[27] The eumelanin pigments in the hair are easily bleached by hydrogen peroxide, but the pheomelanins are somewhat resistant. This accounts for the increased difficulty in bleaching the hair of persons with reddish hair. It is difficult to formulate a solution strong enough to degrade hair pigment without damaging the hair keratin structure.

Some patients do not wish to lighten the hair on the entire scalp. For example, if only selected hairs are lightened in color, a technique known as ''highlighting,'' a cap with holes is applied to the scalp and only certain hairs are pulled through and exposed to the bleaching and dyeing process. If only the tips of selected locks of hair are treated, the process is known as ''tipping,'' whereas ''streaking'' involves treating the entire hair shaft of certain locks of hair. ''Frosting'' the hair entails bleaching a larger proportion of entire hair shafts than streaking. Fashion trends dictate the proportion of bleached to unbleached hairs in the scalp.

There is no doubt that two-step processing is the most damaging form of hair coloring. Hair that has been bleached is extremely porous and as a result is brittle, hard to untangle, and lacking in luster. Conditioners can do very little to improve the appearance of hair that has sustained damage this severe. Most patients with double-processed hair who are dissatisfied with the appearance and texture of their hair are best advised to cut the damaged portion of the hair shafts and await new growth. Unfortunately, once the hair has been bleached many shades lighter than the natural hair color, the proximal dark regrowth is cosmetically unattractive. This further encourages the patient to reprocess the hair. Perhaps patients can be encouraged to change to a shorter hair style or wear a wig during the regrowth period. Another alternative is to use a semipermanent dye to blend the bleached and naturally colored areas of the hair shaft, but if a color difference of more than three shades is present, the result will be suboptimal. Two-step processing should be minimized. It is recommended that patients stay within their own color group to maintain a natural appearance and prevent extensive hair shaft damage. Generally, a patient's natural hair color group will complement the eye color and skin tone for an overall attractive blend. Patients who distort this balance create many cosmetic problems.

Two-step processing, however, can be successful and attractive in the mature patient who had dark brown hair and now has more than 60% gray hair. If the patient does not like the appearance of this hair coloring, some dyeing procedure is required. The patient is faced with the dilemma of whether to restore the original dark brown color or to lighten the remaining dark brown hairs and redye the hair blonde. This is a personal decision, since both hair color changes require permanent dyeing. Restoring the entire scalp to a dark brown might increase the contrast between the lighter scalp and darker hair in a mature woman with female pattern alopecia. In addition, the problem of new hair growth will be magnified due to the color difference between the natural gray color and dark brown dyed color. Lightening the hair by two shades followed by a toner could give the patient dark blonde hair with excellent coverage of the gray hair, minimal scalp contrast, and decreased color difference between dyed hair and new growth.

Melanin pigment is very resistant to reducing agents but is easily degraded by oxidizing agents. Therefore, hair bleaching can be considered an oxidative alkaline treatment. Hydrogen peroxide is the major oxidizer in the process, causing oxygen to be released from the hair keratin. The amount of hair lightening obtained is related to the amount of oxygen released, a quantity expressed as ''volumes'' by the cosmetics industry. The volume of a hydrogen peroxide solution is the number of liters of oxygen released by a liter of the bleaching solution. For example, a 20 volume solution contains 6% hydrogen peroxide and a 30 volume solution contains 9% hydrogen peroxide.[28] Home bleaching products generally contain 6% hydrogen peroxide, and professional bleaching products may contain up to 9% hydrogen peroxide. The hydrogen peroxide solution is mixed with an alkaline ammonia solution immediately prior to application to speed the reaction. The pH of the final solution is between 9 and 11. The amount of alkaline material added must be limited, however, because excess keratin damage and scalp irritation may result.

The hair should not be washed prior to bleaching because scalp sebum provides protection from the harsh chemicals. The hair should be shampooed following the bleaching process to remove excess solution. This is best accomplished with an acid pH shampoo with minimal detergent action. The shampooing should be done gently to avoid scalp irritation.

The ease with which pigment bleaching occurs differs throughout the length of the hair shaft, with the hair near the scalp bleaching more easily than the distal shaft. This is thought to be due to the acceleration of the bleaching process by body heat radiating from the scalp. Proper bleaching requires that the solution be applied at the ends first and then the roots to ensure an even color throughout the hair shaft.

As mentioned previously, bleaching is extremely damaging to the hair shaft. This damage results in a 2% to 3% weight loss from the individual shaft, which causes weakening and promotes increased hair breakage. Small amounts of the amino acids tyrosine, threonine, and methionine are degraded. It is estimated that 15% to 25% of the hair disulfide bonds are degraded during moderate bleaching with up to 45% of the cystine bonds broken during severe bleaching.[29] This weakening of the hair shaft is more pronounced in wet hair; thus the hair should be handled minimally until dry.[30] Bleached hair is also more porous and tends to absorb increased water, making it more susceptible to humidity changes and prolonging the drying time. Decreased overlapping of the cuticular scales also leads to increased hair friction, which allows the hair to tangle more readily. Finally, increased porosity allows better penetration of permanent dyeing and waving preparations, so bleached hair will dye to a darker shade than natural hair and will curl more readily than untreated hair. All further chemical processing requires weaker solutions to obtain desirable results.

HAIR DYE REMOVAL

Method of hair dye removal depends upon the type of coloring process used. As discussed previously, temporary hair dyes are removed with one shampooing, while semipermanent hair dyes are removed in four to six shampooings. The amount of time for a dye to wash out is equal to the time required for the dye to color the hair shaft. For example, if it takes 20 minutes for a semipermanent dye to penetrate from the cuticle to the cortex, then it will also take 20 minutes for the dye to exit the hair shaft. Thus, if the hair is shampooed for 5 minutes, the dye will be removed in 4 shampooings for a total elapsed time of 20 minutes.

Permanent hair dye removal is a much different matter, however. It is actually easier to bleach hair than to remove these unnatural pigments. Permanent dyes can be removed with reducing agents or oxidants, such as high strength peroxide. Reducing agents, such as sodium hydrosulfite or sodium formaldehyde sulfoxylate, are dissolved in water to form a 2% to 5% solution followed by an alkaline rinse.[26] Special salon removal products are available (Clairol, Metalux). Permanent dye removal is extremely damaging to the hair and leaves it largely cosmetically unacceptable. If at all possible, the hair should be appropriately trimmed and possibly toned with other dyestuffs.

Metallic dyes should not be removed with peroxide, as the hair can become darkened or discolored. Sulfonated castor oil with the addition of salicylic acid or chelating agents may be effective.[31]

ADVERSE REACTIONS

Hair coloring is generally regarded as a safe procedure with low risk of mutagenicity and oncogenicity.[32-34] A prospective study of permament hair dye use found no increase in hematopoietic cancers.[35] Furthermore, the skin penetration is minimal and limited to 0.02% to 0.2% of the quantity of dye applied to the head.[36] Gradual and temporary hair dyes represent minimal risk for irritant and allergic contact dermatitis. However, semipermanent dyes can cause contact allergic contact dermatitis since they may contain "para" dyes (diamines, aminophenols, and phenols) or dyes that cross-react with the "para" dyes. *p*-Phenylenediamine (PPD) is the sensitizer in permanent hair dyeing,[37] with an estimated incidence of allergic contact dermatitis of 1 in every 50,000 applications.[38] However, patch testing may overestimate the incidence of reactions to PPD-containing hair dyes. This is due to the limited contact time during dyeing and the less than 3% concentration of PPD. Furthermore, PPD combines with oxidizing agents in hair dyes and quickly react to create a new chemical moiety.[39]

Permanent and semipermanent hair dyes must be tested on the patient prior to use, preferably using a small swatch of hair and skin hidden on the posterior neck. The testing is necessary to avoid the possibility of an overwhelming allergic contact dermatitis to the dyestuff. The hair dye should be tested, in addition to the following substances:[40]

p-Phenylenediamine, 1% in petrolatum
p-Toluylenediamine, 1% in petrolatum
o-Nitroparaphenylenediamine, 1% in petrolatum
m-Toluylenediamine, 1% in petrolatum
    Resorcinol, 2% in petrolatum
m-Aminophenol, 2% in petrolatum
    Hydroquinone, 1% in petrolatum

In addition, the dye should be tested on the hair to prevent undesirable color results. Virgin, untreated hair does not accept the dyestuff as readily as previously treated hair. Untreated hair with an intact cuticle may even be so resistant to coloring as to require an alkaline agent to loosen the cuticle or increase porosity prior to dyeing. This type of hair is termed "dye resistant." Previously treated hair will absorb or "grab" the color readily, which can result in overdyeing if the beautician is careless. Hair previously treated with metallic dyes or conditioners may not respond as expected. A color test area, known as a "strand test," allows the beautician to determine if the appropriate color has been applied to the hair for the appropriate amount of time.

Once the hair has been semipermanently or permanently dyed, it is no longer allergenic.[41] However, all excess dye must be removed with a final acidic shampoo, known as a "neutralizing rinse". Sometimes patients with a tremendous *p*-phenylenediamine allergy, who have previously used home-dyeing preparations, develop swelling and bullae formation immediately upon application of the dye product. In their haste to come to the dermatologist's office, they may neglect to remove all of the excess dye. A chloride peroxide rinse is recommended to neutralize the excess dye, which is formulated as follows:[42]

Sodium chloride, 150 g
Hydrogen peroxide (20 volume), 50 ml
Water, q.s. 1,000 ml

This preparation can be mixed by the pharmacist and applied to the patient's hair to remove any remaining allergen. It is not necessary for the patient to cut his or her hair, but further hair dyeing should be avoided.

Hair bleaching has been reported to cause hair breakage, skin irritation, allergic sensitization, and scarring alopecia.[43] Cutaneous and respiratory allergic reactions have been reported to ammonium persulfate, mentioned previously as a booster in the hair bleaching process. Reported reactions include allergic contact dermatitis, irritant contact dermatitis, localized edema, generalized urticaria, rhinitis, asthma, and syncope.[44,45] Some of the reactions are thought to be truly allergic, while others appear to be due to nonimmunologic histamine release.[46] Patch testing may be performed with a 2% to 5% aqueous solution of ammonium persulfate.[27]

REFERENCES

1. Corbett JF: Hair coloring. Clin Dermatol 6:93, 1988
2. Spoor HJ: Permanent hair colorants: oxidation dyes 1. Chemical technology. Cutis 19:424, 1977
3. Corbett JF: Changing the color of hair. p. 160. In Frost P, Horwitz SN (eds): Principles of Cosmetics for the Dermatologist. CV Mosby Company, St. Louis, 1982
4. Menkart J, Wolfram LJ, Mao I: Caucasian hair, negro hair, and wool; similarities and differences. J Soc Cosmet Chem 17:769, 1966
5. Arakindakshan MI, Persad S, Haberman HF, Kurian CJ: A comparative study of the physical and chemical properties of melanins isolated from human black and red hair. J Invest Dermatol 80:202, 1983
6. Brown KC, Prota G: Melanins: hair dyes for the future. Cosmet Toilet 109:59, 1994
7. Cesarini JP: Hair melanin and hair colour. p. 166. In Orfanos CE, Happle R (eds): Hair and Hair Diseases. In Springer-Verlag, Berlin, 1990
8. Vardy DA, Marcus B, Gilead L, Klapholz L et al: A look at gray hair. J Geriatric Dermatol 1:22, 1993

9. Pohl S: The chemistry of hair dyes. Cosmet Toilet 103:57, 1988

10. Spoor HJ: Part II: metals. Cutis 19:37, 1977

11. O'Donoghue MN: Hair cosmetics. Dermatol Clin 5:619, 1987

12. Casperson S: Men's hair coloring. Comet Toilet 109:83, 1994

13. Spoor HJ: Hair dyes: Temporary colorings. Cutis 18:341, 1976

14. Wilkinson JB, Moore RJ: Harry's Cosmeticology. 7th Ed. Chemical Publishing, New York, 1982

15. Corbett JF: Hair dyes. p. 475. In The Chemistry of Synthetic Dyes. Vol. 5. Academic Press, Inc, New York, 1971

16. Spoor HJ: Semi-permanent hair color. Cutis 18:506, 1976

17. Corbett JF: Hair coloring processes. Cosmet Toilet 106:53, 1991

18. Robbin CR: Chemical and Physical Behavior of Human Hair. 2nd Ed. Springer-Verlag, New York, 1988

19. Zviak C: Hair coloring, nonoxidation coloring. p. 235. In Zviak C (ed): The Science of Hair Care. ed, Marcel Dekker, Inc, New York, 1986

20. Tucker HH: Formulation of oxidation hair dyes. Am J Perfum Cosmet 83:69, 1968

21. Corbett JF, Menkart J: Hair coloring. Cutis 12:190, 1973

22. Zviak C: Oxidation coloring. p. 186. In Zviak C (ed): The Science of Hair Care. Marcel Dekker, Inc, New York, 1986

23. Spoor HJ: Permanent hair colorants: oxidation dyes. Part II. Colorist's art. Cutis 19:578, 1977

24. Corbett JF: Chemistry of hair colorant processes—science as an aid to formulation and development. J Soc Cosmet Chem 35:297, 1984

25. Spoor HJ: Hair coloring—a resume. Cutis 20:311, 1977

26. Zviak C: Hair bleaching. p. 213. In Zviak C (ed): The Science of Hair Care. Marcel Dekker, Inc, New York, 1986

27. Fisher AA, Dooms-Goossens A: Persulfate hair bleach reactions. Arch Dermatol 112:1407, 1976

28. Kass GS: Hair coloring products. p. 841. In deNavarre MG (ed): The Chemistry and Manufacture of Cosmetics. Vol. IV. 2nd Ed. Allured Publishing Corporation, Wheaton, IL, 1988

29. Robbins CR: Amino acid analysis of cosmetically altered hair. J Soc Cosmet Chem 20:555, 1969

30. Robbins CR: Physicial properties and cosmetic behavior of hair. p. 225. In Chemical and Physical Behavior of Human Hair. 2nd Ed. Springer-Verlag, New York, 1988

31. Wall FE: Bleaches, hair colorings, and dye removers. p. 279. In Balsam MS, Gershon SD, Rieger MM et al (eds): Cosmetics Science and Technology. Vol. 2. 2nd Ed. Wiley-Interscience, New York, 1972

32. Marcoux D, Riboulet-Delmas G: Efficacy and safety of hair-coloring agents. Am J Contact Dermatitis 5:123, 1994

33. Morikawa F, Fujii S, Tejima M et al: Safety evaluation of hair cosmetics. p. 641. In Kobori T, Montagna W (eds): Biology and Disease of the Hair. University Park Press, Baltimore, 1975

34. Corbett JF: Hair dye toxicity. p. 529. In Orfanos CE, Montagna W, Stuttgen G (eds): Hair Research. Springer-Verlag, New York, 1981

35. Grodstein F, Hennekens CH, Colditz GA (eds): A prospective study of permanent hair dye use and hematopoietic cancer. J Natl Cancer Inst 86:1466, 1994

36. Kalopissis G: Toxicology and hair dyes. p. 287. In Zviak C (ed): The Science of Hair Care. Marcel Dekker, Inc, New York, 1986
37. Goldberg BJ, Herman FF, Hirata I: Systemic anaphylaxis due to an oxidation product of *p*-Phenylenediamine in a hair dye. Ann Allergy 58:205, 1987
38. Rostenberg A, Kass GS: Hair Coloring. AMA Committee of Cutaneous Health and Cosmetics, 1969
39. Corbett JF: *p*-Benzoquinonediimine—a vital intermediate in oxidative hair dyeing. J Soc Cosmetic Chem 20:253, 1969
40. DeGroot AC, Weyland JW, Nater JP: Unwanted Effects of Cosmetics and Drugs Used in Dermatology. Elsevier, Amsterdam, 1994
41. Reiss F, Fisher AA: Is hair dyed with para-phenylenediamine allergenic? Arch Dermatol 109:221, 1974
42. Calnan C: Adverse reactions to hair products. In Zviak C (ed): The Science of Hair Care. Marcel Dekker, Inc, New York, 1986
43. Bergfeld WF: In Orfanos CE, Montagna E, Stuttgen G (eds): Hair Research. Berlin, Springer-Verlag, 1981
44. Brubaker MM: Urticarial reaction to ammonium persulfate. Arch Dermatol 106: 413, 1972
45. Blainey AD, Ollier S, Cundell D et al: Occupational asthma in a hairdressing salon. Thorax 41:42, 1986
46. Calnan CD, Shuster S: Reactions to ammonium persulfate. Arch Dermatol 88:812, 1963

17

Hair Permanent Waving Agents

The idea of making straight hair permanently curly is appealling to both men and women who want to achieve fashionable hair styles. The entire chemical process is based on the 16% cystine incorporated into disulfide linkages between polypeptide chains in the hair keratin filament. These disulfide linkages are responsible for hair elasticity and can be reformed to change the configuration of the hair shaft. In short, this is the technique of modern permanent hair waving.

HISTORY

Methods of waving and curling straight hair have been practiced since ancient Egyptian times when water and mud were applied to hair wound on sticks and allowed to dry in the sun. The ancient Greeks refined the technique through the use of hot irons that were wrapped with hair. The use of hot irons to curl hair was rediscovered by Marcel in 1872 and is still a popular technique among Black men and women. The first hair waving solution was developed by Nessler in 1906 and consisted of borax paste, which produced longer lasting waves but was very damaging to the hair. This method utilized external heat in the form of either electrically heated hollow iron tubes or, later, a chemical heating pad that was attached to the curling rods with a clamp. Temperatures reached about 115°C, and heating continued for 10 to 15 minutes.[1]

In the 1930s, the first cold wave was introduced, which virtually replaced the heat methods of curling. The solution was based on ammonium thioglycolate containing free ammonia and a controlled pH. The original U.S. patent was granted to E. McDonough on June 16, 1941. Interestingly, this cold wave solution, with slight variations, is still popular today for both salon and home use. It is estimated that more than 65 million permanent waves are sold in salons and 45 million home waves are performed on an annual basis in the United States.[2]

169

CHEMISTRY

Permanent waving utilizes three processes: chemical softening, rearranging, and fixing.[3] The basic chemistry involves the reduction of the disulfide hair shaft bonds with mercaptans.[4] The process can be chemically characterized as follows:[5]

1. Penetration of the thiol compound into the hair shaft
2. Cleavage of the hair keratin disulfide bond (kSSk) to produce a cysteine residue (kSH) and the mixed disulfide of the thiol compound with the hair keratin (kSSR)

$$kSSk + RSH \rightleftharpoons kSH + kSSR$$

3. Reaction with another thiol molecule to produce a second cysteine residue and the symmetrical disulfide of the thiol waving agent (RSSR)

$$kSSR + RSH \rightleftharpoons kSH + RSSR$$

4. Rearrangement of the hair protein structure to relieve internal stress determined by curler size and hair wrapping tension
5. Application of an oxidizing agent to reform the disulfide cross-links

$$kSH + HSk \xrightarrow{\text{oxidizing agent}} kSSk + water$$

APPLICATION TECHNIQUE

Cold permanent waves can be administered at home or in a salon, but involve the same application technique.[6] It usually takes about 90 minutes to complete the entire process, depending on the length of the hair.

The standard procedure involves initial shampooing of the hair to remove dirt and sebum. This wetting process is the first step in preparing the hair for chemical treatment, since the water enters the hair's hydrogen bonds and allows increased flexibility. The hair is then sectioned into 30 to 50 areas, depending on the length and thickness of the hair, and wound on mandrels or rods. The size of the rod determines the diameter of the curl, with smaller rods producing tighter curls. A sufficient amount of tension must be applied to the hair as it is wound around the rod to provide the stress required to encourage bond breaking. If too much tension is applied, the hair can be stretched beyond its elastic range, transforming it into a brittle substance that will easily fracture. Tissue paper squares about 5 × 5 cm, known as "end papers," are applied to the distal hair shafts to prevent irregular wrapping of the ends around the rod. Failure to use end papers can result in a frizzy appearance of the distal hair shaft.

Next, the waving lotion is applied and left in contact with the hair for 5 to 20 minutes, depending on the condition of the hair. The reducing action of the waving lotion is said to "soften" the hair and contains a disulfide bond-breaking agent, such as ammonium or calcium thioglycolate, and an antioxidant, such as sodium hydrosulfite, to prevent the lotion from reacting with air before it reaches the hair. Sequestering agents, such as tetrasodium EDTA, are added to prevent trace metals such as iron in tap water from reacting with the thioglycolate lotion. Other ingredients include pH adjusters, conditioners, and surfactants to remove the remaining sebum from the hair. Coarse hair requires a longer processing time than fine hair, and undyed hair requires a longer processing time than permanently dyed or bleached hair. A "test curl" is then checked to determine if the desired amount of curl has been obtained and overprocessing avoided.

The hair disulfide bonds are subsequently reformed with the hair in the new curled conformation around the perming rods. This process is known as neutralization, fixation, or "hardening." The neutralization procedure, chemically characterized as an oxidation step, should involve two steps. First, two-thirds of the neutralizer should thoroughly saturate the hair with the rods in place and be allowed to set for 5 minutes. The rods are then removed and the remaining one-third of the neutralizer applied for an additional 5 minutes. The hair is then carefully rinsed. Patients who complain of an undesirable odor following permanent waving, especially after shampooing, have undergone incomplete neutralization. Repeating the neutralization process as outlined above will reduce the excessive odor.[7]

The newly curled hair is now ready for drying and styling. Most companies recommend avoiding shampooing or manipulating the hair for 1 to 2 days following the cold wave procedure to ensure long-lasting curls.

A permanent wave is designed to last 3 to 4 months. Curl relaxation occurs with time as the hair returns to its original conformation. Hairdressers generally will therefore select a curl tighter than the patient desires with this fact in mind. Most of the curl relaxation occurs within the first 2 weeks after processing, a fact that is reassuring to the patient who has had an undesirable result. Curl relaxation can be increased slightly by frequent shampooing beginning immediately following the permanenting procedure. Some strong detergent shampoos, such as those recommended for seborrheic dermatitis, will cause curl relaxation more rapidly than conditioning shampoos. New hair growth also decreases the curled appearance of the hair. Patients with rapidly growing hair need to repeat the permanent waving procedure more frequently. Increased hair growth during pregnancy could account for the fact that some hairdressers note that permanent waves do not "take" in pregnant women. Hair at the nape of the neck also has a decreased "take."

FACTORS INFLUENCING COLD WAVING

Several factors determine the success or failure of a cold waving procedure. Most of the suboptimal results that cause patients to seek dermatologic help result from failure to consider the following key points while performing the procedure:[8]

1. The hair must not be wound with excessive tension around the rods, or increased breakage may occur.[9]
2. Smaller rods will produce smaller curls, which are more damaging to the hair shaft.
3. The hair must fit around the rod at least once for complete curl formation in patients with short hair.
4. A stronger waving lotion will not produce a tighter curl. The curl diameter is determined by the rod diameter.
5. Weak waving lotions with shorter processing times should be used for damaged hair.
6. It may be necessary to use different strengths of waving lotions on new proximal growth and previously waved distal growth, especially in patients with bleached hair.
7. A test curl should be performed to avoid over-processing the hair. Long processing times can excessively damage hair, increasing breakage.
8. Discoloration of the hair may occur in patients who have used *p*-phenylene-diamine-based permanent dyes that have been incompletely oxidized.

METHODS OF ASSESSING PERMANENT WAVE EFFECTIVENESS

There are several methods used by manufacturers of cold waving products to determine wave efficiency and degree of hair shaft damage. These are the deficiency in tightness value, the curl length, and the 20% index.[8]

The deficiency in tightness (DIT) value is determined as follows:

$$\text{DIT} = \frac{\text{diameter of curl (mm)} - \text{diameter of rod (mm)}}{\text{diameter of rod (mm)}} \times 100$$

The higher the DIT value, the greater the effectiveness of the curling solution. In other words, weak cold wave solutions have low DIT values.

The curl length is evaluated by suspending a fresh curl and observing the spring of the formed coil. The degree of laxity is indicative of the efficiency of the wave and also of the degree of hair shaft damage. Thus, longer curls are indicative of greater hair shaft damage.

The 20% index is determined by stretching freshly permed hair with a uniformly increasing load. The ratio of the load required after perming to the load required prior to perming to stretch a wet strand of 12 hairs to 20% of their original length is known as the 20% index. The higher the index, the lower the reduction in hair strength due to the cold wave procedure.

Cold wave chemists use these three criteria to determine not only the success of the permanent wave procedure but also the degree of hair shaft damage. Factors affecting the efficacy of a permanent waving product are processing time, processing temperature, concentration of reducing agent, ratio of lotion to hair quantities, penetration of the lotion, pH, and the nature and condition of the untreated hair.[10] A marketable permanent wave solution must produce the best curl with the least amount of hair damage.[11]

HAIR ALTERATIONS FOLLOWING PERMANENT WAVING

Following the permanent waving process, the hair has been irreversibly altered. These changes contribute to some of the dermatologic problems noted in chemically waved hair. First, the dry waved hair shaft is shorter than the original hair shaft.[12] This may account for the perception by many patients that their hair was cut too short following a perming procedure. Second, the chemically treated hair shaft is 17% weaker and thus less able to withstand the trauma of combing and brushing.[13] Patients comment that their hair is falling following permanent waving when in actuality the hair shaft is fracturing more readily. Third, the hair demonstrates more frictional resistance following permanent waving.[14] This means that it is more difficult to comb. Lastly, the hair demonstrates an increased swelling capacity, which is evidence of cortical damage.[15] This swelling accounts for the increased penetration of other chemicals applied to the hair, such as dyes, yielding unexpected results.

TYPES OF PERMANENT WAVES

Waving lotions consist primarily of a reducing agent in an aqueous solution with an adjusted pH.[16] Table 17-1 summarizes waving lotion ingredients and their functions.[1] The most popular reducing agents are the thioglycolates, glycerol thioglycolates, and sulfites. On the basis of waving lotion type, permanent waves can be classified into the following groups:[4,17]

Alkaline Permanents
Buffered alkaline permanents
Exothermic permanents
Self-regulated permanents
Acid permanents
Sulfite permanents

Table 17-1. Permanent Waving Lotion Ingredients

Ingredient	Chemical Examples	Function
Reducing agent	Thioglycolates, sulfites	Break disulfide bonds
Alkaline agent	Ammonium hydroxide, triethanolamine	Adjust pH
Chelating agent	Tretrasodium EDTA	Remove trace metals
Wetting agent	Fatty alcohols	Improve hair saturation with waving lotion
Conditioner	Proteins, humectants, quaternium compounds	Protect hair during waving process
Opacifier	Polyacrylates, polystyrene latex	Opacify waving lotion

(Adapted from Lee et al.,[1] with permission)

Table 17-2 summarizes the differences between each of the permanent wave types.

Alkaline Permanents

Alkaline permanents utilize ammonium thioglycolate or ethanolamine thioglycolate as the reducing agent in the waving lotion. The pH is adjusted to between 9 and 10 since the thioglycolates are not as effective at a lower pH. These products process extremely rapidly and produce a tight, long-lasting curl; however, they are harsh on the hair. The alkalinity allows hair shaft swelling, which can cause problems in individuals with color-treated hair, especially bleached hair. For this reason, the concentration of the thioglycolate waving lotion is

Table 17-2. Permanent Wave Types

Type	Main Ingredient	Effect on Hair	Patient Suitability
Acid cold wave	Thioglycolic acid, uses body heat for processing	pH = 7–8.5 Produces soft, loose curl	Excellent for dyed or bleached hair
Acid heat-activated	Thioglycolic acid, uses hair dryer for processing	pH = 7–8.5 Produces soft, loose curl	Excellent for dyed or bleached hair
Self-regulated	Thioglycolic acid and dithioglycolic acid	Same as acid permanent wave	Will not overprocess
Exothermic	Hydrogen peroxide added to thioglycolic acid to produce heat as by-product	Same as acid permanent wave	May be more comfortable for mature patient, must be properly mixed
Alkaline	Ammonium thioglycolate	pH = 9–10 Produces tighter, longer-lasting curl	Harsh on dyed hair, may leave hair frizzy
Sulfite	Sodium bisulfite	pH = 6–8 Produces loose, short-lived curl	Safely used at home, less harsh on hair

adjusted from the 7% used on natural hair to 1% used on heavily bleached hair.

Buffered Alkaline Permanents

To decrease the hair swelling encountered due to the high pH of alkaline permanent waves, a buffering agent such as ammonium bicarbonate is employed. These products, known as *buffered alkaline permanents,* result in a tight curl at a pH of 7 to 8.5. Their advantage is the production of a tight, long-lasting curl with less hair damage.

Exothermic Permanents

Exothermic permanent waves produce heat as a by-product to increase client comfort, as some individuals may feel chilled during the permanent waving process. The heat is produced when an oxidizing agent, such as hydrogen peroxide, is mixed with the thioglycolate-based waving lotion immediately prior to scalp application. The reaction of the thioglycolate with the peroxide produces dithiodiglycolate (the disulfide of thioglycolate), which limits the extent to which the permanent wave can process. Irreversible hair damage will result if the waving lotion is not mixed with the oxidizing agent before application. For this reason, exothermic permanent waves are mainly available for professional use only.

Self-Regulated Permanents

Self-regulated permanent waves are designed to limit the amount of hair disulfide bond breakage so that irreversible hair damage is prevented. Overprocessing, due to leaving the permanent wave solution on the hair longer than recommended, causes extensive hair breakage, acting like a depilatory. It is not unusual for a busy beautician to have three to four permanent waves processing at the same time. Self-regulated permanent waves are designed to form a chemical equilibrium such that the disulfide bond breakage is stopped. This is accomplished by adding dithioglycolic acid to the thioglycolate-based waving lotion. This is the same chemical reaction discussed for exothermic permanent waves.

Acid Permanents

Acid permanent waves occur in an acidic environment with a pH of 6.5 to 7. They are based on thioglycolate esters such as glycerol monothioglycolate. The lower pH is an advantage since less hair shaft swelling occurs than at higher pH levels; thus hair damage is minimized. These products result in a looser, shorter lasting curl, but leave the hair soft. They are ideal for bleached or color-treated hair. It is possible to achieve a tighter curl if the permanent wave is processed with added heat under a hair dryer, but more hair shaft damage results.

The glycerol monothioglycolate in this type of permanent wave can cause allergic contact dermatitis in both beauticians and clients.[18] Interestingly, the hair may continue to be allergenic even after all products have been thoroughly rinsed from the hair.

Sulfite Permanents

Sulfite permanent waves are mainly marketed for home use and have not found popularity among salons in the United States. These products differ in that the reducing agent is a sulfite or bisulfite instead of a mercaptan. This accounts for their reduced odor, which is their primary advantage. They require a long processing time at a pH of 6 to 8 and result in loose curls. A conditioning agent must be added to the formulation, as the sulfite permanent waves can leave the hair feeling harsh.

Home Permanents

Home permanents are designed for the nonprofessional and are of two types: ammonium thioglycolate permanents and sulfite permanents. The ammonium thioglycolate permanents have the same characteristics as the salon solutions except that they are one-third the strength. This is to prevent excessive hair damage by the novice. Thus, home thioglycolate permanents produce looser curls that are not as long lasting as salon permanents.

As mentioned previously, sulfite permanents are manufactured only for home use and have no professional counterpart. The major advantages of this type of permanent wave is decreased odor. The head is covered with a plastic cap to use body heat for processing, and an alkaline rinse is applied as a neutralizer. The mild curls produced are not long lasting.

NEUTRALIZERS

Neutralizers function to reform the broken disulfide bonds and restore the hair to its original condition. Two methods are available: self-neutralization and chemical neutralization. Both methods rely on oxidation. Self-neutralization allows air to oxidize the permanent wave, but this requires 6 to 24 hours. During this time, the hair must be left on the permanent wave rods. This method is rarely used. Chemical neutralization is more popular, due to its speed, and relies upon the use of an oxidizing agent. The oxidizing agent is usually 2% hydrogen peroxide adjusted to an acidic pH. Bromates may also be used, but are more

Table 17-3. Function of Neutralizer Ingredients

Ingredient	Chemical Example	Function
Oxidizing agent	Hydrogen peroxide, sodium bromate	Reform broken disulfide bonds
Acid buffer	Citric acid, acetic acid, lactic acid	Maintain acidic pH
Stabilizer	Sodium stannate	Prevent hydrogen peroxide breakdown
Wetting agent	Fatty alcohols	Improve hair saturation
Conditioner	Proteins, humectants, quaternium compounds	Improve hair feel
Opacifier	Polyacrylates, polystyrene latex	Make neutralizer opaque

(Adapted from Lee et al.,[1] with permission.)

expensive. The ingredients found in a chemical neutralizer and their functions are summarized in Table 17-3.[1]

ADVERSE REACTIONS

The use of permanent wave solutions is considered safe; however, cases of both irritant and allergic contact dermatitis to thioglycolate-containing waving lotions have been reported.[19] Irritant contact dermatitis is more common and can be avoided by minimizing skin contact with the solution.[20] This is especially important in patients using topical tretinoin, who seem to experience skin irritation more readily with permanent waving. Prior to application of the waving lotion, a layer of petroleum jelly should be applied to the margins of the scalp and covered with a band of absorbent cotton. This provides a protective covering for the nonhair-bearing skin that might come in contact with any waving lotion running over the scalp. Patients with a sensitive scalp can even apply petroleum jelly to the scalp as protection. The petroleum jelly contacts the proximal hair shaft, however, preventing curling in this region.

Allergic contact dermatitis can occur immediately after permanent waving or persist as a result of an allergen in the hair of patients who undergo permanent waving procedures involving glyceryl monothioglycolate (GMTG).[18,21] The North American Contact Dermatitis Group found this chemical to be the fifth most common cause of dermatitis.[22] The substance should be patch tested at a 1% concentration in petrolatum.[23]

REFERENCES

1. Lee AE, Bozza JB, Huff S, de la Mettrie R: Permanent waves: an overview. Cosmet Toilet 103:37, 1988
2. Wickett RR: Disulfide bond reduction in permanent waving. Cosmet Toilet 106: 37, 1991

3. Wickett RR: Permanent waving and straightening of hair. Cutis 39:496, 1987
4. Zviak C: Permanent waving and hair straightening. p. 183. In Zviak C (ed): The Science of Hair Care. Marcel Dekker, New York, 1986
5. Cannell DW: Permanent waving and hair straightening. Clin Dermatol 6:71, 1988
6. Draelos ZK: Hair cosmetics. Dermatol Clin 9:19, 1991
7. Brunner MJ: Medical aspects of home cold waving. Arch Dermatol 65:316, 1952
8. Heilingotter R: Permanent waving of hair. p. 1167. In de Navarre MG (ed): The Chemistry and Manufacture of Cosmetics. Allured Publishing Co, Wheaton, IL, 1988
9. Wortman FJ, Souren I: Extensional properties of human hair and permanent waving. J Soc Cosmet Chem 38:125, 1987
10. Shipp JJ: Hair-care products. p. 80. In Chemistry and Technology of the Cosmetics and Toiletries Industry. Blackie Academic & Professional, London, 1992
11. Szadurski JS, Erlemann G: The hair loop test—a new method of evaluating perm lotions. Cosmet Toilet 99:41, 1984
12. Garcia ML, Nadgorny EM, Wolfram LJ: Letter to the editor. J Soc Cosmet Chem 41:149, 1990
13. Feughelman M: A note on the permanent setting of human hair. J Soc Cosmet Chem 41:209, 1990
14. Robbins CR: Chemical and Physical Behavior of Human Hair. Springler-Verlag, New York, 1988
15. Shansky A: The osmotic behavior of hair during the permanent waving process as explained by swelling measurements. J Soc Cosmet Chem 14:427, 1963
16. Ishihara M: The composition of hair preparations and their skin hazards. p. 603. In Koboir T, Montagna W (eds): Biology and Disease of the Hair. University Park Press, Baltimore, 1975
17. Gershon SD, Goldberg MA, Rieger MM. Permanent waving. p. 167. In Balsam MS, Sagarin E (eds): Cosmetics Science and Technology. Vol. 2. 2nd Ed. Wiley-Interscience, New York, 1972
18. Morrison LH, Storrs FJ: Persistence of an allergen in hair after glyceryl monothioglycolate–containing permanent wave solutions. J Am Acad Dermatol 19:52, 1988
19. Lehman AJ: Health aspects of common chemicals used in hair-waving preparations. JAMA 141:842, 1949
20. Fisher AA: Management of hairdressers sensitized to hair dyes or permanent wave solutions. Cutis 43:316, 1989
21. Storrs FJ: Permanent wave contact dermatitis: contact allergy to glyceryl monothioglycolate. J Am Acad Dermatol 11:74, 1984
22. Adams RM, Maibach HI: A five-year study of cosmetic reactions. J Am Acad Dermatol 13:1062, 1985
23. White IR, Rycroft RJG, Anderson KE et al: The patch test dilution of glyceryl thioglycolate. Contact Dermatitis 23:198, 1990

18

Cosmetic Hair Techniques

Dermatologist may encounter patients in their practice for whom cosmetic advice regarding the use of wigs is required. Furthermore, the patient may request information on maximizing the cosmetic appearance of existing hair. This chapter presents cosmetic techniques appropriate for patients with absent or damaged hair.

HAIR PIECES

The use of hair pieces can restore a positive self-image to those patients who have temporary or permanent hair loss. There are both natural human hair and synthetic fiber types available. The custom-made natural human hair products are more expensive ($100 to $2,000) and have a short life (2 to 3 years) due to hair breakage. Synthetic hair products are less expensive ($10 to $100) and have a longer life (3 to 5 years), but are limited in their styling capabilities. Synthetic fibers are designed to have a permanent curl and require less maintenance than natural fibers.

A hair piece is formed by attaching individual fibers to a meshwork designed to fit a specific scalp location. Two methods of attaching hair fibers to the mesh are used: hand tied and machine wefted. Hand-tied hair pieces are more expensive because the fibers are individually knotted to the mesh. Machine-wefted wigs are made by sewing the fibers onto strips of material and then attaching wefts to the mesh.

Synthetic and natural fiber hair pieces are cleaned in much the same manner as a head of hair. The hair piece is turned inside out and a drop of mild shampoo placed in the center of the hair and gently agitated under a stream of warm water. Once the shampoo is completely removed, a drop of instant conditioner is placed in the wig and again rinsed. The hair piece is allowed to air dry while inside out by attaching it with a clothespin to an indoor clothesline. Once dry, the hair piece may be styled with a specially designed wig brush.

History

The hair piece originated in Egypt in 3000 BC; many of these still survive today. Hair pieces were popular among both ruling men and women and were fashioned from human and vegetable fibers coated with beeswax. Blond wigs were popularized by the Romans in the 1st century BC and made of hair taken from German captives. Eventually, however, blonde wigs became the trademark of Roman prostitutes and were outlawed by the Christian Church. By 1580 AD, wigs were again fashionable due to the influences of the English queens who developed female pattern hair loss. Even Mary, Queen of Scots, wore a wig, a fact unknown by her followers until she was beheaded. The popularity of wigs spread to France by the 18th century such that the French court of Versailles employed 40 resident wigmakers. Today, wigs remain part of the formal attire of some judges.[1]

Hair Piece Types

Hair pieces come in seven basic types, depending on the scalp area to be covered (Fig. 18-1):

1. Wigs: constructed on a flexible cap-shaped mesh designed to cover the entire head
2. Falls: long locks of hair attached to a firm contoured mesh designed to rest on the scalp vertex (Fig. 18-1A)
3. Cascades: curled locks or buns attached to a firm oblong contoured base designed to rest on the posterior scalp (Fig. 18-1B)
4. Toupees: custom-fit hair piece on a silk base to cover the top of the head (Fig. 18-1C)
5. Demiwigs: flexible cap-shaped mesh designed to cover the entire scalp except the front hairline (Fig. 18-1D)
6. Wiglets: localized hair pieces designed to create bangs or add additional hair on the top of the head (Fig. 18-1E)
7. Switches: long strands of hair in the form of braids or ponytails secured together at one end (Fig. 18-1F)

Hair Piece Selection

Patients with severe alopecia areata, alopecia totalis, alopecia universalis, or chemotherapy-induced anagen effluvium require complete wigs. It is recommended that patients select a wig prior to complete hair loss, thus allowing them to adjust emotionally and to aid in selecting a wig that mimics the natural hair color and style. If this is not possible, a picture of the patient prior to hair loss is helpful to the wig artist.

Most patients, however, only require supplementation of their natural hair

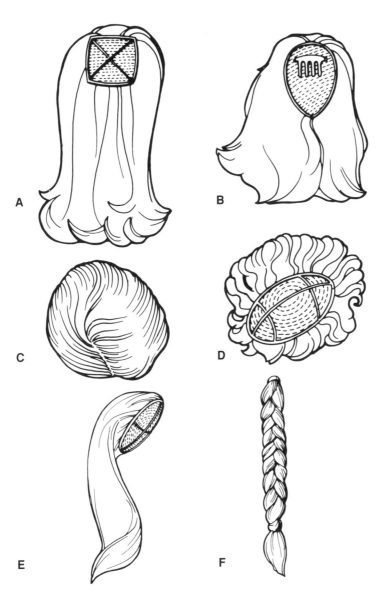

FIG. 18-1. Types of artificial hair pieces. (**A**) Fall. (**B**) Cascade. (**C**) Toupee. (**D**) Demiwig. (**E**) Wiglet. (**F**) Switch.

by a hair piece selected to cover areas of thinning or loss. For example, female pattern alopecia can be covered with a demiwig known as a "hair thickener." This hair piece is attached to a loosely woven mesh through which the patient pulls her own hair, allowing blending of the hair fibers and also firmly securing the hair piece to the scalp. Women who note that their hair will no longer grow to a length desired may wish to consider a fall to add length or a cascade to add a bun or mass of curls.

Toupees are specifically designed for the balding man and are available in a variety of colors with the appropriate percentage of gray hair to match the patient's state of canities. Natural part line toupees, which add a small insert of sheer plastic in the part line to expose the natural color of the underlying scalp, may create a more natural appearance. Some toupees come uncut, allowing the patient to take the toupee to the barber for styling along with the patient's natural hair. Attachment of toupees to the scalp, however, remains poor, relying on clips or adhesives.

Chemotherapy patients with scalp tenderness or patients undergoing immunotherapy utilizing contact sensitization for alopecia may wish to cover their head with a soft terry cloth turban. A more natural appearance can be achieved by adding a wiglet of bangs.

HAIR ADDITIONS

Another semipermanent approach to thinning or locally absent scalp hair is the use of hair additions. Hair additions are worn continuously for approximately 8 weeks, remaining in place while swimming, bathing, sleeping, and exercising. The technique utilizes synthetic or natural human hair fibers to supplement existing hair where needed. Hair additions may be obtained in full-service beauty salons or at salons specializing in the technique. Augmentation of hair through additions is widely used in the entertainment industry, by Black persons who wish to achieve hair length, by men who wish to camouflage androgenetic alopecia, and by women who desire special effect hair styles.

Fiber Types

The fibers used to supplement existing scalp hair can be made of a synthetic fiber or natural human hair. Synthetic fibers are formed from modacrylic, composed of two polymerized monomers: acrylonitrile and vinylchloride. The polymer is drawn through a multihole metal disk, dried, and stretched. The disk design is such that fibers with an irregular cross section and surface variations are produced to mimic natural human hair more closely. Dye may be added to the polymer either before or after extrusion.

Care is taken to mix fibers of varying diameters and color hues, as not all natural hair shafts are of the same thickness or color. Additionally, the fiber thickness can be varied to simulate hair shaft size more accurately in Black, Caucasian and Oriental hair. The modacrylic can also be permanently heat formed to reproduce the appropriate amount and tightness of curl unique to the hair of different ethnic groups.

Synthetic hair offers some advantages over natural human hair for use in hair additions. First, synthetic fibers are lighter weight than natural human hair, thus exerting less pull on existing scalp hairs. Second, synthetic fibers are less expensive than human hair. Third, synthetic fibers can be melted to bond to existing scalp hair.

Human hair obtained from Indian or Chinese women who grow their hair for sale may also be used for hair additions. Indian hair has a fine diameter and a slight natural wave, whereas Chinese hair is coarser and straighter. Usually, the human hair is lightened and redyed to obtain a range of colors and may also be permanently waved to obtain the desired amount of curl. Coloring and curling of hair used in additions may be performed both before and after the added hair is attached to the scalp, using standard salon products.

Human hair does not require the color and fiber diameter mixing of synthetic hair fibers, as natural variations are already present. Thus, the main advantage of human hair additions is their ability to blend with existing scalp hair. Disadvantages include the weight of the natural fibers and the cost, which increases with increasing lengths of hair.

Methods of Hair Attachment

Hair additions use existing scalp hair to anchor the synthetic or natural human hair fibers. The added fibers may be affixed by braiding, sewing, bonding, or glueing. The attachment method selected depends on the amount of natural hair and on the number or length of fibers to be added.

Braiding On the Scalp

The most popular method of hair addition employs braiding on the scalp, adapted from the Black hair style known as ''corn rows.'' Corn rows are plaited on the scalp in geometric designs with tension applied to the hair shafts exposing scalp between the braids. This is a popular hair style among Black individuals as it allows for organization of tightly kinked hair. Individual hair fibers can be woven into the braids to either thicken their appearance or, more commonly, to add length. Wefted hair, or hair fibers sewn together in a strip, can be sewn with a needle and thread to the corn rows to add large amounts of hair quickly.

Braiding Off the Scalp

Braiding off the scalp employs a standard plaiting technique to which individual hair fibers are added. Fibers are attached by working them securely into the braids and leaving the loose ends for curling and styling. This technique is popular among individuals with short kinky hair who wish to have long straight hair.

Bonding

Bonding employs a hot glue gun to fuse individual synthetic hair fibers to the base of clumps of existing scalp hair. Only a few fibers can be attached at a time due to the weight of the additions. This technique is used by both men and women to thicken the hair. The bonds are intended to remain in place for 8 weeks; however, individuals with excessive sebum production may notice early loosening and loss of the added hair.

Glueing

This hair addition technique combines braiding on the scalp with adhesive attachment. The existing hair is initially braided into concentric arcs on the posterior scalp, known as ''tracks.'' These tracks serve as anchors to which wefted hair is glued. The adhesive employed is a cold latex-based glue that is subject to removal by scalp sebum production.

Care of Hair Additions

Hair additions are worn continually for a period of 8 weeks, or less, at which time they must be removed. Individuals with slowly growing hair may wear the hair style longer, while those with rapidly growing hair will notice that the added hair fibers loosen sooner. The additions are shampooed along with the individual's existing hair using the same cleansing products and cleansing frequency. Many individuals are afraid to wash the additions, as they fear loosening will occur, but good hygiene is important.

Removal of Hair Additions

Hair additions must be removed at 8 weeks to avoid hygiene problems and other complications such as traction alopecia. If the hair and scalp have been properly cleansed, hair additions begin to loosen and look ungroomed at 8 weeks. Removal of braided additions simply requires undoing the braid and removing the added strands of hair, which may be reused in later procedures. Bonded additions are removed by melting the hot glue with the tip of the glue gun and pulling out the individual or wefted hair fibers. Peanut oil is then rubbed through the scalp to facilitate removal of any remaining material. Latex-based glue is removed with a specially designed solvent. Lastly, sewn additions can be removed by cutting the attachment thread.

It is understandable that individuals would like to wear the additions as long as possible, since the cost may vary between $250 and $1,000, depending on the complexity of the hair style, the amount and length of the added hair fibers, the salon time required, and whether synthetic or human hair fibers are used. The average hair addition requires 3 to 5 hours in a salon.

Adverse Effects

Successful use of hair additions requires a hair stylist who is trained in the technique and a client who will put forth the effort to maintain the added hair. Braided and sewn hair additions pose the least problems, as no adhesives are used; however, the added hair fibers put increased pull on existing scalp hair, augmenting the pull already exerted by the tight braids. For these reasons, traction alopecia is a problem for individuals who continually wear hair additions. The traction alopecia is identical to that seen in Black patients who wear tightly pulled hair styles. Initially, only loss of the hair shaft is observed, but, with continued traction, the process can result in loss of the follicular ostia and permanent alopecia. Extensive traction alopecia will eventually preclude the use of hair additions, as no existing scalp hair will be available to anchor added hair.

Glued additions employ adhesives that must be patch tested prior to use. Additionally, the hair stylist must take care not to apply glue carelessly throughout the scalp, which may increase hair breakage since hair combing is impeded by glue. The hot bonding gun must be kept from the scalp to avoid scalp burns, which can result in permanent alopecia if severe.

High standards of hygiene must be maintained to prevent inflammation of the scalp, in the form of seborrheic dermatitis, and infection of the scalp, in the form of bacterial folliculitis. The individual who chooses to have hair additions must realize that the new hair style requires more grooming and upkeep than natural scalp hair.

HAIR INTEGRATION SYSTEMS

Hair integration systems are a useful method of allowing the patient to supplement hair loss only where necessary. These hair pieces are custom made by fashioning a loose net to fit the scalp. Synthetic or natural human hair fibers are tied to the meshwork in the desired location, amount, length, color, and texture. Any hair style can be easily created. The patient puts the integration system over the scalp and pulls the existing hair through the fenestrations in the net. This affixes the hair piece securely to the scalp and also allows a natural appearance. Integration systems can be rather costly, depending upon the amount and length of hair attached. They are extremely versatile for patients with alopecia areata, androgenetic alopecia, scarring, or radiation hair loss.

CREPE HAIR TECHNIQUES

Crepe hair can be used temporarily to camouflage very small, localized areas of scalp hair loss. Its utility is for patients who have recent onset alopecia areata with an excellent prognosis for hair regrowth who need an inexpensive, short-term camouflage. Crepe hair is made from wool and purchased as braids in a variety of colors. The wool strands are pulled from the braid and artistically glued to the scalp with adhesive. The process must be re-done with each shampooing and the adhesive removed with a specially formulated product.

SCALP CAMOUFLAGE TECHNIQUES

Many times it is the contrast between the pale bald scalp and the dark hair that accentuates hair loss. This contrast can be minimized by coloring the scalp to match the hair either temporarily with wax crayons or vegetable dyes or permanently with tatoo pigment.

CAMOUFLAGE TECHNIQUES FOR FEMALE PATTERN HAIR LOSS

Female pattern hair loss affects susceptible women beginning at puberty, with noticeable thinning present by age 40. These women present with hair loss over the entire scalp, but the thinning is most prominent over the frontoparietal areas, with sparing of a thin fringe along the anterior hair line. This pattern was first illustrated by Ludwig.[2] Camouflaging hair loss over the top of the scalp presents a greater challenge than camouflaging hair loss over the sides of the scalp. Cosmetic methods of camouflaging female androgenetic alopecia should be combined with appropriate medical treatments.[3] Only cosmetic approaches for androgenetic alopecia are discussed: hair styling, hair styling products, hair permanent waving, hair coloring agents, hair pieces, and hair additions.

Hair Styling

Careful hair style selection can minimize the appearance of female pattern hair loss. Since the hair thins predominantly on the top of the head, styling techniques should be aimed at adding volume and fullness in this area. The perception of thick hair is based on the distance that the hair stands away from the scalp, but hair styling and styling products can create the illusion of fullness.

Two styling techniques are valuable for creating the illusion of hair volume: curling and back combing. Curled hair does not lay as close to the scalp as straight hair and therefore appears fuller. Temporary curls can be created by heat styling with a blow dryer and a round brush, setting wet hair on rollers, wrapping hair around heated rollers or a curling rod, and forming pin curls close to the scalp. Tighter curls will yield more hair fullness.

Back combing involves combing the hair in the opposite direction from which it would normally lay on the scalp. In most females, the hair pattern is such that the hair on the top of the scalp lays forward. Combing the hair backward from the front of the head to the crown lifts the hair, creating the illusion of volume. The hair will not stay in this unnatural position for long; therefore, styling aids are necessary for the hair to hold this shape.

Teasing is another technique, popular in the 1960s "beehive" hair styles, that was used to create volume. Teasing involves combing the hair from the distal to proximal hair shaft using a fine-toothed comb or teasing brush to create tangles between the hair shafts. These tangles, or "rats" as they are known, allow the hair to stand away from the scalp. Teasing, however, can result in disruption of the hair shaft cuticle and accelerate hair breakage. It is important to avoid hair breakage in areas where the hair is already thinned.

Hair-Styling Products

Hair-styling products can aid in creating the illusion of fullness by allowing the hair to stand away from the scalp. Available styling products include styling gels, sculpturing gels, mousses, and hair sprays. Styling gels, sculpturing gels, and mousses are generally applied to towel-dried hair, while hair sprays are used to improve the hold of a finished hair style. Sculpturing gels provide a stiffer hold than styling gels, which provide a better hold than mousses.

A small amount of gel or mousse is massaged into the base of the hair shafts, and then the hair is dried with a blow dryer while combing the hair away from the scalp. This will increase the ability of the hair to stand away from the scalp, creating the illusion of volume. The styling products lose their hold once the hair is combed or wetted, so reapplication is necessary each time the hair is styled.

Hair spray can be used to keep the final hair style in place. For example, after back combing the hair, it can be liberally sprayed to allow the hair to fall backward instead of forward on the forehead.

Permanent Waving

Permanent waving of the hair increases apparent hair volume, allowing less hair to cover more scalp due to increased curl. Thus, a permanent wave in the frontoparietal area can nicely camouflage female pattern hair loss. However, chemical curling damages the hair shaft by decreasing its strength, degrading its structure, and causing protein loss. This damage can be minimized if the permanent wave is performed with care.

Hair shaft damage can be decreased by wrapping the hair loosely around larger curling rods, resulting in a looser curl that is shorter lasting, but also less likely to fracture the hair shaft. Another method of decreasing hair shaft damage is to shorten the processing time, which decreases the degree of bond breaking. It is also advisable to allow as much time as possible between permanent waving procedures.

Dyeing

Hair color lightening can be an effective camouflage technique for female pattern hair loss by providing better blending with a fair scalp. Of all the hair coloring types available, only permanent hair dyes can achieve color lightening, but permanent hair dyes are also the most damaging to the hair shaft.

Hair Pieces

For the female with androgenetic alopecia, a hair piece serves as a hair thickener, which sits on top of the head, to provide additional hair in the frontoparietal region. The hair is wefted to a mesh through which the patient can pull her own hair to both anchor the hairpiece and provide a natural appearance. This type of hairpiece costs between $30 and $100, depending on whether it is constructed of synthetic or natural human hair.

Hair Additions

Hair additions can nicely camouflage frontoparietal thinning, but must be used cautiously as the weight of the hair addition can result in traction alopecia, only augmenting hair loss. Hair additions can be expensive, depending on the time required to complete the hair style, and are not appropriate for all patients.

CAMOUFLAGE TECHNIQUES FOR MALE PATTERN HAIR LOSS

The same basic camouflage techniques described previously for female pattern hair loss also apply to male pattern hair loss. However, male pattern hair loss does not spare a thin strip of hair at the anterior hairline.[4] This makes re-creation of a natural-appearing anterior hairline more challenging.

COSMETIC TECHNIQUES FOR DAMAGED HAIR

Unfortunately, cosmetically damaged hair cannot be repaired by the body. However, cosmetic remedies may allow the hair to assume an acceptable apperance until new growth occurs. Table 18-1 lists cosmetic suggestions for the some common hair problems.

Table 18-1. Cosmetic Techniques for Damaged Hair

Problem	Possible Cosmetic Cause	Possible Cosmetic Solution
Hair texture		
Fine, limp hair	Overconditioning	Use instant oily hair conditioner
Coarse, unmanageable hair	Underconditioning	Use deep conditioner
Fine, frizzy hair	Underconditioning	Use instant conditioner for dry hair
Hair contour		
Too curly	Underconditioning	Use instant conditioner for dry hair
Too straight	Overconditioning	Use instant conditioner for oily hair
Hair color		
Early graying, less than 15%	Normal process	Vegetable or synthetic semipermanent dye or stain
Yellow-gray hair tones	Gradual loss of eumelanin pigments	Temporary rinse applied followind shampooing
Hair grow out	New undyed hair growth	Touch up dye to roots, not entire hair shaft
Undesirable permanent dye hair color	Dyeing of previously chemically treated hair	Use semipermanent dye to tone undesirable shade until grown out
Green hair	Copper in swimming pool water	Wear swim cap, treat pool water, use special shampoo
Hair thinning		
Total scalp	Numerous medical problems	Wig
Top of scalp	Male or female pattern baldness	Partial hair piece, spot permanent wave; use of styling gels, sculpturing gels, or mousse
Decreased length	Slower growth rate, hair breakage	Remove damaged hair to halt inevitable breakage
Hair breakage		
Trichoptilosis	Loss of cuticle on distal hair shaft	Cut damaged hair or use instant conditioner containing hydrolyzed animal protein for temporary repair
Trichoclasis	Styling trauma	Avoid tight hair clasps and use ball-tipped styling combs and brushes
General shaft fragility	Overprocessed hair	Use semipermanent instead of permanent hair dyes, use short permanent wave processing time
Hair appearance		
Dull	Cuticle irregularities	Use styling glaze or leave-in conditioner
Lack of body	Fine hair texture	Hair permanent wave, styling gel, or sculpturing gel to increase hold
Hair texture		
Dry, rough	Overshampooing, permanent wave process time to long	Deep conditioner, shorten permanent wave processing time, do not repeat permanent wave for 3 months
Greasy, slick	Overconditioning or inadequate shampooing	Avoid conditioning shampoos and deep or oily hair conditioners

See glossary for definition of terms.

The initial step in advising a patient on cosmetic remedies for hair problems is to ensure that he or she is using the appropriate shampoo. Patients with light-colored hair may note greenish discoloration following swimming in a pool with copper-contaminated water from copper-containing algicides or copper pipes.[5] Low water pH, chlorinated water, and copper contamination all must be present for the hair discoloration to occur. This problem is most pronounced in individuals with bleached hair, as the copper is readily absorbed due to the increased content of dysteic acid and other anionic sulfonate groups.[6] Special shampoos (Clairol, Metalux) or 2% penicillamine shampoos have been reported to be effective in removing the abnormal color.[7] Green hair may also be seen after using copper-contaminated tap water[8] and some tar-based shampoos. Special shampoos can aid in removing of the undesirable hue.

Shampoo selection is also important for chemically treated hair, which is dry and more subject to static electricity and tangling than healthy hair. Patients can achieve improved feel and manageability if a conditioning shampoo is selected. Patients with fine, chemically treated hair, however, may find that a conditioning shampoo works well for about 1 to 2 weeks and then leaves the hair limp and without ability to hold a curl. This is due to excess conditioner on the hair shaft, which is inadequately removed by the mild shampoo. Shampooing with a deep cleaning detergent shampoo once weekly will prevent conditioner build up. Patients should be encouraged to allow their hair to begin drying prior to combing, since wet hair is more elastic and more subject to fracture.

It is recommended that patients with chemically treated hair use an instant conditioner following shampooing. The optimal instant conditioner should contain hydrolyzed animal protein. For severely damaged hair, a deep conditioner is recommended every 2 weeks, although too frequent application will render the hair limp. Patients who have a permanent wave will note that heavy conditioners tend to relax the curl, which may or may not be desirable.

Damaged chemically treated hair should be subjected to as little physical stress as possible. Permanent waving alone decreases hair strength by 15%. Styling, including combing and brushing, should be kept to a minimum. Tight hair clasps and hair styles that pull on the hair shaft should be avoided. Patients should be encouraged not to sleep with brush-type plastic rollers in their hair. Curling irons that clamp the hair to the heated rod should be avoided. In other words, anything that might result in hair breakage should be minimized, since chemically treated hair is more likely to demonstrate trichoptilosis and trichoclasis. Recommended styling procedures include the use of a round, ball-tipped brush to curl the hair while blow drying and heat set rollers.

Shine, or gloss, can be restored to chemically damaged hair with a hair glaze or leave-in conditioner. Additional shine and hold can be achieved with a styling gel for minimal hold or a sculpturing gel for maximal hold. These products work best when applied sparingly to damp hair and massaged throughout the hair prior to styling.

Many patients undergo another chemical process to improve the appearance of damaged hair. For example, a patient who notes that her permanently dyed hair does not hold a curl may undergo a "conditioning" permanent wave. The end result is more hair damage and further problems. Patients are better advised to opt for an attractive wig, which may cost no more than a permanent wave, until new hair growth occurs.

COSMETIC TECHNIQUES FOR MEDICAL HAIR CONDITIONS

Numerous inherited medical hair conditions (e.g., trichorrhexis nodosa, trichorrhexis invaginata, pili annulati) exhibit a variety of hair shaft defects. The end result of all these conditions is a fragile hair shaft lacking shine or slow growth. Defective hair shafts should not undergo permanent dyeing or waving procedures. The end result will be cosmetically poor, and the hair shaft will fracture more readily. However, temporary or semipermanent hair dyes may be used; these coat or minimally penetrate the hair shaft without causing severe internal shaft damage.

Hair manipulation, including shampooing, combing, brushing, and curling, should be minimized. Patients generally do best with a short, straight hair style. Infrequent shampooing with a conditioning shampoo followed by an instant conditioner decreases breakage and increases manageability.

If the quality of the scalp hair is poor, patients may wish to investigate the possibility of wearing a hair piece.

REFERENCES

1. Panati C: Atop the vanity p. 234. In Extraordinary Origins of Everyday Things. Harper & Row Publishers, New York, 1987
2. Ludwig E: Classification of the types of androgenetic alopecia (common baldness) occurring in the female sex. Br J Dermatol 97:247, 1977
3. Bergfeld WF: Etiology and diagnosis of androgenetic alopecia. Clin Dermatol 6: 102, 1988
4. Hamilton JB: Patterned long hair in man: types and incidence. Ann NY Acad Sci 53:708, 1951
5. Roomans GM, Forslind B: Copper in green hair: a quantitative investigation by electron probe x-ray microanalysis. Ultrastruct Pathol 1:301, 1980
6. Zultak M, Rochefor A, Faiver B et al: Green hair: clinical, chemical, and epidemiologic study. Ann Dermatol Venereol 115:807, 1988
7. Person JR: Green hair: treatment with a penicillamine shampoo. Arch Dermatol 121:717, 1985
8. Nordlund JJ, Hartley C, Fister J: On the cause of green hair. Arch Dermatol 113: 1700, 1977

19

Black Skin and Hair Cosmetics

Black skin and hair present unique cosmetic challenges because of tremendous variation in skin color and hair shape seen in this genetically heterogeneous racial group. Furthermore, Black skin is subtly structurally different from Caucasian skin because of the presence of more mixed apocrine–eccrine sweat glands,[1] increased blood and lymphatic vessels,[2] predisposition to hyperpigmentation,[3] denser and more compact stratum corneum,[4] increased transepidermal water loss after irritation,[5] and possibly increased skin sensitivity to irritants.[6,7]

BLACK SKIN COSMETICS

The formulations and types of facial cosmetics available to patients with darker skin tones are the same as those formulated for lighter skin tones. Some cosmetics companies that traditionally cater to light-skinned customers have now enlarged their color selection to include products for darker skin tones. However, many new cosmetics companies are producing product lines specifically created for women of color. It is estimated that Black Americans spend five times the percentage of their per capita income on personal care products as do Caucasians.[8]

The unique aspect of colored cosmetic formulation for darker skin tones is the blending of pigments with the underlying skin color. Fair-skinned individuals, with little underlying skin pigment, can select a colored cosmetic and expect it to look similar in the packaging and on the skin. However, Black individuals can expect the cosmetic to look entirely different in the package than on the skin. For example, a light pink blush that provides cheek highlights in a Caucasian patient is imperceptible on Black skin. Therefore, Black cosmetics generally contain vivid pigments to provide the desired result.

Facial Foundations

Facial foundations for women of color are found both at the cosmetics counter and in mass merchandisers. It is estimated that there are over 35 different colors of dark skin, requiring tremendous color selection for complexion matching[9] compared with the seven basic colors of Caucasian skin. Black women traditionally wear facial foundations to blend uneven facial tones while fair-skinned individuals wear facial foundations to add color to the skin. Table 19-1 lists some of the foundations available for Black women with various skin types. Greater emphasis is placed on foundations for dry skin, however, as Black skin is more subject to xerosis because of its higher rate of transepidermal water loss.[5,10] Many Black women also consider their skin to be extremely ''sensitive,'' even though studies do not demonstrate a genetic predisposition to contact dermatitis.[11,12]

The description of Black skin requires a more complex discussion of color in terms of value, intensity, and undertone.[13] The value of a color is a measure of its light reflectivity. Dark skin with blue/black or mahogany hues may appear deeper in color due to the low value of these colors. ''Intensity'' refers to the brightness or dullness of a color. True colors, without the addition of white,

Table 19-1A. Facial Foundations for Black Skin Acne/Oily Skin

Name/Company	Type	Cost	Coverage	Wearability	Availability
Maquicontrole (Lancome)	Liquid	+ + + +	Moderate	Moderate	Wide, cosmetics counter
Pore-Minimizer (Clinique)	Shake Lotion	+ + +	Very sheer	Very short	Wide, cosmetics counter
Stay-True (Clinique)	Liquid	+ + +	Sheer	Short	Wide, cosmetics counter
Oil Free Liquid (Fashion Fair)	Liquid	+ + +	Moderate	Moderate	Wide, cosmetics counter
Oil Free Soufflé	Soufflé	+ + + +	Moderate	Moderate	Wide, cosmetics counter
Shades Of You Oil Free Liquid Make-Up (Maybelline)	Liquid	+	Sheer	Short	Wide, non-cosmetics counter
Makeup #3 (Prescriptives)	Liquid	+ + + +	Sheer	Short	Limited, cosmetics counters
Demi-Matte (Estee Lauder)	Liquid	+ + + +	Moderate	Moderate	Wide, cosmetics counter
Oil Free Liquid Foundation (Ebone')	Liquid	+	Sheer	Short	Wide, non-cosmetics counter

Cost: + = $4–5, + + = $5–10, + + + = $10–20, + + + + = $20–30.
Coverage: very sheer = only provides facial color, sheer = minimally evens facial color, moderate = conceals minor blemishes.
Wearability: very short = 2 hours, short = 3 hours, moderate = 4 hours.
Availability: cosmetics counter = available in department stores, non-cosmetics counter = available in drug stores and mass merchandise.

Table 19-1B. Facial Foundations for Black Skin/Normal Skin

Name/Company	Type	Cost	Coverage	Wearability	Availability
Sheer Foundatioñ (Fashion Fair)	Liquid	+ +	Sheer	Short	Wide, cosmetics counter
Balanced Makeup (Clinique)	Liquid	+ + +	Moderate	Moderate	Wide, cosmetics counter
Maquimat Ultra Naturel (Lancome)	Liquid	+ + + +	Sheer	Short	Wide, cosmetics counter
Shades of You 100% Oil-Free Compact Creme Make-Up (Maybelline)	Creme/ powder	+	Moderate	Moderate	Wide, non-cosmetics counter
Makeup #2 (Prescriptives)	Liquid	+ + + +	Moderate	Moderate	Limited, cosmetics counter

brown, or black pigments, tend to have higher intensity than mixed colors. For example, primary red has a greater intensity than brick red produced by the mixing of primary red with brown. This is an important concept in selecting facial foundations for dark skin, since too many pigments can leave the skin muddy appearing due to reduced color intensity. Lastly, ''undertones'' are extremely important. It is the undertone that accounts for the tremendous variation seen in Black skin. Red, yellow, or orange undertones are said to give the skin a warm appearance, while blue, purple, or green undertones are said to give the skin a cool appearance. Based on an analysis of undertones Black skin can be further classified as jet black, blue/black, purple/black, brown/red, bronze, and honey.

Table 19-1C. Facial Foundations for Black Skin/Dry Skin

Name/Company	Type	Cost	Coverage	Wearability	Availability
Maquivelours (Lancome)	Liquid	+ + + +	Moderate	Moderate	Wide, cosmetics counter
Perfect Finish Creme Makeup (Fashion Fair)	Cream	+ +	Moderate	Moderate	Wide, cosmetics counter
Maquidouceur (Lancome)	Liquid	+ + + + +	Moderate	Moderate	Wide, cosmetics counter
Maximum Coverage Cream Foundation (Ebone')	Cream	+	Full	Long	Wide, non-cosmetics counter
Makeup #1 (Prescriptives)	Liquid	+ + + +	Moderate	Moderate	Limited, cosmetics counter

Cost: + = $4–5, + + = $5–10, + + + = $10–20, + + + + = $20–30, + + + + + = $30–40, + + + + + + = $40–50.

Coverage: very sheer = only provides facial color, sheer = minimally evens facial color, moderate = conceals minor blemishes, full = conceals blemishes and minor pigmentation irregularities.

Wearability: very short = 2 hours, short = 3 hours, moderate = 4 hours, long = 8 hours.

Eye and Cheek Cosmetics

Colored cometics applied to the Black face must contain deeper pigments. Popular eye shadow colors include deep blue, lilac, wine, gold, or emerald. Facial highlighter and blush colors for facial contouring in Black skin are deep plum, bronze, deep orange, coral, wine, or burgundy. The color selected depends upon the skin color shade, for example, wine or plum blush for jet-black skin, coral or deep orange for brown skin, and pink or peach for light brown skin. The eye and face contouring methods, however, are the same for light-and dark-skinned patients (discussed earlier).

BLACK NAIL COSMETICS

Black patients also have a more deeply pigmented nail bed than Caucasian patients; thus the same vivid colors found in facial cosmetics are employed. Nail polishes that are deep red, wine, or brown provide the best coverage for nail discolorations such as melonychia striata.

BLACK HAIR COSMETICS

Black hair is unique due to its kinky configuration, deep pigmentation, and easily fractured shafts. It is estimated that the Black hair care industry has annual wholesale revenues in excess of $1.5 billion in the United States.[14] For these reasons, the hair care needs of Black patients require careful dermatologic consideration.

Black Hair Anatomy

Black hair is identical to Caucasian hair in its amino acid content, but has a slightly larger diameter, lower water content, and, most importantly, a different cross-sectional shape.[15] Caucasian hair has a symmetrical circular cross section, allowing the hair to hang straight, while Black hair has a flattened elliptical cross section.[16] It is the asymmetry of this cross section that accounts for the irregular kinky appearance of Black hair. Hair that is wavy or loosely kinked has a cross-sectional shape in between a circle and a flattened ellipse.

However, the cross-sectional shape of the hair fiber accounts for more than the degree of curl; it also determines the amount of shine and the ability of sebum to coat the hair shaft.[17] Straight hair possesses more shine than kinky hair due to its smooth surface, allowing maximum light reflection. The irregularly kinked hair shafts appear duller, even though they may have an intact cuticle. For this reason, Black hair care products contain agents designed to add shine to the finished hair style.

The shape of the hair shaft also determines grooming ease. Straight hair is the easiest to groom since combing friction is low and the hair is easy to arrange in a fashionable style. Kinky hair, on the other hand, demonstrates increased grooming friction, resulting in increased hair shaft breakage. Kinky hair also does not easily conform to a predetermined hair style, unless the shafts are short. This creates a predisposition to trichorrhexis nodosa, trichonodosis, and pseudofolliculitis barbae.[18] Therefore, Black hair requires special grooming tools to minimize friction and unique styling to increase manageability.

Black Hair Cleansing

Hair cleansing needs differ between Caucasian individuals with straight hair and Black individuals with kinky hair. Straight hair is difficult to style and limp if coated with excess sebum, thus encouraging frequent shampooing. Kinky hair, on the other hand, requires sebum to add shine, decrease combing friction, and increase manageability. Kinky hair naturally stands away from the scalp; therefore excess sebum can increase styling ease. This accounts for the preference of individuals with straight hair to shampoo daily or every other day for an optimal appearance while individuals with kinky hair may only require once weekly shampooing, or less, to achieve an optimal appearance.

There are shampoo products specifically designed for the Black patient. These shampoos are known as conditioning shampoos, since they are formulated with both cleaning and conditioning agents, such as wheat germ oil, steartrimonium hydrolyzed animal protein, or lanolin derivatives. They remove sebum from the hair shaft and replace it with a layer of oily conditioner.[19] The conditioner increases manageability, decreases grooming friction, and adds shine.

Black patients can develop seborrheic dermatitis, which can be difficult to treat if the patient shampoos once weekly or once every 2 weeks. Traditional anti-seborrheic shampoos contain tar, sulfur, selenium disulfide, or zinc pyrithione in a detergent shampoo base. These shampoos may be difficult for the Black patient to use as they thoroughly remove hair sebum. This leaves the hair dull, unmanageable, and brittle. A better alternative may be use an overnight scalp treatment containing salicylic acid in an oily base to loosen scale, followed by shampooing in the morning with a medicated shampoo containing ketoconazole.

Black Hair Conditioning

Conditioners are important hair cosmetics for the Black patient to restore shine, increase manageability, add body, improve softness, reduce grooming friction, and decrease hair breakage. There are three types of conditioners valuable to the patient with kinky hair: instant conditioners, leave-in conditioners, and deep conditioners. Instant conditioners are applied to the scalp after shampooing and rinsed following brief contact with the hair. These products aid in detangling, but must be followed by a second leave-in conditioner in most black patients. These products are applied to towel-dried hair prior to styling and may be reapplied daily even though the hair has not been shampooed. They are designed to moisturize the hair and contain both occlusive and humectant agents, such as silicone derivatives, polymers, and quaternized proteins. Deep conditioners are designed for once weekly application and are left on the hair 20 to 30 minutes before shampooing. These moisturizing products are either protein-containing creams, known as protein packs, or hot oil treatments. The protein creams are designed to repair damaged hair shafts minimally while the oil treatments improve shine and lubricity.

Black Hair Styling Products

The goal of grooming for the Black patient is to allow the hair to remain in an organized style dictated by fashion. Hair styles requiring minimal use of styling products are natural "Afros" combed with a wide-toothed pick and closely shaved cuts where the hair shafts are approximately 1/4 inch long and require no combing. Most other Black hair styles require maintenance with special grooming products.

Black styling products are designed both to straighten and to add shine to the hair (Table 19-2). Pomades, which are now called "cream brilliantines" by some manufacturers, are anhydrous products containing petrolatum, waxes, lanolin, and vegetable or mineral oils.[20] They combine conditioning and styling properties, but can also contain sulfur or tar derivatives to aid in the treatment of seborrheic dermatitis. The pomade adds shine, lubrication, and hold to allow the hair to remain close to the scalp with some curl reduction. These products are preferred by Black men who wear close-cropped hair cuts. Pomade acne,

Table 19-2. Black Hair Styling Products

Styling Product	Type	Main Ingredients	Purpose
Pomade	Cream	Petrolatum, wax, lanolin, mineral oil, vegetable oils	Moisturize hair, add shine, decrease breakage, aid in straightening hair
Gel curl activator	Gel	Glycerin	Moisturize hair, add shine
Brilliantine	Liquid	Vegetable oils, mineral oil, silicone	Moisturize hair, add shine
Oil sheen spray	Aerosol	Vegetable oils, mineral oil, silicone	Moisturize hair, add shine
Hair spray	Aerosol	Film-forming polymer and hair conditioners	Hold finished style

as reported by Plewig et al.,[21] is comedonal acne along the hair line that is frequently seen in patients using olive oil–containing pomades. Some of the newer glycerin-based products can be substituted for a petrolatum or olive oil pomade without producing acne. These are known as "gel curl activators," but they do not repel moisture or moisturize the hair quite as well as the traditional pomades.

Liquid brilliantines are popular for maintaining natural, kinky hairstyles. These products allow ease of styling and provide shine without causing an oil build up. Traditionally they contain mineral and vegetable oils.[22] Newer formulations contain silicone to add lubricity, castor oil to aid in manageability, and soluble glycoprotein to maintain proper moisture balance and enhance shine.[23] If the product is sprayed on to the hair, it is known as an oil sheen spray. In general, these products are less comedogenic than the older pomades.

Hair sprays for Black hair must also contain additional moisturizing and shine agents such as glycerin. The main holding ingredient in most products are the polyvinyl polymers, but steartrimonium hydrolyzed animal protein may be added for conditioning and moisturizing, and a difatty cationic amino acid derivative or a silicone derivative may be added for both shine and additional moisturizing. Alcohol concentrations must be kept to a minimum to prevent further hair dryness.

Black Hair-Styling Techniques

Several physical hair styling options are available to the Black patient.[24] Fashion and personal style dictate the popularity of the techniques.

Natural Styles

Black hair cutting techniques are designed to control the tightly kinked hair so it can be arranged into a fashionable hair style. Natural Black hair styles involve trimming all hairs at an even distance from the scalp. If the hairs are shaved 1/4 inch from the scalp, the hair requires no combing. Variety can be introduced into the close-cropped hair styles by shaving all the hair in certain areas to create patterned designs. If the hair is allowed to grow longer, the style is known as an "Afro" and is groomed with a broad-toothed pick. Hair-styling techniques where the hair is longer on top and shorter on the sides is known as "fading."

Braided Styles

Another manner of organizing kinky hair is twisting or braiding. A popular hair style in young Black children involves sectioning the hair into quadrants on the top, sides, and posterior scalp. The hair is then gathered in each quadrant and secured with a rubber band or clasp and twisted or braided. This is an easy method of styling the hair that does not require chemical processing. Problems arise if the hair is repeatedly pulled too tightly, resulting in traction alopecia, or if the hair is sectioned in the same location for a prolonged period of time, resulting in increased localized hair breakage.[25]

Braiding can also be performed on the scalp in a technique known as "corn rowing." The hair is pulled tightly to form continuous braids on the scalp in various patterns. Beads or other jewels can be woven into the hair style as fashionable. Usually the hair style is worn for 2 to 4 weeks and then undone and rebraided, if desired. This continuous tension on the hair shaft can result in traction alopecia, especially at the temples.[26-29] Even though the hair is shampooed with the braids in place, thorough cleansing of the scalp is not possible and seborrheic dermatitis may occur.

Hair Additions

The hair addition techniques most popular among Black patients are hair extensions and hair lacing. Hair extensions are natural or synthetic hair fibers braided along with the patient's natural hair initially on the scalp and then off the scalp (see Ch. 18). The extensions create the illusion of long braided hair and can be woven in many patterns and adorned with beads or jewels. The hair style remains in place for 2 to 8 weeks and is shampooed, but requires minimal grooming. Traction alopecia and seborrheic dermatitis may result.[30]

Another related technique is hair lacing. Hair lacing involves braiding the patient's natural hair with synthetic or natural hair fibers except that the braids are stopped 1 to 2 inches from the scalp and the added hair allowed to flow freely. The hair can then be styled as desired. It is difficult for the Black patient with tightly kinked hair to grow long hair due to hair breakage, accounting for the popularity of hair lacing.

Thread Wrapping

A style adapted from Africa is the tight wrapping of black cotton thread around strands of hair. The hair is then parted in various manners to fashion elaborate interlocking arcs. Traction alopecia is also seen with this technique.

Hair Straightening Techniques

Kinky hair can be straightened with mechanical, heat, or chemical techniques (Table 19-3). Straightening of the hair is popular among Black individuals for the following reasons:

1. Hair manageability is improved.
2. The hair can be more easily combed and styled.
3. Hair breakage may be decreased due to less combing friction.
4. Hair shine is improved with a straighter hair shaft.
5. Fashion may dictate the need for straight hair.

Table 19-3. Hair-Straightening Techniques

Technique	Main Ingredient	Effect on Hair	Comments
Hot pressing or hot combing	Pressing cream and metal hot comb heated to 300–500°F	Temporary straightening reversed with water contact	Inexpensive, easy to burn scalp and hair
Bisulfite relaxer	Ammonium bisulfite	Moderately permanent chemical hair straightener	Least damaging to hair and scalp, popular home product
Thioglycolate relaxer	Thioglycolate	Moderately effective permanent chemical hair straightener	Can cause damage to hair and scalp, extremely drying to hair, least popular
Lye relaxer	Sodium hydroxide	Maximally effective permanent chemical hair straightener	Can cause severe corneal and scalp burns, most damaging to hair, salon use only, most popular product
No-lye relaxer	Guanidine hydroxide Lithium hydroxide	Effective permanent chemical hair straightener	Must be properly mixed, can cause corneal and scalp burns

See glossary for definition of terms.

Mechanical Straightening

Mechanical hair straightening employs heavy cream pomade hair dressings. The weight of the cream adheres the hair shaft to the scalp and provides minimal straightening.[31]

Heat Straightening

Heat straightening techniques, including hot combing and hair pressing, were developed by Madame C. J. Walker, who is credited with originating the ethnic hair care industry.[14] Hot combing employs a metal comb that is heated to a minimum of 300°F and drawn through the hair. This breaks the water-reformable bonds (hydrogen bonds and salt linkages) and allows the hair to be pulled straight. The change is temporary, however, as moisture from perspiration, humidity, or shampooing allows the bonds to reform and the hair returns to its natural kinky state.[32] Thus, heat straightening techniques are temporary, but can be improved if a pressing oil is added to the hair prior to hot combing or ironing between hot metal plates. The pressing oil improves water resistance and contains oily substances such as petrolatum, mineral oil, ceresin wax, or cetyl alcohol. It also, however, contributes to hot comb alopecia resulting in eventual follicular destruction.[33] There is some controversy as to whether all cases of scarring alopecia in Black patients who use heat straightening represent hot comb alopecia or the newly described follicular degeneration syndrome.[34] Temporary heat straightening remains popular since it is inexpensive and can be performed at home.

Chemical Straightening

Chemical hair straightening, also known as "hair relaxing" or "lanthionization," uses substances to break disulfide bonds in the hair shaft. The first hair relaxers were developed around 1940 and consisted of sodium hydroxide or potassium hydroxide mixed into potato starch. Once the disulfide bonds are broken, the hair is pulled straight and the disulfide bonds reformed in their new configuration. This technique is popular due to its versatility; the hair can be completely straightened, minimally straightened, texturized, or straightened and recurled.

Application technique   The basic application technique for chemical hair straightening is as follows:[35]

1. The hair should *not* be shampooed.
2. The scalp is coated with a petrolatum base for protection.
3. The hair is sectioned into quadrants.
4. For previously untreated hair, the chemical straightener is applied from root to end, beginning at the nape of the neck and moving forward to the anterior hairline. For previously treated hair, the chemical straightener is applied to the new growth only, taking care to minimize scalp contact.
5. The chemicals are left on the hair from 10 to 30 minutes during which time the hair is gently combed straight.
6. The hair is rinsed with water.
7. A neutralizer is smoothed on the hair, taking care to keep it straight and untangled.
8. The hair is shampooed with a nonalkaline shampoo, conditioned and styled.

The key to successful hair relaxing is an experienced beautician who can quickly apply and remove the chemicals and determine when the desired degree of disulfide bond breaking has occurred. It is estimated that virgin hair loses about 30% of its tensile strength following a properly performed chemical straightening procedure.

Types Chemical relaxing can be accomplished with lye-based, lye-free, ammonium thioglycolate, or bisulfite creams.[36] Lye-based, or sodium hydroxide, straighteners are alkaline creams with a pH of 13. Sodium hydroxide is a caustic substance that can damage hair, produce scalp burns, and cause blindness if it contacts the eye. These products are generally restricted to professional or salon use and may contain up to 3.5% sodium hydroxide. The straightening occurs as one-third of the hair cystine content is changed to lanthionine along with minor hydrolysis of the peptide bonds.[37]

They are available in two forms: "base" and "no-base" relaxers. The "base" relaxers contain between 1.5% and 3.5% sodium hydroxide and therefore require that the scalp and hairline be coated with a petrolatum base prior to application. These products are necessary for hard to straighten hair. "No-base'' relaxers, on the other hand, contain 1.5% to 2.5% sodium hydroxide and only require base application to the hairline.[38] They are more popular since it is time consuming for the beautician to apply the base to the scalp, and most individuals are re-straightening hair that has already been chemically weakened.

Other strong alkali chemicals sometimes used in place of sodium hydroxide are guanidine hydroxide and lithium hydroxide, which are known as "no-lye" chemical hair straighteners. These relaxing kits contain 4% to 7% cream calcium hydroxide and liquid guanidine carbonate. The guanidine carbonate activator is then mixed into the calcium hydroxide cream to produce calcium carbonate and guanidine hydroxide, the active agent. These products do not require basing of either the scalp or the hairline.

Thioglycolate straighteners are identical to permanent wave solutions except that they are formulated as thick creams, rather than lotions, to add weight and aid in holding the hair straight. They are extremely harsh on the hair, however, and the least popular of all the relaxing chemicals. The thioglycolate cream has a pH of 9.0 to 9.5, which removes the protective sebum and facilitates hair shaft penetration. Chemical burns can also occur with this straightener.[39]

The least damaging hair straightening products are the ammonium bisulfite creams. These products contain a mixture of bisulfite and sulfite in varying ratios depending on the pH of the lotion. Many of the home chemical straightening products are of this type, but produce the least permanent straightening of all the chemicals discussed. As a general rule, the chemicals that produce the greatest, longest-lasting hair straightening are also the most damaging to the hair shaft.

Adverse reactions Kinky hair that has been overprocessed by use of strong chemical straightener or an excessively long processing time will lose its elastic properties. The hair shaft then becomes brittle, fracturing with minimal combing trauma usually at the scalp, where stress is maximal. Patients frequently comment that their hair is falling out following an aggressive chemical straightening. Unless a severe chemical burn has occurred, which is unusual, straightening procedures do not damage the hair follicle. Hair breakage is most commonly the cause of hair loss. The dermatologist can verify hair breakage by noting that the lost hairs do not include the hair bulb. Unfortunately, if the hair has been appropriately neutralized, there is nothing that can be done to repair the damaged disulfide bonds. The brittle hair must be trimmed, and overprocessing of the new growth should be avoided. Hair breakage can be minimized by combing or styling the hair as little as possible, applying moisturizing conditioning agents, and avoiding any further chemical treatments such as permanent hair dyeing or bleaching.[40]

Hair straightening chemicals are all known cutaneous irritants; thus the base cream applied to the scalp and surrounding skin is extremely important. Irritant contact dermatitis is frequently seen in patients even when care has been taken to protect the skin.

Permanent Waving Techniques

Some Black patients may wish to curl or wave the hair permanently. These products are similar to Caucasian permanent waves in that they are based on thioglycolic acid neutralized with ammonium hydroxide or a primary amine. The main difference is the level of the active ingredients and the application steps. Application is as follows:

1. The hair is rinsed or shampooed.
2. The hair is sectioned into quadrants.
3. Rearranger (reducing agent) is applied to the hair from root to end or virgin hair starting at the nape of the neck proceeding to the anterior hair line. In previously chemically treated hair, the rearranger is only applied to new growth.
4. The rearranger is rinsed and a booster applied from the root of the hair to the end.
5. The hair is then sectioned and placed in rods for 15 to 20 minutes under a hooded hair dryer.
6. A test curl is performed to determine that the desired amount of curl has been obtained.
7. The hair is thoroughly rinsed.
8. Neutralizer (oxidizing agent) containing sodium bromate is applied for each rod for 10 to 20 minutes.
9. The rods are removed.
10. The hair is thoroughly rinsed.
11. A moisturizer is applied to the hair for 10 to 20 minutes.
12. A curl activator is applied and the hair is styled.

These products were introduced in the late 1970s, but have recently lost some of their original appeal. The curling procedure is extremely damaging to Black hair, leaving it frizzy, dry, and brittle. Furthermore, daily use of propylene glycol and glycerin curl activators is required prior to styling to maintain the hair style and decrease breakage.

Hair Coloring Techniques

Hair coloring techniques available to the Black patient are the same as those discussed for the Caucasian patient (Ch. 16). Many dyes in temporary, semipermanent, and permanent formulations are available for darkening the hair color of the Black patient. This can be done for fashion reasons or to cover gray hair. Darkening the hair color is not as damaging as lightening the hair color, but may result in excessive hair breakage if permanent hair coloring is combined with chemical straightening. However, if bleaching or lightening of the hair is desired, high volume peroxide is required, which can be extremely damaging to the hair shaft. If Black hair is lightened, it usually bleaches to a red color as the pheomelanins are not easily removed. If hair bleaching is combined with hair straightening, the hair can be so severely damaged that it cannot withstand the trauma of routine grooming. The hair breaks at its exit point from the scalp, leaving the patient with thin, ungroomable hair.

REFERENCES

1. Anderson KE, Maibach HI: African-American and white skin differences. J Am Acad Dermatol 1:276, 1979
2. Montagna W, Carlisle K: The architecture of black and white facial skin. J Am Acad Dermatol 24:929, 1991
3. McLaurin DI: Unusual patterns of common dermatoses in blacks. Cutis 32:352, 1983
4. Weigand DA, Haygood C, Baylor JR: Cell layers and density of negro and caucasian stratum corneum. J Invest Dermatol 62:563, 1974
5. Wilson D, Berardesca E, Maibach HI: In vitro transepidermal water loss: differences between black and white human skin. Br J Dermatol 119:647, 1988
6. Stephens TJ, Oresajo C: Ethnic sensitive skin. Cosmet Toilet 109:75, 1994
7. Berardesca E, Maibach HI: Sensitive and ethnic skin. A need for special skin care agents? Dermatol Clin 9:89, 1991
8. Chester J, Dixon M: Ethnic market feels growth. Manufacturing Chemist 59:32, 1988
9. McLaurin CI: Cosmetic for blacks a medical perspective. Cosmet Toilet 98:47, 1983
10. Hood HL, Wickett RR: Racial differences in epidermal structure and function. Cosmet Toilet 107:47, 1992
11. Maibach HI: Racial and skin color differences in skin sensitivity. Cosmet Toilet 105:35, 1990
12. E Berardesca E, Maibach HI: Racial differences in sodium lauryl sulphate induced cutaneous irritation: black and white. Contact Dermatitis 18:65, 1988
13. Patton JE: Color to Color. Fireside, New York, 1991
14. Syed AN: Ethnic hair care. Cosmet Toilet 108:99, 1993
15. Brooks G, Lewis A: Treatment regimes for styled Black hair. Cosmet Toilet 98:59, 1983
16. Lindelof B, Forslind B, Hedblad M et al: Human hair form: morphology revealed by light and scanning electron microscopy and computer-aided three-dimensional reconstruction. Arch Dermatol 124:1359, 1988
17. Johnson BA: Requirements in cosmetics for black skin. Dermatol Clin 6:409, 1988
18. Dawber RPR: Knotting of scalp hair. Br J Dermatol 91:169, 1974
19. Brooks G, Burmeister F: Black hair care ingredients. Cosmet Toilet 103:93, 1988
20. Goode ST: Hair pomades. Cosmet Toilet 94:71, 1979
21. Plewig G, Fulton JE, Kligman AM: Pomade acne. Arch Dermatol 101:580, 1970
22. Balsam MS, Sagarin E: Hair grooming preparations. p. 119. In Cosmetics: Science and Technology. Vol. 2. 2nd Ed. Wiley-Interscience, New York, 1972
23. Wells FV, Lubowe II: Hair grooming aids. Part II. Cutis 22:270, 1978
24. Vaughan-Richards A: Black and Beautiful. Published in association with Johnson Products Co., Collins Publishing, 1986

25. Rollins TG: Traction folliculitis with hair casts and alopecia. Am J Dis Child 101: 639, 1961
26. Scott DA: Disorders of the hair and scalp in blacks. Dermatol Clin 6:387, 1988
27. Rudolph RI, Klein AW, Decherd JW: Corn-row alopecia. Arch Dermatol 108:134, 1973
28. Morgan HV: Traction alopecia. Br Med J 1:115, 1960
29. Slepyan AH: Traction alopecia. Arch Dermatol 78:395, 1958
30. Harman RRM: Traction alopecia due to hair extension. Br J Dermatol 87:79, p. 302. 1972
31. McDonald CJ: Special requirements in cosmetics for people with black skin. p. 302. In Frost P, Horwitz SN (eds): Principles of Cosmetics for the Dermatologist. CV Mosby, St. Louis, 1982
32. Grimes PE, Davis LT: Cosmetics in blacks. Dermatol Clin 9:53, 1991
33. LoPresti P, Papa DM, Kligman AM: Hot comb alopecia. Arch Dermatol 98:234, 1968
34. Sperling LC, Sau P: The follicular degeneration syndrome in black patients. Arch Dermatol 128:68, 1992
35. Brooks G: Treatment regimes for styled black hair. Cosmet Toilet 59, 1983
36. Cannell DW: Permanent waving and hair straightening. Clin Dermatol 6:71, 1988
37. Hsuing DY: Hair straightening. p. 1155. In deNavarre MG (ed): The Chemistry and Manufacture of Cosmetics. 2nd ed. Allured Publishing Corp, Wheaton, IL
38. Khalil EN: Cosmetic and hair treatments for the black consumer. Cosmet Toilet 101:51, 1986
39. Bulengo-Ransby, Bergfeld WF: Chemical and traumatic alopecia from thioglycolate in a black woman. Cutis 49:99, 1992
40. Burmeister F, Bollatti D, Brooks G: Ethnic hair: moisturizing after relaxer use. Cosmet Toilet 106:49, 1991

20

Skin Cleansers

Much attention has recently been directed toward cleansing of the skin, especially facial skin, in order to remove sebum and environmental dirt thoroughly while not overdrying the skin to accentuate wrinkles. This marketing approach the spurred the development of new cleansing methods by the cosmetics industry. Cleansing is now part of a daily ''skin treatment'' routine incorporating a variety of products and application methods, depending upon current marketing trends. Nevertheless, the cleansing products in all cosmetics lines can be classified into the following categories: soaps and cleansing bars, lipid-free cleansers, cleansing creams, astringents and toners, exfoliants, abrasive scrubbers, and masks.

SOAPS AND CLEANSING BARS

History

Soap has been a cleansing staple for 4,000 years, ever since the Hittites of Asia Minor cleaned their hands with the ash of the soapwort plant suspended in water and the Sumerians of Ur produced alkali solutions for washing. Neither of these products, however, is chemically similar to soap as it is known today. The actual modern soap preparation was developed about 600 bc by the Phoenicians, who first saponified goat fat, water, and potassium carbonate-rich ash into a solid, waxy product. The popularity of soap has waxed and waned over the years. During the Middle Ages, soap was outlawed by the Christian Church, which believed that exposing the flesh, even to bathe, was evil. Later, when the idea of bacteria-induced infection surfaced, the sale of soap soared.

The first widely marketed soap was developed in 1878 by Harley Procter, who decided that his father's soap and candle factory should produce a delicately scented, creamy white soap to compete with imported European products. He accomplished this feat with the help of his cousin chemist, James Gamble, who made a richly lathering product called ''White Soap.'' By accident, they discovered that whipping air into the soap solution before molding resulted in a floating soap that could not be lost in the bath.[1] This resulted in a product known as Ivory soap, still manufactured today.

Manufacture

Soap functions by employing a surfactant to lower the interskin tension between the nonpolar soil and the rinsing water, which floats away the dirt in the lather. The manufacturing stages in a typical bar soap are as follows:

1. Saponification of natural fats and preparation of milling chips
2. Blending of soap chips with other ingredients
3. Milling and shredding
4. Extrusion into long strips, known as "billets," and cutting into appropriate lengths
5. Stamping into the final shape
6. Ageing and wrapping

Formulation

In basic chemical terms, soap is a reaction between a fat and an alkali, resulting in a fatty acid salt with detergent properties.[3] Modern refinements have attempted to adjust its alkaline pH, possibly resulting in less skin irritation,[4] and incorporate substances to prevent precipitation of calcium fatty acid salts in hard water, known as "soap scum."[5] Nevertheless, modern soap is basically a blend of tallow and nut oil, or the fatty acids derived from these products, in a ratio of 4:1. Increasing this ratio results in "superfatted" soaps designed to leave an oily film behind on the skin. Bar soaps can be divided into three basic types:

1. True soaps composed of long-chain fatty acid alkali salts with a pH between 9 and 10
2. Combars composed of alkaline soaps to which surface active agents have been added also with a pH of 9 to 10
3. Syndet (synthetic detergent) bars composed of synthetic detergents and fillers that contain less than 10% soap and have an adjusted pH of 5.5 to 7.0[6]

The purpose in developing new synthetic detergents over traditional soaps was to provide a product less irritating to the skin. Commonly used detergents in bar type cleansers are sodium cocoate, sodium tallowate, sodium plam kernelate, sodium stearate, sodium palmitate, triethanolamine stearate, sodium cocoyl isethionate, sodium isethionate, sodium dodecyl bezene sulfonate, and sodium cocoglyceryl ether sulfonate. Detergents in liquid formulations are sodium laureth sulfate, cocoamido propyl betaine, lauramide DEA, sodium cocoyl isethionate, and disodium laureth sulfosuccinate. The normal pH of the skin is acidic, between 4.5 and 6.5. Applying an alkali soap theoretically raises the pH of the skin, allowing it to feel dry and uncomfortable.[7] However, healthy skin rapidly regains its acidic pH.[8] The effects and measurement of surfactant-induced irritation remains a controversial area under investigation.[9]

Several methods are used to evaluate the effects of various soap and detergent formulations on the skin. One method of measuring the effects of cleansers on the skin is the soap chamber test developed by Frosch and Kligman.[10] An 8% soap solution is applied under occlusion to the volar surface of the forearm in human volunteers. The site is evaluated for scaling and erythema several days later.[11] This technique has been expanded to include measurements of transepidermal water loss with an evaporimeter. As expected, soaps induce more transepidermal water loss than the synthetic detergents listed previously. A modified chamber test is also used where a 5% solution of the soap or detergent is applied to the forearm and covered with an aluminum chamber for 18 hours. These tests exaggerate cleanser contact with the skin; thus actual use is required. This is accomplished by having human volunteers wash their forearms for a 2 minute duration four times per day for a week. Visual and evaporimeter assessments are used to evaluate the skin effect.

Special additives to the previously discussed formulations allow the tremendous variety of soaps marketed today (Table 20-1). Lanolin and paraffin may be added to a moisturizing syndet soap to create a superfatted soap, while sucrose and glycerin can be added to create a transparent bar. Adding olive oil instead of another form of fat distinguishes a Castile soap. Medicated soaps

Table 20-1. Specialty Soap Formulations

Type of Soap	Unique Ingredients
Superfatted	Increased oil and fat, fat ratio up to 10%
Castile	Olive oil used as main fat
Deodorant	Antibacterial agents
French milled	Additives to reduce alkalinity
Floating	Extra air trapped during mixing process
Oatmeal	Ground oatmeal added (coarsely ground to produce abrasive soap, finely ground for gentle cleanser)
Acne	Sulfur, resorcinol, benzoyl peroxide, or salicylic acid added
Facial	Smaller bar size, no special ingredients
Bath	Larger bar size, no special ingredients
Aloe vera	Aloe vera added to soap, no special skin benefit
Vitamin E	Vitamin E added, no special skin benefit
Cocoa butter	Cocoa butter used as major fat
Nut or fruit oil	Nut or fruit oils used as major fat
Transparent	Glycerin and sucrose added
Abrasive	Pumice, coarse oatmeal, maize meal, ground nut kernels, dried herbs or flowers added
Soap-free	Contains synthetic detergents (syndet bar)

may contain benzoyl peroxide, sulfur, resorcinol, or salicylic acid. Deodorant bars have an added antibacterial agent, such as triclocarban or triclosan. Triclocarban is excellent at eradicating gram-positive organisms, but triclosan eliminates both gram-positive and gram-negative bacteria. These soaps have a pH between 9 and 10 and may cause skin irritation. Moisturizing syndet bar soaps contain sodium lauryl isethionate with a pH adjusted to between 5 and 7 by lactic or citric acid. These products are less irritating to the skin and are sometimes labeled "beauty bars." Most bar soaps marketed by cosmetic companies are of this type.

Additives to soap are also responsible for a characteristic appearance, feel, and smell. Titanium dioxide is added in concentrations of up to 0.3% to opacify the bar and increase its optical whiteness. Pigments, such as aluminium lakes, can color the bar without producing colored foam, a characteristic considered undersirable. Foam builders, such as sodium carboxymethylcellulose and other cellulose derivatives, can make the lather feel creamy. Lastly, perfume in concentrations of 2% or more can be added to ensure that the soap bar retains its smells until completely used.[2]

LIPID-FREE CLEANSERS

Lipid-free cleansers are liquid products that clean without fats. They are applied to dry or moistened skin, rubbed to produce a lather, and rinsed or wiped away. These products may contain water, glycerin, cetyl alcohol, stearyl alcohol, sodium laurel sulfate, and occasionally propylene glycol. They leave behind a thin moisturizing film and can be used effectively to remove facial cosmetics and dirt in persons with sensitive or dermatitic skin. Lipid-free cleansers have been shown to cause less cutaneous irritation in photoaged skin.[12] It should be recognized, however, that propylene glycol can cause cutaneous stinging, and sodium laurel sulfate is a detergent.

CLEANSING CREAMS

Cleansing creams are applied to the face to both clean and moisturize. They are composed of water, mineral oil, petrolatum, and waxes.[13] The classic cream for facial cleansing was known as "cold cream." Cold creams combine the effect of a lipid solvent such as beeswax and mineral oil with detergent action from borax, also known as decaydrate of sodium tetraborate.[14] These products are popular to remove cosmetics and provide cleansing for patients with dry skin.

ASTRINGENTS AND TONERS

The terms *astringent* and *toner* are synonymous and refer to a fragranced alcohol solution used to remove oil and produce a "tight" skin feeling. Most cosmetics cleansing routines recommend that an astringent be used after washing with a syndet soap. Astringents had their greatest utility when traditional alkaline soaps were used for cleansing with hard well water. The astringent functioned to remove any remaining soap film from the face. but most homes now use detergent cleansers and public water sources. Cosmetics companies have given their astringent products a variety of names, including clarifying lotions, controlling lotions, protection tonics, skin fresheners, and toning lotions.

Astringent formulations are available for all skin types (oily, normal, and dry), which is amazing considering the product was designed for oil and soap film removal. Oily skin astringents contain a high concentration of alcohol, thus removing any sebum left behind following prior cleansing and producing a clean, tight feeling many patients find desirable. Medicated astringents for acne patients may contain menthol or camphor to create a tingling feeling when applied to the skin. Astringents for normal skin contain lower alcohol concentrations, while those for dry skin are labeled alcohol-free. Dry skin formulations contain largely propylene glycol and water to act as a humectant moisturizer. Soothing agents may also be added such as allantion, guaiazulene, and quaternium-19.[15]

A variation on astringents are products known as *T-zone controllers*. The *T-zone* refers to the central face (forehead, nose, and central chin) with the most prominent sebaceous glands and increased sebum production. These products claim to decrease oil production and absorb excess oil. Some products are formulated as shake lotions with clay suspended in alcohol, while others are gels that contain vitamins or specialty additives.

EXFOLIANTS

Exfoliants are basically astringents with the addition of substances such as witch hazel or salicylic acid to encourage stratum corneum desquamation. The idea is to remove the "dead" skin surface cells and uncover "new" skin that looks cleaner, fresher, and finer. Exfoliants are also said to "speed" the natural renewal of skin cells and "aid" in the treatment of acne by alleviating comedones. Exfoliants are designed for oily skin and are used in place of astringents in most cleansing routines for acne-prone persons.

ABRASIVE SCRUBBERS

Abrasive scrubbers are mechanical exfoliants that use an abrasive sponge or abrasive scrubbing granules in a creamy base to remove skin scale. They do not contain the irritating chemicals present in exfoliants. The claims made for abrasive scrubbers are the same as for exfoliants as far as uncovering "new" skin to reveal a cleaner, fresher look. Many cosmetics companies' skin treatment and cleansing routines use an abrasive scrubber once weekly for patients with oily skin.

Abrasive scrubbing creams incorporate polyethylene beads, aluminum oxide, ground fruit pits, or sodium tetraborate decahydrate granules to remove desquamating stratum corneum from the face.[16] Sibley et al.[17] consider abrasive scrubbing creams effective in controlling excess sebum and removing desquamating tissue. However, they can cause epithelial damage if used too vigorously. This view is held by Mills and Kligman,[16] who noted that the products produced peeling and erythema without a reduction in comedones. Aluminum oxide and ground fruit pits provide the most abrasive scrub, followed by polyethylene beads, which are softer. Sodium tetraborate decahydrate granules become softer and dissolve during use, providing the least abrasive scrub.

Another method of abrasive scrubbing has been labeled "epidermabrasion" by Durr and Orentreich,[18] who examined the use of a nonwoven polyester fiber web sponge. They and others have concluded that physical–mechanical exfoliation with the nonwoven polyester fiber web sponge was valuable in the removal of keratin excrescences and trapped hairs in pilosebaceous ducts.[19,20] Some sponges come impregnated with detergents.

FACIAL MASKS

Facial masks, also known simply as "facials," claim to produce skin tightening, deep cleaning of the pores, and acne treatment, depending on the mask type. There are four basic mask formulations: wax-based, vinyl- or rubber-based, hydrocolloid, and earth-based.

Wax-Based Masks

Wax-based masks are popular among women for their warm, esthetically pleasing feel. They are composed of beeswax or, more commonly, paraffin wax to which petroleum jelly and cetyl or stearyl alcohols have been added to provide a soft, pliable material for facial application with a soft brush. The wax is heated and sometimes applied directly to the face or at other times applied over a thin gauze cloth draped over the face. Gauze is used to enable the facial technician to remove the wax in one piece. Clients are then sometimes given the wax mold of their face to take home.

Wax-based face masks are most frequently recommended for individuals with dry skin due to their temporary ability to impede transepidermal water loss. This effect is indeed temporary and limited only to the time the mask is in direct contact with the face unless a suitable occlusive moisturizer is applied immediately following mask removal.

Vinyl- and Rubber-Based Masks

Vinyl- and rubber-based masks are popular masks for home use since they are easily applied and removed. Rubber-based masks are usually based on latex, while vinyl-based masks are based on film-forming substances such as polyvinyl alcohol or vinyl acetate. They are squeezed premixed from a tube or pouch and applied with the fingertips to the face. Upon evaporation of the vehicle, a thin flexible vinyl or rubber film remains behind on the face. The mask is generally left in contact with the skin for 10 to 30 minutes and then removed in one sheet by loosing at the edges.

Vinyl and rubber masks are appropriate for all skin types. The evaporation of the vehicle from the wet mask creates a cooling sensation and the shrinking of the mask with drying may give the impression that the skin is actually tightening. These masks can temporarily impede transepidermal water loss while they are in contact with the skin.

Hydrocolloid Masks

Hydrocolloid masks are used both in professional salons and at home. Hydrocolloids are substances, such as oatmeal, that are of large molecular weight and thus interfere with transepidermal water loss. These masks are formulated from gums and humectants and enjoy tremendous popularity since many specialty ingredients are easily incorporated into their formulation. They are marketed in the form of dry ingredients in a sealed pouch that must be mixed with warm water prior to application. The resulting paste is then smeared over the face with the hands and allowed to dry.

Hydrocolloid masks also leave the skin feeling smooth and create the sense of skin tightening as the water evaporates and the mask dries. Temporary moisturization can occur while the mask is on the skin. Specialty additives such as honey, almond oil, zinc oxide, sulfur, avocado, and witch hazel, may be used to customize the mask.

Earth-Based Masks

Earth-based masks, also known as ''paste masks'' or ''mud packs,'' are formulated of absorbent clays such as bentonite, kaolin, or china clay. The clays produce an astringent effect on the skin, making this mask most appropriate for oily-complected patients. The astringent effect of the mask can be enhanced through the addition of other substances such as magnesium, zinc oxide, or salicylic acid. The versatility of paste masks is tremendous and the number of additives unlimited.

REFERENCES

1. Panati C: Extraordinary Origins of Everyday Things. Perennial Library, Harper & Row Publishers, New York, 1987
2. Van Abbe NJ, Spearman RIC, Jarrett A: Pharmaceutical and Cosmetic Products for Topical Administration. William Heinemann Medical Books Ltd, London, 1969
3. Willcox MJ, Crichton WP: The soap market. Cosmet Toilet 104:61, 1989
4. Wortzman MS: Evaluation of mild skin cleansers. Dermatol Clin 9:35, 1991
5. Jackson EM: Soap: a complex category of products. Am J Contact Dermatitis 5: 173, 1994
6. Wortzman MS, Scott RA, Wong PS et al: Soap and detergent bar rinsability. J Soc Cosmet Chem 37:89, 1986
7. Prottey C, Ferguson T: Factors which determine the skin irritation potential of soap and detergents. J Soc Cosmet Cem 26:29, 1975
8. Wickett RR, Trobaugh CM: Personal care products. Cosmet Toilet 105:41, 1990
9. Wilhelm KP, Freitag G, Wolff HH: Surfactant-induced skin irritation and skin repair. J Am Acad Dermatol 30:944, 1994
10. Frosch PJ, Kligman AM: The soap chamber test. A new method for assessing the irritancy of soaps. J Am Acad Dermatol 1:35, 1979
11. Frosch PJ: Irritancy of soaps and detergents. p. 5. In Frost P, Horwitz SN (eds): Principles of Cosmetics for the Dermtologist. CV Mosby Company, St. Louis, 1982
12. Mills OH, Berger RS, Baker MD: A controlled comparison of skin cleansers in photoaged skin. J Geriatr Dermatol 1:173, 1993
13. deNavarre MG: Cleansing creams. p. 251. In deNaarre MG (ed): The Chemistry and Manufacture of Cosmetics. Vol. III. 2nd Ed. Allured Publishing Corporation, Wheaton, IL, 1975
14. Jass HE: Cold creams. p. 237. In deNaarre MG (ed): The Chemistry and Manufacture of Cosmetics. Vol III. 2nd Ed. Allured Publishing Corporation, Wheaton, IL, 1975
15. Wilkinson JB, Moore RJ: Astringents and skin toners. p. 74. In Harry's Cosmeticology. 7th Ed. Chemical Publishing, New York, 1982
16. Mills OH, Kligman AM: Evaluation of abrasives in acne therapy. Cutis 23:704, 1979
17. Sibley MJ, Browne RK, Kitzmiller KW: Abradant cleansing aids for acne vulgaris. Cutis 14:269, 1974
18. Durr NP, Orentreich N: Epidermabrasion for acne. Cutis 17:604, 1976
19. Mackenzie A: Use of Buf-Puf and mild cleansing bar in acne. Cutis 20:170, 1977
20. Millikan LE, Ameln R: Use of Buf-Puf and benzoyl peroxide in the treatment of acne. 28:201, 1981

21

Personal Care Products

The major personal care products marketed in the United States are antiperspirants, deodorants, and shaving preparations. Personal care products are designed to promote better hygiene.

ANTIPERSPIRANTS AND DEODORANTS

The words "antiperspirant" and "deodorant" invariably appear together on the packaging of products designed to diminish axillary wetness. However, the meaning of these two words is not synonymous. An antiperspirant is an astringent designed to decrease the secretions of the eccrine and apocrine sweat ducts, while a deodorant is designed to remove odor from the axilla. Most antiperspirants, however, also act as deodorants, but most deodorants do not act as antiperspirants.

Antiperspirants are considered over-the-counter drugs in the United States because their mode of action alters a body function, while deodorants are considered cosmetics.

History

Bathing and perfumes were probably the first two measures developed for the control of body odor. However, as personal hygiene sophistication developed, so did products designed to change normal body odor into something that is perceived as more desirable by modern society. The original deodorant appeared on the United States market in 1888. Later, in 1919, advertising first introduced the notion that body odor was offensive, thus creating a market for deodorants and antiperspirants. Present popularity of such products can be attributed to social consciousness of body odor and development of nonirritating germicides and products that do not contribute to fabric deterioration.[1]

Mechanism of Odor Production

Axillary odor is caused by the action of bacteria on sterile eccrine and apocrine sweat. The apocrine sweat is responsible for a large part of the odor, as it is rich in organic material ideal for bacterial growth. Eccrine sweat, on the other hand, is more dilute and does not provide a high concentration of bacterial nutrients. However, eccrine sweat indirectly promotes odor by dispersing the apocrine sweat over a larger area and providing the moisture necessary for bacterial growth. Axillary hair also contributes to odor by acting as a collecting site for apocrine secretions and increasing the surface area suitable for bacterial proliferation.[2]

Each person has a unique odor due to sebaceous gland secretions, the combined effect of the foods last eaten, and the physical or psychological body state. Therefore, two women may smell completely differently even though they are wearing the same perfume.

Taking these factors into account, it is then possible to list methods available to reduce axillary odor: reduce apocrine perspiration, reduce eccrine perspiration, remove the apocrine and eccrine gland secretions as they are produced, or decrease bacterial growth.[3]

Mechanism of Action of Antiperspirants

There are 25,000 eccrine glands per axiallary vault capable of producing large quantities of perspiration in response to heat and emotional stimuli. The following chemicals can function as antiperspirants to reduce axillary moisture:[4]

Metal salts (aluminum chlorohydrate, aluminium zirconium chlorohydrate)
Anticholingeric drugs
Aldehydes (formaldehyde, glutaraldehyde)
Antiadrenergic drugs
Metabolic inhibitors
Miscellaneous (various alcohols, other organic acids)

Several theories have been advanced regarding the mechanism of sweat reduction due to axillary application of metal salts. Papa and Kligman[5] originally proposed that the metal salts damaged the sweat duct, causing the secreted sweat to diffuse into the interstitial space; they have since retracted that theory. Shelley and Hurley[6] proposed that the metal salts combine with intraductal keratin fibrils to cause eccrine duct closure and formation of a horny plug to obstruct sweat flow to the skin surface.[6] A second paper by Holzle and Kligman[7] also provided evidence that the metal salts cause a physical obstruction of the duct opening.[7]

Anticholinergic drugs are the most effective antiperspirant agents known. Blockage of the cholinergic innervation of the eccrine sweat glands effectively stops sweating. Agents such as scopolamine and atropine have been studied in this regard; however, skin penetration is poor unless administered via injection or iontophoresis. Furthermore, their action is nonspecific, allowing for side affects such as dry mouth, urinary retention, and mydriasis. No antiperspirants containing anticholinergic drugs are available for over-the-counter purchase in the United States at this time.

Aldehydes, such as formaldehyde and glutaraldehyde, can effectively decrease axillary sweating.[8,9] It is believed that these chemicals also result in blockage of the eccrine sweat duct. They are not popular at this time due to the sensitizing potential of formaldehye and the brownish-yellow skin staining associated with glutaraldehye.

Antiadrenergic drugs theoretically could also decrease sweating. Adrenergic neurotransmitters, such as epinephrine and norepinephrine, have been shown to decrease sweating in humans when they are injected intradermally. This is perhaps due to some adrenergic nerve fibers providing dual innervation to the sweat glands in addition to the cholinergic fibers. But this aspect of sweating is poorly understood. There are no commercially marketed antiperspirants of this type in the United States.

Lastly, metabolic inhibitors may decrease perspiration. Since the process of sweating is dependent upon a supply of energy, drugs that interrupt Na^+/K^+-ATPase, such as ouabain, might also be effective. These substances are only of academic interest.

Formulation of Antiperspirants

Metal salts of aluminum, zirconium, zinc, iron, chromium, lead, and mercury have astringent properties on the skin. The only two metal salts that are presently used in antiperspirants are aluminum and zirconium.[10] Zirconium salts, however, have had an interesting safety profile over the last 35 years. In 1955, sodium zirconyl lactate was used in deodorant sticks, but was found to cause axillary granuloma formation.[11,12] In 1973, aerosol zirconium-based products were voluntarily removed from the market by several manufacturers who had received reports of skin irritation. Aerosol zirconium-based products were banned by the FDA in 1977, but no such products were left on the market at that time. Nonaerosol formulations at concentrations less than 20% are still allowed, but the incidence of axillary granulomas has greatly decreased.[13,14]

The original antiperspirant formulation developed in 1914 was a 25% solution of aluminum chloride hexahydrate in distilled water.[15] This solution was so effective that every second or third day application reduced axillary moisture. However, the solution is extremely irritating to skin and its high acidity damaging to clothing. Newer, less irritating aluminum formulations are more popular today, but they are also less effective. The FDA did express some concern in 1978 regarding long-term inhalation of aluminum-containing aerosol preparations.[16]

Commonly used active agents in antiperspirants include aluminum chloride (concentration of 15% or less in an aqueous nonaerosol dosage form), aluminum chlorohydrate (concentration of 25% or less in an aerosol and nonaerosol dosage form), aluminum zirconium chlorohydrate (concentration of 20% or less or a nonaerosol dosage form), and buffered aluminum sulfate (concentration of 8% or less aluminum sulfate buffered with an 8% concentration of sodium aluminum lactate in a nonaerosol dosage form).[17] Other additives are employed to package the product as a stick, roll-on, or spray antiperspirant. Stick antiperspirants are packaged in a roll-up tube and consist of waxes, oils, volatile silicones, antibacterials, and aluminum or aluimum/zirconium complexes. Roll-on products are an emulsion or clear liquid applied with a rolling ball mechanism to the armpits. These consist of aluminum chlorohydrate as the active ingredient in combination with gelling agents, emollients, and antibacterials. The spray antiperspirants are aluminum chlorohydrate complexes, oils, solvents, and antibacterials propelled by hydrocarbon gases.[18,19]

Effectiveness of Antiperspirants

To be effective, an antiperspirant must reduce axillary sweating by 20% or more. Interestingly, antiperspirant effectiveness is dependent upon both the formulation and the form in which the product is applied, as demonstrated in Table 21-1. "Efficacy" is defined as the percentage reduction in the rate of sweating achieved after application of the antiperspirant product. The percentage of sweating reduction can be determined gravimetrically, where a human volunteer holds an absorbant pad in the armpit while in a hot room, or hygrometrically, where the water content of dry gas sprayed in the armpit of a human volunteer is measured and the rate of sweating calculated.[3]

Mechanism of Action of Deodorants

Deodorants function either by masking the axillary odor with a perfume or by decreasing axillary bacteria, such as *Staphylococcus aureus, Corynebacteria,* and *Aerobacter aerogenes.* Therefore, many deodorant's are antibacterials that function by decreasing the axillary pH to 4.5 or less.[20]

Table 21-1. Antiperspirant Effectiveness by Form (U.S. FDA Over-the-Counter Antiperspirant Review Panel)

Dosage Form	Average Reduction (%)
Aerosols	20–33
Creams	35–47
Roll-ons	14–70
Lotions	28–62
Liquids	15–54
Sticks	35–40

Formulation of Deodorants

Many antibacterial agents are suitable for formulation as deodorants: quaternary ammonium compounds (benzethonium chloride) and cationic compounds (chlorhexidine, triclosan). A popular additive of deodorants and deodorant soaps, hexachlorophene, was banned by the FDA in all nonprescription products in September 1972. Many companies were forced to reformulate their deodorant products at that time, since it had been shown that brain lesions were produced in test animals fed high doses of hexachlorophene.[1]

Sometimes the vehicle of a product can act as an antibacterial such as ethyl alcohol. Additionally, certain botanicals such as thyme oil (thymol) and clove oil (eugenol) have antibacterial properties.

Deodorant Effectiveness

The effectiveness of a deodorant can be measured in two ways: bacterial culture plates and the sniff test. Application of a proposed deodorant formulation to a culture plate swabbed with human perspiration can determine the percent reduction of bacterial growth, but this is not the best method to evaluate consumer acceptability of a deodorant product. Most companies retain several individuals with highly trained noses to "sniff" armpits before and after application of a deodorant. Perspiration is usually induced by placing the subject in a hot room, and a cupped hand is waved across the armpit to bring the odor to the trained nose.[3]

Application

Antiperspirants and deodorants are designed for application to a clean, dry armpit. All products contain warnings stating that use should be discontinued if irritation develops.

Adverse Reactions

The major drawback of aluminum and zirconium salt antiperspirants is their acidic pH (pH 1.8 to 4.2), which can irritate the skin, cause clothing discoloration, and weaken natural fabrics such as linen and cotton. Aluminum and zirconium chlorhydrates have the least skin irritancy. The sulfate forms are intermediate, and chloride forms are the most irritating. Zinc oxide, magnesium oxide, aluminum hydroxide, and triethanolamine may be added to reduce irritancy in some products.

Many patients who develop underarm irritation to aerosol antiperspirants/deodorants find that they can tolerate the roll-on type better or possibly need a product designed for sensitive skin in a cream or stick form. Certainly, these products are a common cause of irritant contact dermatitis in abraded underarm skin.[21] A variety of different ingredients in antiperspirants and deodorants have been reported as causes of dermatitis: vitamin E,[22] propantheline,[23] quaternary ammonium compounds,[24] and so forth. These products are open patch tested "as is."

SHAVING PREPARATIONS

Shaving preparations are intended to decrease the amount of trauma that results from using a sharp metal blade to remove hair from the body. They are available as preshave products, shaving products and aftershave products.

History

The development of shaving products was necessary when the practice of shaving increased in popularity. Alexander the Great is credited with popularizing shaving among the Greeks in order to prevent the beard from being used as an aid for throat slashing or decapitation. From the 14th century to World War I, shaving soaps were the main preparation available. Lathering shaving creams were introduced in 1936 and continue in popularity.[25]

Formulation

Preshave Products

Preshave products, popular among men who use an electric razor, are designed to reduce friction between the shaver and the beard, thus allowing greater pressure to be applied on the shaver. This allows a closer shave, but with reduced irritation. These are mainly fragranced alcoholic solutions that reduce surface friction by reducing surface moisture and dry the hair, allowing it to stand more upright. Some products also contain volatile silicones to function as lubricants.[26]

Shaving Products

Shaving products may be formulated as soaps, sticks, powders, and creams. However, aerosol shaving creams have virtually replaced the other forms.[27] Shaving creams are essentially a modern version of fatty acid shaving soaps, but with an increased amount of water and additives to ensure stability. The goal of a shaving cream is to allow a close shave without removing excess stratum corneum or promoting corrosion of the razor blade. This can only be accomplished if the hair is softened through adequate hydration and the skin lubricated. The force required to cut water-saturated beard hair is about 65% less than that for dry hair.[28,29] Thus, an effective shaving cream should possess low solution viscosity, high foam density, small molecular diameter, low solute concentration, good detergent action, low film strength, and high diffusivity.[25]

Shaving creams are formulated as foaming shaving creams and postfoaming shave gels. There is some evidence that postfoaming shave gels are superior lubricants over shave foams. The reason for this is not clear, but may be related to the orientation of the fatty acids into the lamellar layers necessary to form a gel.[30]

Shaving creams contain either sodium or potassium hydroxide, a superfatting agent (stearic acid, vegetable oils, mineral oil, or lanolin) and glycerol or propylene glycol to allow the cream to remain soft and improve lather by aiding moisture retention. Menthol is added to some preparations to provide both fragrance and a cooling effect on the skin. Beard softeners are wetting agents such as sulfuric acid esters of lauryl alcohol or fatty acid amides.

Aftershave products

Aftershave products function to relieve the discomfort induced by shaving. They are designed to sooth and cool the skin while imparting a feeling of well-being. The fragranced alcoholic lotions are the most popular. Other additives may include menthol for its cooling effect, an antibacterial to prevent infection, and glycerol or propylene glycol to act as an emollient and humectant.[31] These products have enjoyed a renewed popularity as they are now formulated to cross over into the fragrance market for men.

Application

Proper shaving cream application is important in patients who are prone to develop irritant contact dermatitis. These patients generally do not allow the skin and hair shaft to absorb sufficient moisture prior to shaving. A shaving cream left in contact with the skin for at least 4 minutes will decrease razor trauma in most patients. Some patients will require additional lubrication and softening, which can be provided by applying a lipid-free cleanser to the area for an additional 15 minutes followed by shaving cream application. A more detailed discussion regarding shaving techniques is found in Chapter.

Adverse Reactions

Preshave, shaving, and aftershave preparations may cause irritant contact dermatitis since they are used on skin that may not possess an intact stratum corneum. Patients with easily irritated skin should avoid preshave and aftershave lotions that contain high alcohol concentrations. Shaving creams, on the other hand, are necessary to reduce razor burn and should be used by all individuals. Reports of allergic and irritant contact dermatitis reactions to these products, aside from fragrance allergies, are rare. The products may be open patch tested "as is."

REFERENCES

1. Mueller WH, Quatrale RP: Antiperspirants and deodorants. p. 205. In deNavarre MG (ed): The Chemistry and Manufacture of Cosmetics. Allured Publishing Corporation, Wheaton, IL, 1975
2. Plechner S: Antiperspirants and deodorants. p. 373. In Balsam MD, Safarin E (eds): Cosmetics, Science and Technology. Vol. 2, 2nd Ed. Wiley-Interscience, New York, 1972
3. Wilkinson JB, Moore RJ: Harry's Cosmeticology. 7th Ed. Chemical Publishing, New York, 1982
4. Quatrale RP: The mechanism of antiperspirant action in eccrine sweat glands. p. 89. In Ladan K, Felger CB (eds). Antiperspirants and Deodorants. Marcel Dekker, Inc., New York, 1988
5. Papa CM, Kligman AM: Mechanisms of eccrine anhidrosis: II. The antiperspirant effects of aluminum salts. J Invest Dermatol 49:139, 1967
6. Shelley WB, Hurley HJ Jr: Studies on topical antiperspirant control of axillary hyperhidrosis. Acta Dermatol Venereol 55:241, 1975
7. Holzle E, Kligman AM: Mechanism of antiperspiration action of aluminum salts. J Soc Cosmet Chem 30:279, 1979
8. Juhlin L: Topical glutaraldehyde for plantar hyperhidrosis. Arch Dermatol 97: 327,1968
9. Sato K, Dobson RL: Mechanism of the antiperspirant effect of topical glutaraldehyde. Arch Dermatol 100:564, 1969
10. Jass HE: Rationale of formulations of deodorants and antiperspirants. p. 98. In Frost P, Horwitz SN (eds): Principles of Cosmetics for the Dermatologist. CV Mosby Company, St. Louis, 1982
11. Rubin L, Slepyan H, Weber LF et al: Granulomas of the axilla caused by deodorants. JAMA 162:953, 1956
12. Shelled WB, Hurley KJ: The allergic origin of zirconium deodorant granulomas. Br J Dermatol 70:75, 1958
13. Lisi DM: Availability of zirconium in topical antiperspirants. Arch Intern Med 152:421, 1992
14. Skelton HG, Smith KJ, Johnson FB et al: Zirconium granuloma resulting from an aluminum zirconium complex. J Am Acad Dermatol 28:874, 1993
15. Emery IK: Antiperspirants and deodorants. Cutis 39:531, 1987
16. Klepak PB: Aluminum and health: a perspective. Cosmet Toilet 105:53, 1990
17. Morton JJP, Palazzolo MJ: Antiperspirants. p. 221. In Whittam JH (ed): Cosmetic Safety: a Primer for Cosmetic Scientists. Marcel Dekker, Inc, New York, 1987
18. Calogero AV: Antiperspirant and deodorant formulation. Cosmet Toilet 107:63, 1992
19. Walder D, Penneys NS: Antiperspirants and deodorizers. Clin Dermatol 6:29, 1988
20. Chavkin L: Antiperspirants and deodorants. Cutis 23:24, 1979
21. Mukin W, Cohen HJ, Frank SB: Contact dermatitis from deodorants. Arch Dermatol 107:775, 1973
22. Aeling JL, Panagotacos PJ, Andreozzi RJ: Allergic contact dermatitis to vitamin E in aerosol deodorant. Arch Dermatol 108:579, 1973
23. Hannuksela M: Allergy to propantheline in an antiperspirant. Contact Dermatitis 1:244, 1975

24. Shmunes E, Levy EJ: Quaternary ammonium compound contact dermatitis from a deodorant. Arch Dermatol 105:91, 1972
25. Saute RE: Shaving preparations. p. 1313. In deNavarre MG (ed): The Chemistry and Manufacture of Cosmetics. Allured Publishing Corporation, Wheaton, IL, 1975
26. Brooks GJ, Burmeister F: Preshave and aftershave products. Cosmet Toilet 15:67, 1990
27. Flaherty FE: Updating the art of shaving. Cosmet Toilet 91:23, 1976
28. Deem DE, Rieger MM: Observations on the cutting of beard hair. J Soc Cosmet Chem 27:579, 1976
29. Breuer MM, Sneath RL, Ackerman CS: Perceptual evaluation of shaving closeness. J Soc Cosmet Chem 40:141, 1989
30. Wickett RR: The effect of gels and foams on shaving comfort and efficacy. Skin Care 2:1, 1993
31. Bell SA: Preshave and aftershave preparations. p. 13. In Balsam MD, Safarin E (eds): Cosmetics, Science and Technology. Vol. 2. 2nd Ed. Wiley-Interscience, New York, 1972

22

Perfumes and Fragrances

Perfumes and fragrances are of paramount importance in the formulation of cosmetics for their intrinsic value of imparting a pleasant smell to the body and for their ability to mask undesirable raw material odors. A perfume may enhance the perception of product performance or act as a preservative. The use of fragrance to affect mood or induce relaxation is known as "aromatherapy."[1] Perfumery is certainly an art of blending and mixing, with more than 6,000 possible ingredients to obtain a special scent.

HISTORY

Originally, perfume was used in the form of incense for religious purposes. The word itself is Latin for "through the smoke."[2] Incense was thus a deodorizer to mask the smell of burning flesh when an animal was sacrificed to the gods. The transition from incense to perfumes for adornment occurred about 6,000 bc in both the Far East and the Middle East. By 3,000 bc, the Sumerians and Egyptians were bathing in oils and alcohols of jasmine, iris, hyacinth, and honeysuckle. Cleopatra is said to have anointed her hands with an oil of roses, crocus, and violets and her feet with a lotion of almond oil, honey, cinnamon, orange blossoms, and tinting henna. Greek and Roman men both embraced perfumes to the point where a soldier was considered unfit for battle unless he was duly anointed with fragrances. As the Roman Empire conquered other lands, they introduced their own perfumes and acquired new fragrances.

The concept of cologne was introduced by an Italian barber, Jean-Baptiste Farina, who arrived in Cologne, Germany, in 1709 to develop a fragrance trade. He concocted an alcoholic blend of lemon spirits, orange bitters, and mint oil from the bergamot fruit that became the first cologne. Soon perfume meant any mixture of ethyl alcohol with 25% or more essential fragrant oils, toilet water with 5% essential oils, and cologne with 3% essential oils.

FORMULATION

The raw materials for perfume formulation fall into two categories: natural and synthetic. Natural components are of animal or plant origin, while synthetic ones are produced from a wide range of raw materials. The use of animal extracts in perfumery has declined because of animal rights issue; however, animal-derived products still include musk from the musk deer, castoreum from the beaver, civet from the civet cat, and ambergris from the sperm whale. Most of these substances have been chemically analyzed and are now synthesized.[3]

Plant products comprise the majority of substances used within perfumery. These extracts can be obtained through steam distillation, expression, and extraction. Distillation is the method used for removal of geranium, lavender, rose, and orange blossom (known as neroli) scents. Expression is used to squeeze the oil from the peeling of begamot, lemon, lime, and other citrus fruits. If the aromatic substance is unstable at the higher temperatures required for distillation or the yield of the oil minimal through expression, then extraction is employed.

Extraction can be accomplished by enfleurage, maceration or the use of volatile solvents. Enfleurage involves the use of animal fats or vegetable oils to extract the scent at room temperature. The flower petals are sprinkled on glass plates encased in wooden frames that have been brushed with fats or oils. The wooden frames are then stacked to sandwich the petals between two glass plates. Fresh petals are added daily until the grease, known as a pomade, absorbs a sufficient amount of perfume. This method is used for extracting the perfume of jasmine, orange blossom, jonquil, and lily.[4] If heat is added, then the extraction technique is termed *maceration*. Here the flowers are mixed with hot liquid fats or oils at 60° to 70°C and stirred until the cells containing the fragrance

Table 22-1. Common Fragrance Materials

Fragrance Material	Characteristics
Benzyl acetate	Light floral, slightly fruity
Benzyl salicylate	Warm, balsamic
Iso-bornyl acetate	Fresh, piney
P-t-butyl cyclohexyl acetate	Soft, woody
Cedryl acetate	Sharp, woody
Citronellol	Rosy
Dihydro myrcenol	Citrus
Geraniol	Floral, rosy
Heliotropine	Sweet, floral, powdery
Hexyl cinnamic aldehyde	Light, delicate
Indole	Floral, animalic
Gamma-methyl ionone	Woody, floral
Musk ketone	Musky, animalic, warm
Phenyl ethyl alcohol	Floral
Vanillin	Sweet, powdery, vanilla

(Adapted from Dallimore,[7] with permission.)

rupture. The mixture is then poured on a screen allowing the scented grease to drain. Rose, acacia, and violet perfumes are obtained in this manner. Volatile solvents and percolators are used to extract the essential oils of mimosa, carnation, heliotrope, stock, and oakmoss.[5]

Steam distillates are termed *essential oils,* while solvent extracts result in a nearly solid perfume wax referred to as *concretes.* Ethanolic extractions of concretes yields *absolutes,* but if raw materials are subjected to ethanolic extraction *tinctures* are produced. Organic solvent extraction yields *resinoids,* which can be further extracted with ethanol to yield *resin absolutes.*[6] All parts of the plant, including roots, fruits, leaves, flowers, bark, and rind, can be used in perfume production. Of the 250,000 species of flowering plants, only 2,000 contain essential oils appropriate for fragrance production.

Synthetic fragrances are becoming more popular due to cost and inability to obtain natural animal and plant sources. Table 22-1 lists some of the more common aroma chemicals used in perfumery today.[7]

A special vocabulary is use to describe fragrances as briefly outlined in Table 22-2. The perception of smell is very subjective, accounting for the tremendous

Table 22-2. Odor Descriptors

Odor	Description
Aldehydic	Sharp, fatty or soapy
Amber	Sweet, warm
Animalic	Redolent of animal odors
Balsamic	Warm, sweet and resinous
Camphoraceous	Medicated
Chemical	Harsh, aggressive and basic
Citrus	Fresh, tangy and zesty
Earthy	Green, rooty and dank
Fatty	Odor of animal or vegetable oil
Floral	Odor of flowers
Fresh	Used subjectively
Fruity	Odor of natural fruit
Green	Odor of grass or leaves
Herbal	Odor of fresh plants
Leather	Phenolic, warm and animalic
Light	Discrete
Medicinal	Pungent
Mossy	Earthy, mossy, phenolic or green
Nutty	Odor of natural nuts
Pine	Odor or fine wood, needles and resin
Powdery	Soft, gentle
Resinous	Warm, sweet, balsamic
Spicy	Pungent, hot, culinary
Sweet	Heavy, cloying
Warm	Ambery, animalic, sweet
Woody	Odor of natural wood

(Adapted from Dallmore,[7] with permission.)

number of popular perfumes presently on the market. A successful formulation is a prized secret among fragrance manufacturers. Generally, perfumes fall into three categories:

Simple notes representing naturally occurring aromas, such as fruits, herbs, spices, flowers, and animal smells

Complexes representing combinations of odors, such as green floral, spicy citrus, and fruity floral

Multicomplexes representing up to 12 identifiable fragrance themes

Perfumes are further described by the manner in which their smell changes with time.[8] The top note of a perfume refers to the rapidly evaporating oils that are discernible when the bottle is opened, but disappear shortly after skin application. The middle note is the smell of the dried perfume on the skin, and the end note is the ability of the perfume to diffuse fragrance over time.[9]

ADVERSE REACTIONS

Irritant and allergic contact dermatitis reactions to perfumes and fragrances are well-known phenomena.[10–13] In fact, fragrances have been reported as the most common cause of cosmetics–related allergic contact dermatitis.[14] The North American Contact Dermatitis Group reported that cinnamic aldehyde, a fragrance material, was one of the 10 most common allergens on the standard dermatology patch test tray.[15] Table 22-3 lists some of the more common fragrances and their irritancy potential as represented in the fragrance literature.[16] Table 22-4 lists some of the common fragrances and their allergenic potential as represented in the dermatologic literature.[17] The North American Contact Dermatitis Group found the following fragrance materials to be sources of allergic contact dermatitis, in order of decreasing frequency: cinnamic alcohol, hydroxycitronellal, musk ambrette, isoeugenol, geraniol, cinnamic aldehyde, coumarin, and eugenol.[18] Certainly, patients with fragrance sensitivities require special counseling.[19]

Fragrance sensitivities can be detected by patch testing with a fragrance mixture containing the most common fragrance allergens. It consists of a 2% concentration of cinnamic alcohol, cinnamic aldehyde, eugenol, isoeugenol, hydroxycitronellal, oakmoss absolute, geraniol, and alpha-amyl cinnamic alcohol in petrolatum.[20] Unfortunately, irritant reactions can occur.[21] This mixture detects approximately 70% to 80% of fragrance sensitivities.[17] Further evaluation of the allergic contact dermatitis needs to be evaluated with individual fragrances.[22] The patient's perfume can also be used for patch testing if diluted to a 10% to 30% concentration in alcohol or petrolatum. Interestingly, Balsam of Peru, one of the standard substances on a patch test tray, serves as a marker for fragrance sensitivity and is patch test positive in about 50% of cases of

Table 22-3. Irritant Potential of Perfumes

Irritating perfumes
    Benzylidene acetone
    Methyl heptin carbonate
    Methyl octin carbonate
Moderately irritating perfumes
    Cyclamen aldehyde
    Ethyl methylphenyl glycinate
    Eugenols gamma-nonyl lactone
    Balsam of peru
    Phenylacetaldehyde
    Vanillin
Least irritating perfumes
    Benzaldehyde
    Benzoin resin
    Benzyl benzoate
    Cinnamic acid and cinnamates
    Citrus oils
    Cresol and methyl cresol
    Diethyl phthalate
    Heliotropin
    Higher aliphatic aldehydes
    Hydroxycitronellal
    Menthol
    Salicylates

(Adapted from Wells and Lubowe,[16] with permission.)

Table 22-4. Allergic Potential of Perfumes

Perfume	Allergic Potential	Patch Test Concentration in Petrolatum
Cinnamic alcohol	High	5%
Cinnamic aldehyde	High	1%
Hydroxycitronellal	High	4%
Isoeugenol	High	5%
Eugenol	High	5%
Oakmoss absolute	High	5%
Alpha-amyl cinnamic alcohol	Moderate	5%
Geraniol	Moderate	5%
Benzyl salicylate	Moderate	2%
Sandalwood oil	Moderate	2%
Anisyl alcohol	Moderate	5%
Benzyl alcohol	Moderate	5%
Coumarin	Moderate	5%
Musk ambrette	Photoallergen	5%

(Adapted from Larsen,[17] with permission.)

perfume allergy. More extensive information regarding patch testing for perfumes can be obtained in the text by DeGroot et al.[23]

Determining the source of fragrance allergies can be quite complex.[24] The average soap contains 50 to 150 fragrance ingredients, the average cosmetic contains 200 to 500 fragrance ingredients, and the average perfume contains 700 fragrance ingredients.[25] The concentration of fragrance ingredients also varies. Fine perfumes contain 15% to 30% fragrance, colognes contain 5% to 8% fragrance, scented cosmetics contain 0.1% to 1% fragrance, while masking fragrances are used at concentrations below 0.1%.[26] Most cosmetics houses are able to provide fragrance products for testing, or fragrance fractions can be analyzed through gas chromatography or infrared spectroscopy.[27]

REFERENCES

1. Jackson EM: Aromatherapy. Am J Contact Dermatitis 4:240,1993
2. Panati C: Extraordinary Origins of Everyday Things. Perennial Library, Harper & Row, Publishers, New York, 1987
3. Launert E: Scent & Scent Bottles. Barrie & Jenkins, London, 1974
4. Guin JD: History, manufacture, and cutaneous reactions to perfumes. p. 111. In Frost P, Horwitz SN (eds): Prinicples of Cosmetics for the Dermatologist. CV Mosby Company, St. Louis, 1982
5. Ellis A: The Essence of Beauty. The Macmillan Company, New York, 1960
6. Balsam MS: Fragrance. p. 599. In Balsam MD, Gerson SD, Rieger MM et al. (eds): Cosmetics Science and Technology. 2nd Ed. Wiley-Interscience. New York, 1972
7. Dallimore A: Perfumery. p. 258. In Williams DF, Schmitt WH (eds): Chemistry and Technology of the Cosmetics and Toiletries Industry. Blackie Academic & Professional, London, 1992
8. Jellinek JS: Evaporation and the odor quality of perfumes. J Soc Cosmet Chem 12:168,1961
9. Poucher WA: A classification of odours and its uses. J Soc Cosmet Chem 6:80,1955
10. Rothengorg HW, Hjorth N: Allergy to perfumes from toilet soaps and detergents in patients with dermatitis. Arch Dermatol 97:417, 1963
11. Maibach HI: Fragrance hypersensitivity. Cosmet Toilet 106:25,1991
12. Maibach HI: Fragrance hypersensitivity, part II. Cosmet Toilet 106:35,1991
13. Larsen WG, Maibach HI: Fragrance contact allergy. Semin Dermatol 1:85,1982
14. Eiermann HJ, Larsen WG, Maibach HI, Taylor JS: Prospective study of cosmetic reactions, 1977–1980. J Am Acad Dermatol 6:909,1982
15. Storrs FJ, Rosenthal LE, Adams RM et al: Prevalence and relevance of allergic reactions in patients patch tested in North America. J Am Acad Dermatol 20:1038,1989
16. Wells FV, Lubowe II: Cosmetics and the Skin. Reinhold Publishing Corporation, New York, 1964
17. Larsen WG: Perfume dermatitis. J Am Acad Dermatol 12:1,1985
18. Adams RM, Maibach HI: A five-year study of cosmetic reactions. J Am Acad Dermatol 13:1062,1985

19. Larsen WG: How to instruct patients sensitive to fragrances. J Am Acad Dermatol 21:880,1989
20. Larsen WG: Perfume dermatitis: a study of 20 patients. Arch Dermatol 113: 623,1977
21. Calnan CD, Cronin E, Rycroft R: Allergy to perfume ingredients. Contact Dermatitis 6:500,1980
22. Fisher AA: Patch testing with perfume ingredients. Contact Dermatitis 1:166,1975
23. DeGroot AC, Weyland JW, Nater JP: Unwanted Effects of Cosmetics and Drugs Used in Dermatology. Elsevier, Amsterdam, 1994
24. Larsen WG: Cosmetic dermatitis due to a perfume. Contact Dermatitis 1:142,1975
25. Jackson EM: Substantiating the safety of fragrances and fragranced products. Cosmet Toilet 108:43,1993
26. Marks JG, DeLeo VA: Contact and Occupational Dermatology, Mosby Yearbook, St. Louis, 1992
27. Yates RL: Analysis of perfumes and fragrances. p. 126. In Senzel AJ (ed): Newburger's Manual of Cosmetic Analysis. 2nd Ed. Published by the Association of Official Analytical Chemists, Inc, Washington, DC, 1977

23

Photoaging, Sunscreens, and Cosmeceuticals

It is well recognized that sun exposure can prematurely age the skin, as well as induce carcinogenesis. Nevertheless, the practice of obtaining a tan from the sun remains popular, and the development of tanning salons has now made light exposure accessible year around to individuals in all locations. Tanning probably remains popular since there is a 20 to 30 year delay between the cutaneous injury and the onset of visible effects, such as wrinkling, dyspigmentation, telangiectasia, and so forth. While the young are tanning, mature individuals are in search of sunscreens and cosmeceuticals to undo actinic damage. This chapter examines photoaging, sunscreens, and cutaneous cosmeceuticals.

PHOTOAGING

Aging of the skin can be classified into two components: Intrinsic and extrinsic aging. As the names imply, intrinsic aging is due to genetically controlled senescence, and extrinsic aging is due to environmental factors superimposed on intrinsic aging. Environmental factors known to accelerate extrinsic aging are sun exposure and cigarette smoking. Cutaneous aging due to sun exposure is known as "photoaging."[1]

Youthful skin is characterized by its unblemished, evenly pigmented, smooth, pink appearance. This is in contrast to intrinsically aged skin, which is thin, inelastic, and finely wrinkled with deepening of facial expression lines.[2] These changes are evident histologically as a thinned epidermis and dermis with flattening of the rete pegs at the dermoepidermal junction.[3] Extrinsically aged, sun-exposed skin appears clinically as blemished, thickened, yellowed, lax, rough, and leathery.[4] These changes may begin as early as the second decade[5]

Table 23-1. Glogau Classification of Photoaging Groups

Group 1, mild
    No keratoses
    Little wrinkling
    No scarring
    Little or no make-up
    Usually aged 28–35 years
Group 2, moderate
    Early actinic keratoses
    Slight yellow skin discoloration
    Early wrinkling (parallel smile lines)
    Mild scarring
    Little make-up
    Usually aged 35–50 years
Group 3, advanced
    Actinic keratoses
    Obvious yellow skin discoloration with telangiectasia
    Wrinkling present at rest
    Moderate acne scarring
    Always wears make-up
    Usually aged 50–65
Group 4, severe
    Actinic keratoses and skin cancers have occurred
    Wrinkling of actinic gravitational and dynamic origin
    Severe acne scarring
    Wears make-up, but does not cover well
    Usually aged 60–75 years

and can be used to divide photoaged skin into the four groups of the Glogau Classification (Table 23-1). It may also contain precancerous and cancerous growths, as well as telangiectasias and lentigines.[6] Some of the propensity toward cancerous growths may be due to a decrease in Langerhans cells and their function.[7] Photoaged skin is characterized histologically by epidermal dysplasia with varying degrees of cytologic atypia, loss of keratinocyte polarity, an inflammatory infiltrate, decreased collagen, increased ground substance, and elastosis. Elastosis is the degradation of elastic material, which, in early photoaging, is increased in amount and seen microscopically as thickened, twisted, degraded elastic fibers.[8] These fibers degenerate into an amorphous mass as photoaging progresses.[9] Thus, intrinsic aging of the skin results in atrophy, while extrinsic photoaging results in hypertrophy. This distinction is not always clinically apparent, but in ideal cases intrinsically aged skin has fine wrinkling, while photoaged skin demonstrates coarse wrinkling and furrowing.[10]

Cutaneous sun exposure accelerates and exaggerates the clinical changes associated with advanced age.[11] Thus, individuals turn to cosmetics that can aid in the camouflage of telangiectasias and lentigines, but they cannot conceal the deep wrinkling caused by photoaging. Facial foundations become difficult to apply evenly and tend to migrate into cutaneous furrows. The yellow skin hue imparted by elastosis can be improved by use of a purple undercover cosmetic, but, again, uniform application is difficult. The patient may attempt to solve these problems by using a high-coverage cream foundation. Unfortunately, thicker facial foundations, which can cover skin color abnormalities, only accentuate the deep wrinkling and furrows. One possible cosmetic solution is to use a white eyeliner pencil to line the depths of each furrow followed by application of a moderate-coverage facial foundation appropriate for the patient's skin type (see Tables 1-3 to 1-6). The white pigment placed at the depth of each furrow will make the recessed skin less shadowed, based on the concepts presented in Chapter 7. Lining each furrow is time-consuming but can improve, although not eliminate, the photoaged skin appearance.

SUNSCREENS

The recognition that sun protection can decrease and possibly reverse the effects of photoaging of the skin has led to the inclusion of sunscreens in suntan preparations, facial foundations, facial moisturizers, and hair care preparations. These items are sometimes labeled treatment products, antiaging products, protective products, or defense products based on their inclusion of sunscreens. This class of over-the-counter drug is of particular importance to the dermatologist.

History

The first sunscreen was marketed in the United States in 1928 and consisted of an emulsion of benzyl salicylate and benzyl cinnamate. *p*-Aminobenzoic acid (PABA) was introduced in 1943, which initiated many new sunscreen formulations. Physical agents, such as red petrolatum, were used by the military during World War II.[12] In 1978, the RDA reclassified sunscreens from cosmetics to over-the-counter drugs designed to protect ''the structure and function of the human integument against actinic damage.''[13]

Formulation

Sunscreens can be divided into two types: chemical sunblocks and physical sunblocks. Chemical sunblocks such as the PABA esters, cinnamates, benzophenones, salicylates, and anthranilates contain molecules that absorb the radiant light energy, while physical sunblocks such as titanium dioxide, magnesium oxide, magnesium silicate, zinc oxide, iron oxide, red veterinary petrolatum, and kaolin place a coating on the skin that reflects the light. Sun-protective clothing can also act as a physical sunscreen.[14]

Chemical Sunscreens

Chemical sunscreens function by absorbing photons of light energy. They are generally aromatic compounds based on the benzene ring's ability to transform high energy ultraviolet radiation into harmless long wave radiation above the 380 nm range. This phenomenon is accomplished via resonance delocalization. The long wave radiation is emitted from the skin as heat.[15]

Chemical sunscreens absorb 95% of the UV radiation within wavelengths of 290 to 320 nm. This is the UVB spectrum, known as the sunburn range since these wavelengths of light energy produce skin erythema and wrinkling. Most current chemical sunscreens do not block light energy from 320 to 400 nm, the UVA range. UVA exposure can produce direct tanning of the skin without the preceding erythema produced by UVB exposure. It is known, however, that UVA exposure can produce elastic tissue damage, actinic skin damage, and contribute to the formation of skin cancer.

The FDA has rated the chemicals listed in Table 23-2 as safe, effective sunscreening agents to be used in over-the-counter products.[16,17] There are many more chemicals presently available and in use in Europe. Among the many chemicals listed, PABA derivatives, benzophenones, and cinnamates are the most popular.

Table 23-2. Sunscreening Agent Concentrations Allowed in the United States (FDA-OTC Panel)

UBV absorbers	
Aminobenzoic acid	5–15%
Amyl dimethyl PABA	1–5%
2-Ethoxyethyl p-methoxycinnamate	1–3%
Diethanolamine p-methoxycinnamate	8–10%
Digalloyl trioleate	2–5%
Ethyl 4-bis (hydroxypropyl) aminobenzoate	1–5%
2-Ethylhexyl-2-cyano-3,3-diphenyl-acrylate	7–10%
Ethylhexyl p-methoxycinnamate	2–7.5%
2-Ethylhexyl salicylate	3–5%
Glyceryl aminobenzoate	2–3%
Homomenthyl salicylate	4–25%
Lawsone with dihydroxyacetone	0.25%, 3%
Octyl dimentyl PABA	1.4–8%
2-Penylbenzimidazole-5-sulfonic acid	1.4%
Triethanolamine salicylate	5–12%
UVA absorbers	
Oxybenzone	2–6%
Sulisobenzone	5–10%
Dioxybenzone	3%
Menthyl anthranilate	3.5–5%
Physical agents	
Red petrolatum	3–100%
Titanium dioxide	2–25%

Table 23-3. UVA Chemical Sunscreening Agents

Anthranilates
Benzophenones (oxygenzone, sulisobenzone, dioxybenzone)
Eusolex 2020
Parsol 1789

PABA esters, such as octyl dimethyl PABA (padimate O), have replaced pure PABA because of lower skin sensitization and less irritation. The PABA esters also do not stain cotton and synthetic fibers, such as polyester or nylon. Their substantivity to the stratum corneum is high, allowing long-standing photoprotection that may be somewhat waterproof. Usually concentrations of 5% to 15% are employed.[18] Their absorption spectrum is in the UVB range, with maximum absorption at 296 nm.

Some chemical sunscreens, however, such as the benzophenones (oxybenzone, dioxybenzone) and anthranilates (menthyl anthranilate), provide coverage partially extending into the UVA range (Table 23-3).[19] These chemicals are incorporated into products that provide broad spectrum coverage.

Many cosmetics companies are now incorporating the cinnamates into their products since the popular press has publicized the possibility of cutaneous allergy to PABA derivatives. The most popular of the cinnamate derivatives is ethylhexyl *p*-methoxycinnamate. Unfortunately, this group of chemicals binds poorly to the stratum corneum, resulting in decreased substantivity. Careful selection of vehicles can overcome this shortcoming, however. The cinnamates absorb light energy primarily at 305 nm.[20]

Mention should be made of the salicylates, one of the first UV filters developed, currently enjoying a renewed popularity. Octyl salicylate, also known as 2-ethyl hexyl salicylate, and homosalate, also known as homomenthyl salicylate, are the two most popular derivatives. They absorb in the range of 300 to 310 nm and are easily incorporated into cosmetics preparations with other chemical sunscreening agents, such as the benzophenones.[12]

Physical Sunscreens

Physical sunscreening agents are opaque formulations containing particulate matter that is able to reflect and scatter light energy. The only sunscreening agents that can completely block UVB, UVA, visible, and infrared light wavelengths are physical sunblocks (Table 23-4).[21] The best UVA protection, however, is obtained by combining a physical sunscreening agent with a broad spectrum UVA sunscreening agent.[22]

Efficacy

Sunscreen products are rated according to their sun protection factor (SPF). The SPF is calculated according to the FDA formula as follows:

UV energy required to produce minimal erythema dose (MED) on protected

Table 23-4. Physical Sunscreening Agents

Kaolin
Magnesium silicate
Magnesium oxide
Red petrolatum
Titanium dioxide
Iron oxide
Zinc oxide
Red veterinary petrolatum

skin/UV energy required to produce a minimal erythema dose (MED) on unprotected skin.

Thus, a patient who experiences reddening of the skin in 10 minutes of sun exposure without protection would be able to stay in the sun 60 minutes before the same degree of erythema developed while wearing a sunscreen with an SPF of 6. Many dermatologists feel that patients should wear a sunscreen with an SPF of 15 or higher to obtain adequate sun protection. Unfortunately, SPF is mainly an evaluation of the UVB light effects on the skin and does not account for the UVA light effects. Methods have been proposed to define a protection factor for UVA (PFA).[23]

The performance of a sunscreen depends on the concentration of the sunscreening agent and its ability to remain on the skin. Increasing the concentration of a sunscreen chemical can increase the SPF; for example, 3% octyl dimethyl PABA has an SPF of 4, while 4% octyl dimethyl PABA has an SPF of 5. Better performance can be obtained with the octyl dimethyl ester of PABA since it is less water soluble than PABA, accounting for its use in waterproof sunscreens and superior performance under humid conditions. Other factors important in sunscreen performance that cannot be controlled are environmental factors such as heat, wind, humidity, perspiration, and thickness of sunscreen film application.[24] Higher SPF sunscreens are not necessarily more irritating than lower SPF varieties.

A superior sunscreen can also be produced by combining sunscreening agents. A sunscreen containing only 8% octyl dimethyl PABA has an SPF of 8, while a sunscreen combining 8% octyl dimethyl PABA with 3% oxybenzone has an SPF of 20. Some sunscreens will also combine chemical and physical sunscreening agents.

Parsol 1789 and Eusolex 2020 are two newer substances active as chemical sunscreens with extended UVA protection. These have recently entered the U.S. market. Other substances under investigation include iron chelators, such as 2-furildioxime,[25] melanin,[26] and beta-carotene.[27]

Adverse Reactions

Sunscreening chemicals are a more common source of irritant than allergic contact dermatitis,[28] but distinguishing dermatitis from solar-induced phenomena can occasionally be difficult.[29,30] Reports of contact urticaria have also been published, but again the urticas may be solar induced rather than sunscreen induced.[31]

PABA is a known sensitizer at a 5% concentration,[32] but few presently marketed sunscreen formulations contains PABA, but rather PABA esters, such as padimate A and padimate O. These PABA esters have a lower sensitization potential.[18]

The cinnamates are also sensitizers even though they are commonly incorporated into hypoallergenic sunscreen formulations. They interact with balsam of Peru, coca leaves, cinnamic acid, cinnamic aldehyde, and cinnamon oils.[33] Both the salicylates[34] and anthranilates are rare sensitizers.[35,36] Photoallergic reactions have been reported with the benzophenones.[37,38]

The physical sunscreening agents are not sensitizers, but are occlusive and can produce miliaria. It has been reported that the inclusion of titanium dioxide in sunscreen formulations reduces the incidence of photoallergic contact dermatitis, possibly due to its ability to reflect ultraviolet radiation.[31]

COSMECEUTICALS

The relatively new term "cosmeceuticals" is designed to describe prescription pharmaceuticals designed to enhance the cosmetic appearance of the body. The only product approved by the FDA for this purpose is 2% minoxidil (Rogaine, Upjohn), marketed to treat both male and female pattern hair loss. Topical tretinoin (Retin-A, Ortho), designed to improve the appearance of photoaged skin, is pending approval at the time of this writing.

Retinoids

While sun avoidance can halt and possibly reverse the effects of cutaneous photoaging, studies have demonstrated that reversal of photoinduced skin changes can be accelerated by topical application of tretinoin, chemically known as all-trans retinoic acid (Retin-A, Ortho).[39–41] Tretinoin is one of many synthetic vitamin A derivatives known collectively as "retinoids."[42] Tretinoin has been shown to transform an atrophic epidermis into a hyperplastic, thicker epidermis, resulting in improvement of skin wrinkling. Wrinkling associated with lines of facial expression is not improved, however. Tretinoin-treated facial skin also demonstrates new papillary dermal collagen synthesis, new blood vessel formation, increased glycosaminoglycan deposition, and exfoliation of retained stratum corneum.[43,44] These histologic changes translate clinically into skin with less yellow and more pink hues accompanied by increased tactile smoothness.[45]

Changes may be perceived in 4 months in some patients who use topical tretinoin daily, but more improvement is seen with longer therapy. Naturally, more improvement is visible in patients with severe photoaging, but results are also seen in non-sun-exposed elderly skin.[46] It is interesting to note improved psychosocial status in patients who undergo topical tretinoin therapy.[47] At present, the effects of tretinoin on intrinsic aging are unknown.

Tretinoin must be applied daily to the face to achieve reversal of photoaging. Patients who initiate treatment may experience varying degrees of erythema and dermatitis for the first 2 to 6 weeks of therapy. It is thought that the skin eventually "hardens" to the irritating effect of the tretinoin, with the disappearance of burning, pruritus, and desquamation.[48] This hardening effect is lost when application is discontinued. There is some disagreement as to whether irritation is required to achieve the beneficial effects. Weiss and Ellis[41] recommend that the strongest concentration of tretinoin be selected and used virtually to the point of intolerance. Severe cases of retinoid dermatitis can be treated with topical corticosteroids.

Tretinoin is photoinactivated and increases cutaneous photosensitivity, so application at night is recommended. Patients should be encouraged to wear a sunscreen to prevent accelerated sun burning and also further photoaging. Application of the tretinoin on a dry face, 20 to 30 minutes after facial cleansing, is recommended to minimize irritation.[49] Sensitive mucous membranes such as the nose and mouth should be avoided, as well as the eyes, although no ill effects other than irritation have been noted following accidental application to these areas.

The long-term effects of topical tretinoin are not known, although no side effects other than dermatitis have been reported to date. The histologic changes previously described are only present during use; the skin assumes its pretreatment appearance 6 weeks after therapy is stopped.

Topical tretinoin treatment may require the patient to change his or her cosmetic routine. During the phase of retinoid dermatitis, a mild cleansing bar may need to be substituted for a deodorant soap to prevent further xerosis and irritation. The use of all drying agents such as astringents and toners, exfoliants, abrasive scrubbers, and cleansing masks should be discontinued unless deemed necessary by the physician. Oil-free or water-based facial foundations will tend to adhere preferentially to facial scale, necessitating the use of an appropriate moisturizer to smooth the desquamating stratum corneum prior to application of foundation. Where possible, foundation with higher oil content can be selected (see Tables 1-3 to 1-6). Cream formulations of tretinoin can be placed under a facial foundation while gel formulations will decrease the foundation wear time. It is recommended, however, that the tretinoin be applied at night when a facial foundation is not worn. Once the retinoid dermatitis has resolved, patients may return to their usual cosmetic routines.

Table 23-5. pH of Glycolic Acid

Concentration (%)	pH
5	1.7
10	1.6
20	1.5
30	1.4
40	1.3
50	1.2
60	1.0
70	0.6

Alpha-hydroxy acids

Alpha-hydroxy acids represent the oldest facial cosmeceuticals, but have recently gained new popularity. It is said that Cleopatra used the debris at the bottom of the wine barrels to massage her face. Chemically, this represented tartaric acid; thus Cleopatra was the first woman recorded to apply facial alpha-hydroxy acids routinely. Alpha-hydroxy acids represent a group of chemicals consisting of organic carboxylic acids in which a hydroxy group is at the alpha position. Members of this group include glycolic, lactic, citric, malic, mandelic, and tartaric acids. Glycolic acid is derived from sugar cane, lactic acid is derived from fermented milk, citric acid is found in citrus fruits, malic acid is found in unripened apples, mandelic acid is an extract of bitter almonds, and tartaric acid is found in fermented grapes.[50] The acids are now produced synthetically for cosmetic use.

Glycolic acid is the most popular of the alpha-hydroxy acids for antiaging purposes available in over-the-counter and physician-dispensed products. Its pH varies with concentration, as demonstrated in Table 23-5. This acidic pH is sometimes buffered for facial application with phosphoric acid and monosodium phosphate or neutralized with sodium hydroxide.[51] A desirable pH for facial application lies between 2.8 and 4.8. Glycolic acid is finding its way into formulations for facial moisturizers, cleansers, and toners. Additionally, it is used alone, or in combination with other chemicals, at various concentrations for facial peels.[52–54] The epidermal effects of glycolic acid are manifested by decreased keratinocyte cohesion, which may be due to alterations in ionic bonding,[55] while the dermal effects result in increased mucopolysaccharide and collagen synthesis.[56] Visibly this translates into less cutaneous wrinkling and dyspigmentation.[57] Furthermore, glycolic acid may act as an antioxidant, as demonstrated by its ability to alleviate the erythema observed after ultraviolet radiation exposure to the skin.[58]

Alpha-hydroxy acids and tretinoin can be combined as therapy for photoaged skin since the combination is well tolerated and the effects may be additive.[59] They act very different chemically since the hydrophilic alpha-hydroxy acids diffuse freely throughout the watery intercellular phase while the hydrophobic retinoids require proteins in the plasma and skin to act as carriers.[42] Current trends use an 8% glycolic acid moisturizer in the morning accompanied by bedtime use of the highest strength of tretinoin tolerated. This treatment can be supplemented with biweekly to monthly glycolic acid face peels in concentrations of 20%, 35%, 50%, and 70%. More well-controlled clinical studies with histologic evaluation are required before the optimum therapy for photoaged skin emerges.

REFERENCES

1. Gilchrest BA: Cellular and molecular changes in aging skin. J Geriatr Dermatol 2:3, 1994
2. Hurley HJ: Skin in senescence: a summation. J Geriatr Dermatol 1:55, 1993
3. West MD: The cellular and molecular biology of skin aging. Arch Dermatol 130:87, 1994
4. Griffiths CEM, Wag TS, Hamilton TA et al: A photonumeric scale for the assessment of cutaneous photodamage. Arch Dermatol 128:347, 1992
5. Kligman AM: Early destructive effects of sunligt on human skin. J Am Med Assoc 210:2377, 1969
6. Majmudar G, Nelson BR, Mazany KD et al: Cutaneous aging and collagen. J Geriatr Dermatol 2:36, 1994
7. Suader DN: The immunology of aging skin. J Geriatr Dermatol 2:15, 1994
8. Kligman LH, Kligman AM: Ultraviolet radiation-induced skin aging. p. 55. In Lowe NJ, Shaath NA (eds): Sunscreens Development, Evaluation and Regulatory Aspects. Dekker, Inc., New York, 1990
9. Braverman IM, Fonferko E: Studies in cutaneous aging. I. The elastic fiber network. J Invest Dermatol 78:434, 1982
10. Uitto JJ: Intrinsic aging changes in the dermis. J Geriatr Dermatol 2:7, 1994
11. Gilchrest BA: Overview of skin aging. J Cutan Aging Cosmet Dermatol 1, 1988
12. Shaath NA: Evolution of modern chemical sunscreens. p. 3. In Lowe NJ, Shaath NA (eds): Suncreens Development, Evaluation and Regulatory Aspects. Marcel Dekker, Inc., New York, 1990
13. Food and Drug Administration: Sunscreen drug products for over the counter human drugs: proposed safety, effective and labeling conditions. Fed Regul 43:38206, 1978
14. Sayre RM, Hughes SNG: Sun protective apparel: advancements in sun protection. Skin Cancer J February-March 1993
15. Shaath NA: The chemistry of suncreens. p. 223. Lowe NJ, Shaath NA (eds): Suncreens development, evaluation and regulatory aspects. Marcel Dekker, Inc., New York, 1990
16. Murphy EG: Regulatory aspects of sunscreens in the United States. p. 127. In Lowe NJ, Shaath NA (eds): Sunscreens Development, Evaluation and Regulatory Aspects. Marcel Dekker, Inc., New York, 1990
17. Lowe NJ: Sun protection factors: comparative techniques and selection of ultraviolet sources. p. 161. In Lowe NJ (ed): Physician's Guide to Sunscreens. Marcel Dekker, Inc., New York, 1991

18. Fisher AA: Sunscreen dermatitis: para-aminobenzoic acid and its derivatives. Cutis 50:190, 1992
19. Menter JM: Recent developments in UVA photoprotection. Int J Dermatol 29:389, 394, 1990
20. Fisher AA: Sunscreen dermatitis: part II, the cinnamates. Cutis 50:253, 1992
21. Sterling GB: Sunscreens: a review. Cutis 50:221, 1992
22. Roelandts R: Which components in broad-spectrum sunscreens are most necessary for adequate UVA protection? J Am Acad Dermatol 25:999, 1991
23. Cole C: Multicenter evaluation of sunscreen UVA protectiveness with the protection factor test method. J Am Acad Dermatol 30:729, 1994
24. Geiter F, Bilek PK, Doskoczil S: History of sunscreens and the rationale for their use. p. 187. In Frost P, Horwitz SN (eds): Principles of Cosmetics for the Dermatologist. CV Mosby, St. Louis, 1982
25. Bissett DL, Oelrich DM, Hannon DP: Evaluation of a topical iron chelator in animals and in human beings: short-term photoprotection by 2-furildioxime. J Am Acad Dermatol 31:572, 1994
26. Kollias N, Bager AH: The role of human melanin in providing photoprotection from solar mid-ultraviolet radiation (280–320 nm). J Soc Cosmet Chem 39:347, 1988
27. Mathews-Roth MM, Pathak MA, Parrish JA et al: A clinical trial of the effects of oral beta-carotene on the response of skin to solar radiation. J Invest Dermatol 59: 349, 1972
28. Foley P et al: The frequency of reactions to sunscreens: results of a longitudinal population-based study on the regular use of sunscreens in Australia. Br J Dermatol 128:512, 1993
29. Freeman S, Frederiksen P: Sunscreen allergy. Am J Contact Dermatitis 1:240, 1990
30. Thompson G, Maibach HI, Epstein J: Allergic contact dermatitis from sunscreen preparations complicating photodermatitis. Arch Dermatol 113:1252, 1977
31. Dromgoole SH, Maibach HI: Sunscreening agent intolerance: contact and photocontact sensitization and contact urticaria. J Am Acad Dermatol 22:1068, 1990
32. Mathias CGT, Maibach HI, Epstein J: Allergic contact photodermatitis to paraaminobenzoic acid. Arch Dermatol 114:1665, 1978
33. Thune P: Contact and photocontact allergy to sunscreens. Photodermatology 1:5, 1984
34. Rietschel RL, Lewis CW: Contact dermatitis to homomenthyl salicylate. Arch Dermatol 114:442, 1978
35. Fisher AA: Sunscreen dermatitis: part IV the salicylates, the anthranilates and physical agents. Cutis 50:397, 1992
36. Menz J, Muller SA, Connolly SM: photopatch testing: a six year experience. J Am Acad Dermatol 18:1044, 1988
37. Knobler E, Almeida L, Ruzkowski A et al: Photoallergy to benzophenone. Arch Dermatol 125:801, 1989
38. Ramsay DL, Cohen HS, Baer RL: Allergic reaction to benzopenone. Arch Dermatol 105:906, 1972
39. Kligman AM, Grove GL, Hirose R, Leyden JJ: Topical tretinoin for photoaged skin. J Am Acad Dermatol 15:836, 1986
40. Weiss JS, Ellis CN, Headington JT et al: Topical tretinoin improves photoaged skin. JAMA 259:527, 1988

41. Weiss JS, Ellis CN, Headington JT, Voorhees JJ: Topical tretinoin in the treatment of aging skin. J Am Acad Dermatol 19:169, 1988
42. Hermittte R: Aged skin, retinoids, and alpha hydroxy acids. Cosmet Toilet 107: 63, 1992
43. Goldfarb MT, Ellis CN, Weiss JS, Voorhees JJ: Topical tretinoin therapy: its use in photoaged skin. J Am Acad Dermatol 21:645, 1989
44. Bhawan J, Gonzalez-Serva A, Nehal K et al: Effects of tretinoin on photodamaged skin. Arch Dermatol 127:666, 1991
45. Olsen EA, Katz HI, Levine N et al: Tretinoin emollient cream: a new therapy for photodamaged skin. J Am Acad Dermatol 26:215, 1992
46. Kligman AM, Dogadkina D, Lavker RM: Effects of topical tretinoin on non-sun-exposed protected skin of the elderly. J Am Acad Dermatol 29:25, 1993
47. Gupta MA, Goldfarb MT, Schork NJ et al: Treatment of mildly to moderately photoaged skin with topical tretinoin has a favorable psychosocial effect: a prospective study. J Am Acad Drmatol 24:780, 1991
48. Weinstein GD, Nigra TP, Pochi PE, Savin RC: Topical tretinoin for treatment of photodamaged skin. Arch Dermatol 127:659, 1991
49. Kligman AM: Topical tretinoin for photoaging, tips from the top. J Geriatr Dermatol 1:A14, 1993
50. Rosan AM: The chemistry of alpha-hydroxy acids. Cosmet Dermatol Suppl October, p. 4, 1994
51. Yu RJ, Van Scott EJ: Alpha-hydroxy acids: science and therapeutic use. Cosmet Dermatol Suppl October, p. 12, 1994
52. Moy LS, Murad H, Moy RL: Glycolic acid peels for the treatment of wrinkles and photoaging. J Dermatol Surg Oncol 19:243, 1993
53. Moy LS, Murad H, Moy RL: Glycolic acid therapy: evaluation of efficacy and techniques in treatment of photodamage lesions. Am J Cosmet Surg 10:9, 1993
54. Elson ML: The art of chemical peeling. Cosmet Dermatol Suppl October p. 24, 1994
55. Van Scott JE, Yu RJ: Hyperkeratinization, corneocyte cohesion and alpha hydroxy acids. J Am Acad Dermatol 11:867, 1984
56. Van Scott JE, Yu RJ: Alpha hydroxyacids: therapeutic potentials. Can J Dermatol 1:108, 1989
57. Van Scott EJ, Yu RJ: Alpha hydroxy acids: procedures for use in clinical practice. Cutis 43:222, 1989
58. Perricone NV: An alpha hydroxy acid acts as an antioxidant. J Geriatr Dermatol 1:101, 1993
59. Kligman AM: Compatibility of a glycolic acid cream with topical tretinoin for the treatment of the photo damaged face of older women. J Geriatr Dermatol 1:179, 1993

24

Cosmetic Formulation

Cosmetic formulation involves the careful selection of ingredients to produce a safe elegant, efficacious product suitable for patient purchase.[1] Many substances must be combined to produce such a cosmetic, and consideration must be given to moisture barrier effects, pH, lubricating action, soothing effects, osmotic effects emolliency, and percutaneous absorption.[2] This chapter discusses the dermatologic concerns of key ingredients found in many cosmetic formulations, including preservatives, biological additives, herbal additives vitamin additives, color additives, liposomes, and niosomes.

PRESERVATIVES

Preservatives are the second most common allergenic group of substances, fragrances being the first. However, the number of cases of irritant and allergic contact dermatitis are indeed small compared with the two necessary functions preservatives perform in cosmetics: prevention of spoilage before purchase and prevention of contamination after purchase.[4,5] In short, preservatives reduce the likelihood of infection from cosmetics use. An independent survey of 250 cosmetics covering a wide range of products revealed a 24.4% contamination rate in unused products primarily by *Pseudomonas* species and other gram-negative rods.[6] The most frequently contaminated products were hand and body lotions, liquid eye liners, and cake eye shadows.

Unfortunately, the ideal preservative does not exist.[7] Valuable qualities in a cosmetic preservative include[8]

Lack of irritation
Lack of sensitization
Stability at a wide range of temperatures and pHs
Stability for extended periods of time
Compatibility with numerous ingredients and packaging materials
Effectiveness against numerous microorganisms
No odor or color

An important function of the cosmetics chemist and the microbiologist is to select the preservative that most closely meets all of the aforementioned needs in a given product. Additionally, the preservative must undergo rigorous dermatologic testing to ensure that it is safe for use on human skin.[9,10]

Types

Numerous preservatives are available for incorporation into cosmetics. Table 24-1 lists some of the preservative substances organized into chemical classes. Each of these chemicals has certain advantages and disadvantages, which are summarized in Table 24-2. There is no perfect preservative substance for cosmetics on the market. Some of the more popular preservatives in use today, due to their relatively low irritancy and allergenicity, include paraben esters, imidazolidinyl urea, phenoxyethanol, quaternium-15, and kathon CG.[11] The

Table 24-1. Some Preservatives Used in Cosmetics

Organic acids	Alcohols
Benzoic acid	b-Phenoxyethylalcohol
Sorbic acid	b-p-Chlorphenoxyethylalcohol
Monochloroacetic acid	b-Phenoxypropylalcohol
Formic acid	Benzyl alcohol
Salicylic acid	Isopropyl alcohol
Boric acid	Ethyl alcohol
Propionic acid	Phenolic compounds
Sulfurous acid	Phenol
Citric acid	o-Phenylphenol
Dehydroacetic acid	Chlorothymol
Parabens	Methylcholorthymol
Methyl p-hydroxybenzoate	Dichlorophene
Ethyl p-hydroxybenzoate	Hexachlorophene
Propyl p-hydroxybenzoate	Quaternary ammonium compounds
Butyl p-hydroxybenzoate	Benzethonium chloride
Benzyl p-hydroxybenzoate	Benzalkonium chloride
Mercurial compounds	Cetyltrimethyl ammonium bromide
Phenyl mercury acetate	Cetylpyridinium chloride
Phenyl mercury borate	Miscellaneous
Phenyl mercury nitrate	5-Bromo-5-nitro-1,3-dioxan (Dioxin)
Essential oils	2-Bromo-2-nitropropane-1,3-diol
Eucalyptus	(Bronopol)
Origanum	Imidazolidinyl urea (Germall-115)
Thyme	Trichlorsalicylanilide
Savory	Trichlorcarbanilide
Lemongrass oil	5-Chloro-2-methyl-4-isothiazolin-3-
Aldehydes	one and
Formaldehyde	2-methyl-4-isothiazolin-3-one (Kathon CG)

(Adapted from Wilkinson and Moore,[15] with permission.)

Table 24-2. Comparison of Preservatives

Preservative	Advantage	Disadvantage
Alcohols	Broad coverage, inexpensive	Volatile, high concentration required
Quaternium-15 (Dowicil 200)	Broad coverage (bacteria, yeasts, molds)	Ineffective against some *Pseudomonas* species, formaldehyde releaser
Formaldehyde	Broad coverage (fungicide and bactericide)	Irritant, allergen, concentration regulated, unpleasant odor
Quaternary ammonium compounds	Mainly gram-positive bacteria, some gram negative	Incompatible with anionics and proteins
Parabens	Moderate coverage (fungi, gram-positive bacteria), low allergenicity, low irritancy	Poor against gram-negative bacteria, incompatible with nonionics and cationics, effective only at acidic pH
Organic mercurials	Broad coverage	High toxicity, high irritancy
Phenolics	Broad coverage, effective over wide pH range	High irritancy, volatile
2-Bromo-2-nitropropane-1,3-diol (Bronopol)	Moderate coverage (bacteria)	Formaldehyde releaser, least effective against yeast and fungi
Methylisothiazolinone and methylchloroisothiazolinone (Kathon CG)	Broad coverage (bacteria, yeasts, fungi)	Allergenicity, irritancy, inactivated at high pH
Imidazolidinyl urea (Germall-115)	Moderate coverage (gram-negative bacteria)	Best used combined with parabens and antifungals to obtain broader coverage
Diazolidinyl urea (Germall-II)	Moderate coverage (gram-negative bacteria, *Pseudomonas* species)	Best used combined with parabens and antifungals to obtian broader coverage
Organic acids	Broad coverage (bacteria, yeasts)	Irritating, effective only at acidic pH
Dimethyloldimethyl hydantoin (Glydant)	Broad coverage, effective over wide pH range	Less active against yeasts

(Adapted from Wilkinson and Moore,[15] with permission.)

most commonly used preservative in cosmetics in the United States are the paraben esters, followed by imidazolidinyl urea.[12]

Some of the essential oils and fragrances retain antimicrobial capabilities, such as oil of clove, cinnamon, eucalyptus, rose lavender, lemon, thyme, rosemary, and sandalwood.[13] Products that claim to be preservative-free may actually incorporate one of these aromatic preservatives.

Efficacy

The complexity of cosmetics formulations requires a preservative to function under a variety of conditions. Microorganisms tend to proliferate in the aqueous phase of cosmetics. Under these circumstances the preservative selected must have a high water solubility and low oil solubility to function.

Furthermore, care must be taken to ensure that other ingredients in the formulation do not inactivate the preservative either by binding to active sites or altering the effective pH range. Some solid substances such as talc, kaolin, titanium dioxide, and zinc oxide actually adsorb the preservative, thus lowering its effective concentration.[14]

Organisms that frequently contaminate cosmetics include gram-positive bacteria (*Staphylococcus aureus, Streptococcus species*), gram-negative bacteria (*Pseudomonas aeruginosa, Escherichia coli, Enterobacter aerogenes*), fungi (*Asperigillus niger, Penicillium* species, *Alternaria* species), and yeasts (*Candida* species).[15]

Adverse Reactions

Adverse reactions caused by the preservatives in cosmetics are rare. Paraben esters are the most popular preservatives used in cosmetics, as their sensitization potential is low and they infrequently cause irritancy when applied to healthy skin.[16] They are usually found in concentrations of 0.5% or less in the United States, but concentrations up to 5% have been shown to produce minimal irritation. Some individuals who are allergic to parabens may actually tolerate cosmetics containing them, a phenomenon known as the "paraben paradox."[17] Tolerance is related to application site, concentration, duration, and status of the skin.[18] Since they are most effective against gram-positive organisms and fungi, paraben esters are sometimes used in combination with phenoxyethanol to provide better gram-negative coverage.[19] Parabens and imidazolidinyl urea (Germall 115) or diazolidinyl urea (Germall II) also act synergistically.[20]

Some preservatives, such as imidazolidinyl urea (Germall 115), 2-bromo-2-nitropropane-1,3-diol (Bronopol),[21,22] quaternium-15 (Dowicil 200),[23] and dimethylol dimethyl hydantoin (Glydant), are formaldehyde releasers. This means that free formaldehyde is produced in the presence of water. However, the concentration of formaldehyde is usually too low to cause irritancy or allergenicity. Nevertheless, patients who are allergic to formaldehyde may have difficulty with these preservatives.[24]

Kathon-CG, the CG standing for cosmetic grade, is a relatively new preservative in the United States.[25] It is a source of sensitization and thus recommended for use in products that are rinsed off the skin, such as hair conditioners and shampoos, in concentrations of less than 5 ppm.[26,27] It is used, however, in some leave-on products, such as hand creams, in low concentration. Kathon-CG and quaternium-15 were found to be the most allergic preservatives in a patch testing study.[28]

Some patients may also develop allergic contact dermatitis or contact urticaria to sorbic acid, but this is a less frequently used preservative in cosmetics.[29] It is patch tested at a 2% concentration in petrolatum.[30]

Preservatives can be difficult to patch test due to their inherent irritancy. Excellent articles exist discussing patch testing methods and concentrations.[31] Table 24-3 lists the patch test concentrations of some of the more commonly used preservatives and their typical concentration in cosmetic formulations. It is interesting to note that there is some variability in recommended patch concentrations depending on the reference used.[32,33]

BIOLOGICAL ADDITIVES

Biological additives are substances derived from the extracts and hydrolysates of glands and tissues of animals of different species. Animal organ extracts can be formulated as aqueous, hydroglyceric, hydroalcoholic, hydroglycolic, and oily. Examples of biological additives are collagen, elastin, hyaluronic acid,

Table 24-3. Patch Test and Use Concentrations

Preservative	Use Concentration (%)	Patch Test Concentration
Quaternium-15 (Dowicil 200)	0.02–0.3	2% in petrolatum
Formaldehyde	0.05–0.2	1% Aqueous
Parabens	0.1–0.8	3% in petrolatum if tested individually, otherwise use 12% in petrolatum of paraben mixture[a]
2-Bromo-2-nitropropane-1,3-diol (Bronopol)	0.01–0.1	0.5% in petrolatum
Methylisothiazolinone and methylchloroisothiazolinone (Kathon CG)	3–15 ppm	100 ppm aqueous
Imidazolidinyl (Germall-115)	0.05–0.5	1% in petrolatum or aqueous
Diazolidinyl urea (Germall-II)	0.1–0.5	1% Aqueous
Dimethylol dimethyl hydantoin (Glydant)	0.15–0.4	1–3% Aqueous

[a] Paraben mixture contains 3% each of methyl-, ethyl-, propyl-, and butylparaben.

keratin, placenta, amniotic fluid, pancreas, egg extract, blood derivatives, and extracts of the brain and aorta.

Topically applied biological additives, also known as biofactors, are thought by the cosmetics community to function as active ingredients due to the presence of "intrinsic factors."[34] Intrinsic factors are as of yet unidentified chemicals that have physiologic effects on the human body.

Collagen

Collagen is a biological additive found in moisturizers, hair conditioners, hair shampoos, and nail polishes. It is also available in a form suitable for cutaneous and subcutaneous injection. Collagen is a large molecule composed of three twisted alpha-helical peptide chains. It is usually obtained from shredded calf skin that is carefully handled to eliminate denaturation. Injectable collagen is processed to separate the chains through hydrolysis. The nonhelical end of the chains, known as the telopeptide, is also removed since it is responsible for the antigenicity of bovine collagen experienced in humans.[34]

Injectable collagen is a filler substance used to improve cosmetically the appearance of facial depressions due to scarring or wrinkling. Topical collagen, on the other hand, can be used in its microfibrillar form for hemostasis or in its hydrolyzed form as a protein humectant in moisturizers. Collagen can absorb up to 30 times its weight in water. Hydrolyzed collagen protein can also be used in hair products, especially instant conditioners, as it can reversibly penetrate chemically treated or damaged hair.

Elastin

Elastin is a structural component of the dermis responsible for the ability of the skin to regain its original configuration following stretching and other deformation. The elastin used topically in cosmetic preparations is obtained from bovine neck ligaments, but most preparations contain some collagen contamination. The elastin is usually added in the form of a hydrolysate consisting of a clear yellow liquid with a pronounced odor. It is added for its ability to function as a humectant; however, collagen has a greater water-binding capacity than elastin.

Hyaluronic Acid

Hyaluronic acid is a component of the dermis that has a great cosmetic potential for water retention. In other words, hyaluronic acid can function as a humectant when topically applied. It also can facilitate penetration of other substances through the stratum corneum, since a hydrated epidermis is more permeable. For this reason, hyaluronic acid has been termed a "transdermal delivery system" by some cosmetics manufacturers.

Hyaluronic acid is a glycosaminoglycan, as are chitin, chondroitin sulfate, and heparin. It falls into the broad category of mucopolysaccharides, which are hexosamine-containing polysaccharides of animal origin occurring in their pure state or as protein salts. Hyaluronic acid is obtained from animal sources such as avian combs, calf connective tissue, umbilical cord, and synovia.

Keratin

Keratin, a protein component of the stratum corneum, is used in cosmetics as a humectant moisturizer and to deposit a thin film on the hair and nails. It allows longer curl retention in hair-setting products and can minimally penetrate chemically treated or damaged hair temporarily to replace removed hair proteins. Keratin in found in nail polishes to improve nail hardness. Keratin is a scleroprotein and usually obtained from hydrolyzed bovine horn, horse hair, and boar bristles. It is a brown powder that can be readily added to gels, solutions, and emulsions, thus facilitating its addition to many cosmetics products.

Placenta

Placenta, as used in cosmetics preparations, is a complex mixture of proteins and enzymes such as alkaline phosphatase, lactate dehydrogenase, malate dehydrogenase, glutamate oxalacetate transaminase (GOT), and glutamate pyruvate transaminase (GPT). The number of substances present within the extract depends upon the care with which the placenta was handled. Human and animal placentas are used as sources. In general, the placenta is frozen, ground, and rinsed with sterile deionized water to remove any blood products. The cells are then lysed. The preparation can be treated further, depending on the needs of the cosmetics chemist. In the cosmetics literature, placenta extract is thought to accelerate cellular mitosis, enhance blood circulation, and stimulate cellular metabolism.[34] It is used in a variety of cosmetics, from facial moisturizing creams to hair conditioners.

Amniotic Fluid

Amniotic fluid is used in cosmetics as a moisturizer and a purported "epidermal growth enhancer." It is found in facial and body moisturizers, bust creams, hair lotions, and scalp treatments. Amniotic fluid is formed by the secretions of the amnion and the vascular transudate. The origin of the fluid used for cosmetics purposes is pregnant cows at 3 to 6 months gestation. The fluid is withdrawn from the amniotic sac through a hollow needle. It is a sterile yellow liquid of pH 7 that can be supplied as a water-soluble additive or a sterile powder.

Egg Extract

The whole egg extract and the egg yolk extract are used in shampoos, face masks, hair conditioners, and moisturizers. Egg extract is obtained from chicken eggs in the form of a hydrolyzed transparent, yellow liquid. An extract can also be prepared from the egg yolk alone. This extract is a viscous, opalescent, gold liquid-containing fats, lecithin, and sterols.

Blood Derivatives

There are several cosmetics extracts obtained from bovine blood: blood extract, serum albumin, fetuin, and fibronectin. Pure bovine blood extract is obtained by treating the blood to remove unwanted substances, histamines, and pyrogens. The remaining product is then dried to yield a water-soluble yellow powder. It is thought that this extract stimulates oxygen absorption and is therefore used in shampoos, conditioners, revitalizing creams, and aftershave products.

Bovine serum albumin is the fluid that remains after the fibrin and blood cells have been removed. It is available as a liquid and a freeze-dried powder. Since bovine serum albumin is used as a growth factor in cultured skin cells, it is thought to increase epidermal cell renewal rate. It is a common additive in creams that ''revitalize'' the skin.

HERBAL ADDITIVES

The most confusing area of speciality additives in cosmetics is plant derivatives. This list is almost endless and can only be appreciated by reading chemical company advertisements in cosmetics and toiletries trade journals. Most cosmetics manufacturers do not formulate their own additives, but rather buy them in bulk from wholesalers. Table 24-4 contains a few of the many herbal additives and their purported benefit.[35]

The area of plant additives is made more confusing by the mystery that has for centuries surrounded herbal medicine, still actively practiced, and herbal estheticians, who are making a resurgence with aromatology. There is no doubt that many of the plant additives impart a pleasing smell and color to the cosmetic.[36] Plant additives can be obtained as hydroglycolic extracts, essential oils, and whole plant extracts.[37] Hydroglycolic extracts are a combination of propylene glycol and water that yield the water-soluble plant constituents, but not the oil-soluble aromatic fragrances. These extracts are formulated into finished cosmetics in a 3%–10% concentration. Essential oils, extensively discussed in Chapter 22, yield the volatile nonaqueous constituents but no tannins, flavonides, carotenoids, or polysaccharides. These extracts are formulated into cosmetics in a 2%–5% concentration. Lastly, whole plant extracts, also known as ''aromaphytes,'' are produced by double extraction and contain all the con-

Table 24-4. Herbal Additives

Plant Derivative	Purported Function
Allantoin	Anti-irritating
Almond oil	Emollient
Aloe vera	Skin soother, moisturizer
Avocado oil	Skin soother
Camomile (Bisabolol)	Skin soother
Camphor	Skin refresher
Cypress	Skin refresher
Elder	Skin toner
Gernium	Skin softener
Hawthorne	Astringent
Hazelnut oil	Emollient
Horse tail	Skin toner
Hypericum	Skin refresher
Jojoba	Humectant, moisturizer
Licorice	Skin soother, softener
Linden flower	Skin soother
Lotus	Skin soother, softener
Marigold	Decrease skin edema
Marjoram	Skin toner
Myrrh	Nail strengthener
Sage	Skin toner
Seaweed	Skin soother
Sesame oil	Emollient
Shea butter	Moisturizer
Wheat germ oil	Emollient
Witch hazel	Astringent

stituents of the plant. They are usd at a 5%–20% concentration in cosmetic formulations.

Some of the currently popular herbal additives include aloe, avocado oil, sesame oil, and tea tree oil. Aloe is derived as a gelatinous substance squeezed from the leaf of the *Aloe arborescens* Miller.[38] It is thought to be of benefit in healing burns and enhancing skin repair, although no published wound healing studies have confirmed this belief.[39] It has been shown, however, to induce capillary vasodilation and to act as an antimicrobial in concentrations greater than 70%.[40] Avocado, sesame, and tea tree oils are used in moisturizers as emollients. But tea tree oil, also known as "melaleuca" oil, is derived from the *Melaleuca alternifolia* Cheel and thought to be effective in the treatment of furuncles, psoriasis, and fungal infections. These claims have not been proven, but cases of allergic contact dermatitis to *d*-limonene, a constituent of tea tree oil, have been documented.[41]

Other plant additives, such as witch hazel, are well-established astringents, while allantoin and alpha-bisabolol, a chamomile extract, have been used for years in cosmetics designed for sensitive skin due to their anti-inflammatory

Table 24-5. Vitamin Additives

Vitamin	Purported Function
Beta-carotene	Antioxidant
Biotin	Improve fat metabolism
Panthenol	Hair conditioner
Riboflavin	Maintain healthy skin
Vitamin A	Promote skin elasticity, smoothness
Vitamin C	Antioxidant
Vitamin E	Antioxidant
Vitamin E (essential fatty acids)	Skin nourishing

properties. There is no doubt that many of the original dermatologic medications had their origin as herbal derivatives.

VITAMIN ADDITIVES

Vitamin additives have become popular due to the recognition that beta-carotene, vitamin C, and vitamin E can act as antioxidants. Table 24-5 summarizes some of the currently used vitamins and their purported cosmetic value.[42]

Further study is required before it can be stated that topical vitamin C, vitamin E, and beta-carotene can function as antioxidants, quenching oxygen radicals that can damage structures within the dermis.[43] Nevertheless, some interesting preliminary work has been published in this area. Vitamin C is a hydrophilic substance that can function as an antioxidant, or an oxidant if combined with iron.[44] It has been shown to protect porcine skin from UVB- and UVA-induced phototoxic reactions when topically applied.[45] Thus, it may act as a broad specturm photoprotectant by enhancing cutaneous levels of vitamin C.[46] Studies have demonstrated the value of alpha-tocopherol, also known as vitamin E, as a lipid-soluble chain-breaking antioxidant in erythrocyte membranes.[47] Topically applied alpha-tocopherol has also been shown to inhibit UVB-induced edema and erythema conferring an SPF of 3.[48] This is thought to be due to its ability to absorb light marginally and function as a free radical–quenching, lipid-soluble antioxidant.[49] Carotenoids, of which beta-carotene is an example, have been shown to function as antioxidants in hydrophobic compartments not accessible to tocopherols due to unique solubility properties.[50]

COLOR ADDITIVES

Color additives comprise an important aspect of colored cosmetics and account for the perceived benefits of other cosmetic preparations. The use of synthetic organic colors for cosmetic purposes has been regulated since 1938.[51]

Table 24-6. Frequency of Cosmetic Color
Additive Use (In Order of
Decreasing Frequency)

Titanium dioxide
Iron oxides
Mica
FD&C yellow No. 5
Ultramarine blue
FD&C blue No. 1
D&C red No. 7 calcium lake
Bismuth oxychloride
FD&C red No. 4
FD&C yellow No. 6

The coloring agents most frequently used in cosmetics are listed in Table 24-6.[52] A more complete listing of colors can be found in the *CTFA International Color Handbook* published by the Cosmetics, Toiletry and Fragrance Association, Inc.

There are 116 permitted certified colors available for the cosmetics chemist to combine; they are divided into three classes:

1. FD&C colorants, permitted for use in food, drugs, and cosmetics
2. D&C colorants, permitted for use in drugs and cosmetics
3. External D&C colorants, permitted for use in externally applied drugs and cosmetics, but the lips and any body surface area covered by mucous membranes are excluded

Cosmetic coloring additives can be divided into those that are soluble or insoluble.[53] Soluble colors may be soluble in a variety of substances, including water, alcohol, and oil. These colors are almost all synthetic organic dyestuffs that impart color only when in solution. These soluble synthetic dyestuffs can be further divided into acid dyes, mordant dyes, basic dyes, vat dyes, solvent dyes, and xanthene dyes. Acid dyes are used in the dyeing of many items, such as cosmetics, textiles, food, inks, wood stains, and varnishes. The dyestuffs of this category used in cosmetics are FD&C Blue Nos. 1, 2; FD&C Green Nos. 1, 2, 3; FD&C Red Nos. 2, 3, 4; FD&C Violet No. 1; FD&C Yellow Nos. 5, 6; D&C Blue No. 4; D&C Green No. 5; D&C Orange Nos. 4, 11; D&C Red Nos. 22, 23, 28, 33; D&C Yellow Nos. 7, 10; and Ext. D&C Yellow No. 7. Mordant dyes, basic dyes, and vat dyes are not generally used in cosmetics.

Solvent dyes listed for use are D&C Green No. 6; D&C Red Nos. 17, 37; D&C Violet No. 2; and D&C Yellow No. 11. Xanthene dyes, such fluorescein, are used in the coloring of lipsticks. Dyes of this group approved for use are the acid forms of D&C Orange Nos. 5, 6, 7, 10; D&C Red Nos. 21, 27; and D&C Yellow No. 7. These xanthene dyes are used in their water-soluble form: FD&C Red No. 3; D&C Orange Nos. 11, 12; and D&C Red Nos. 22, 23, 28.

Insoluble coloring matters consist of inorganic and organic substances. The organic materials are lakes of soluble dyes and pigments, while the inorganic materials are largely oxides and metals. The lakes are soluble dyestuffs that are rendered insoluble by precipitation onto a base. Pigments are usually dyes of the azo type. Oxide pigments that are naturally occurring include iron oxides known as ochre, raw and burnt siennas, red oxides, and raw and burnt umbers. Synthetic oxides and ochres are also available to yield shades of red and yellow. Blues are produced as ultramarines, greens formed from chrome oxide, and Guignet's green, while blacks are available as carbon black, vegetable black, bone black, and black oxide of iron. Metallic colors include aluminum powders and bronze powders.

Other popular colorants that do not fit into the above classification include pearl essences, formed from fish scale or bismuth oxychloride, and manganese violet.

Color additives are rarely a cause of dermatitis in cosmetics, but reports of dermatitis caused by coal tar dyes exist.[54] Additionally, the D&C Red dyes have been shown to be comedogenic.[55]

LIPOSOMES AND NIOSOMES

Liposomes were initially discovered in the 1960s and reported by A.D. Bangham in 1965 in the *Journal of Molecular Biology*. His discovery centered on the observation that phospholipids could be dispersed in an aqueous solution to spontaneously form hollow vesicles, or liposomes, containing the dispersing medium.[56] This observation received immediate attention from the pharmaceutical industry, which theorized that liposomes could be used as a delivery system for aqueous solutions of active agents. Later, the cosmetics industry adapted the technology for the delivery of nonprescription items to the skin.

Chemistry

Liposomes are spherical vesicles with diameters between 25 and 5,000 nm formed from membranes that consist of a bilayer of amphiphilic molecules.[57] *Amphiphilic* refers to the fact that the molecules have both polar and nonpolar ends. The polar heads are directed toward both the inside of the vesicle and its outer surface. The nonpolar, or lipophilic, tails are directed toward the middle of the bilayer. This unique structure thus allows the sustained release of water-soluble chemicals from the liposome structure. Liposomes may be one double layer (unilamellar), two to four double layers (oligolamellar), or multilayered (multilamellar) vesicles.

The bilayer that forms the liposome and separates its interior compartment from the external environment is remarkably similar to the cell membrane of mammalian cells. This membrane structure has been highly conserved through evolutionary change. Advocates of liposomes argue that this allows biocompatibility with cells, minimizing adverse reactions.[58]

The primary substances used to form liposomes are phospholipids such as phosphatidylcholine. Other minor components may include phosphatidylethanolamine, phosphatidylinositol, and phosphatidic acid. Vegetable phospholipids are also used due to their high concentration of the essential fatty acids linoleic and linolenic acids. Parameters that influence the function of liposomes in topical preparations include chemical composition, vesicle size, shape, surface charge, lamellarity, and homogeneity. Liposome function is also dependent upon where the active agent is trapped (inside the vesicles, in the membrane, or on the outer surface of the vesicle) and the chemical nature of the active agent (hydrophilic, amphiphilic, or lipophilic).

Niosomes are a specialized form of liposomes composed of nonionic surfactants. Their main components are ethoxylated fatty alcohols and synthetic polyglycerol ethers (polyoxyethylene alkyl ester, polyoxyethylene alkyl ether).

Function

Theoretically, liposomes offer the cosmetics chemist new formulations with new physical properties, a new transport system for active agents, and possibly increased efficacy of active agents. Liposomes, however, are somewhat unstable as they are readily deformed and possibly lysed by the weight of a glass coverslip when viewed under the microscope. They are also subject to fusion, aggregation, and precipitation. The vesicular structure can be stabilized by cholesterol and incorporation of an ionic charge, but they remain fragile.[59]

The mechanism of action of liposomes and niosomes on the skin remains controversial. Many articles in cosmetics trade publications have tried to use radiolabeled substances and freeze fracture electron microscopy to observe their interaction with the stratum corneum and papillary dermis. It is unlikely that liposomes and niosomes are able to diffuse intact intercellularly across the stratum corneum. The corneocytes are embedded in lipids, such as ceramides, glycosylceramides, cholesterol, and fatty acids, which are structurally different from the phospholipids and nonionic surfactants.[60] It is possible that they may enter the skin through appendageal structures, but this accounts for only a small proportion of the skin surface area. Thus, absorption through this route is small.

There is evidence, however, that the components of liposomes and niosomes are able to interact with skin lipids, even if they are not in an intact vesicular form.[61] They may be able to reduce transepidermal water loss by supplementing missing substances within the skin lipid barrier. Furthermore, liposomes, and niosomes can form chemical associations with keratin proteins.

Use and Efficacy

Liposomes were originally developed as a novel drug delivery system. The first pharmaceutical liposome delivery system was for 1% econazole, but this product was only marketed in Switzerland. Data indicated that there was a four fold higher concentration of the antimycotic in the stratum corneum with liposomal delivery.[62] Other dermatologicals suitable for liposomal delivery include hydrocortisone, triamcinolone, topical antibiotics, and retinoids. It is theoretically possible to obtain active ingredient dermal concentrations with liposomes 9 to 14 times greater than with standard water-in-oil emulsions. Researchers have even experimented with the delivery of liposomal encapsulated interferon in animal models.[63] Certainly, more liposome preparations will be introduced.[64]

Liposomes can also be incorporated into cosmetics, bath products, moisturizers, and sunscreens. Empty liposomes have possibilities as bath oils, emollients and wound healing aids due to their rich concentration of phospholipids. Loaded liposomes can be devised to release their contents at specific temperatures or specific pH levels, a concept known as "triggering." These liposomes can be loaded with sunscreens to enhance distribution within the stratum corneum or moisturizers to reduce transepidermal water loss. The liposome concentration in such formulations is usually 1% to 10%.

REFERENCES

1. Kabara JJ: Cosmetic preservation. p. 3. In Kabara JJ (ed): Cosmetic and Drug Preservation. Marcel Dekker, Inc, New York, 1984
2. Van Abbe NJ, Spearman RIC, Jarrett A: Pharmaceutical and Cosmetic Products for Topical Administration. William Heinemann Medical Books Ltd, London, 1969
3. Adams RM, Maibach HI: A five-year study of cosmetic reactions. J Am Acad Dermatol 13:1062, 1985
4. Orth DS: Handbook of Cosmetic Microbiology. Marcel Dekker, Inc., New York, 1993
5. Parsons T: A microbiology primer. Cosmet Toilet 105:73, 1990
6. Wolven A, Levenstein I: TGA Cosmet J 1:34, 1969
7. Smith WP: Cosmetic preservation: a survey. Cosmet Toilet 108:67, 1993
8. Wells FV, Lubowe II: Cosmetics and the Skin. Reinhold Publishing Corporation, New York, 1964
9. Bronaugh RL, Maibach HI: Safety evaluation of cosmetic preservatives. p. 503. In Kabara JJ (ed): Cosmetic and Drug Preservation. Marcel Dekker, Inc, New York, 1984
10. Eiermann HJ: Cosmetic product preservation: safety and regulatory issues. p. 559. In Kabara JJ (ed): Cosmetic and Drug Preservation. Marcel Dekker, Inc, New York, 1984
11. Steinberg DC: Cosmetic preservation: current international trends. Cosmet Toilet 107:77, 1992
12. Frequency of preservative use in cosmetic formulas as disclosed to the FDA-1990. Cosmet Toilet 105:45, 1990
13. Kabara JJ: Aroma preservatives: essential oils and fragrances as antimicrobial agents. p. 237. In Kabara JJ (ed): Cosmetic and Drug Preservation. Marcel Dekker, Inc, New York, 1984
14. McCarthy TJ: Formulated factors affecting the activity of preservatives. p. 359. In

Kabara JJ (ed): Cosmetic and Drug Preservation. Marcel Dekker, Inc, New York, 1984

15. Wilkinson JB, Moore RJ: Harry's Cosmeticology. 7th Ed. Chemical Publishing, New York, 1982

16. Schorr WF, Mohajerin AH: Paraben sensitivity. Arch Dermatol 93:721, 1966

17. Fisher AA: The paraben paradoxes. Cutis 12:830, 1973

18. Fisher AA: The parabens: paradoxical preservatives. Cutis 51:405, 1993

19. Hall AL: Cosmetically acceptable phenoxyethanol. p. 79. In Kabara JJ (ed): Cosmetic and Drug Preservation. Marcel Dekker, Inc, New York, 1984

20. Rosen WE, Berke PA: Germall 115: a safe and effective preservative. p. 191. In Kabara JJ (ed): Cosmetic and Drug Preservation. Marcel Dekker, Inc, New York, 1984

21. Croshaw B, Holland VR: Chemical preservatives: use of Bronopol as a cosmetic preservative. p. 31. In Kabara JJ (ed): Cosmetic and Drug Preservation. Marcel Dekker, Inc, New York, 1984

22. Frosch PJ, White IR, Rycroft RJG et al: Contact allergy to Bronopol. Contact Dermatitis 22:24, 1990

23. Marouchoc SR: Dowicil 200 preservative. p. 143. In Kabara JJ (ed): Cosmetic and Drug Preservation. Marcel Dekker, Inc, New York, 1984

24. Fransway AF: The problem of preservation in the 1990s. Am J Contact Dermatitis 2:6, 1991

25. DeGroot AC, Weyland JW: Kathon CG: a review. J Am Acad Dermatol 18:350, 1988

26. Law AB, Moss JN, Lashen ES: Kathon CG: a new single-component, broad-spectrum preservative system for cosmetics and toiletries. p. 29. In Kabara JJ (ed): Cosmetic and Drug Preservation. Marcel Dekker, Inc, New York, 1984

27. DeGroot AC, Liem DH, Weyland JW: Kathon CG: cosmetic allergy and patch test sensitization. Contact Dermatitis 12:76, 1985

28. DeGroot AC, Liem DH, Nater JP, Van Ketel WG: Patch tests with fragrance materials and preservatives. Contact Dermatitis 12:87, 1985

29. Luck E, Remmert IK: Sorbic acid the preservation of cosmetic products. Cosmet Toilet 108:65, 1993

30. Marks JG, DeLeo VA: Contact and Occupational Dermatology. Mosby Yearbook, St. Louis, 1992

31. Andersen KE, Rycroft RJG: Recommended patch test concentrations for preservatives, biocides and antimicrobials. Contact Dermatitis 25:1, 1991

32. DeGroot AC, Weyland JW, Nater JP: Unwanted Effects of Cosmetics and Drugs Used in Dermatology. 3rd Ed. Elsevier, Amsterdam, 1994

33. Fisher AA: Contact Dermatitis. 3rd Ed. Lea & Febiger, Philadelphia, 1986

34. Hermitte R: Formulating with selected biological extracts. Cosmet Toilet 106:53, 1991

35. Dweck AC, Black P: Natural extracts and herbal oils: concentrated benefits for the skin. Cosmet Toilet 107:89, 1992

36. Purohit P, Kapsner TR: Natural essential oils. Cosmet Toilet 109:51, 1994

37. Bishop MA: Botanicals in bath care. Cosmet Toilet 104:65, 1989

38. McKeown E: Aloe vera. Cosmet Toilet 102:64, 1987

39. Jackson EM: Natural ingredients in cosmetics. Am J Contact Dermatitis. 5:106, 1994

40. Waller T: Aloe vera in personal care products. Cosmet Toilet 107:53, 1992

41. Knight TE, Hausen BM: Melaleuca oil dermatitis. J Am Acad Dermatol 30:423, 1994
42. Der Marderosian ARA, Liberti L: Natural products as cosmetics. p. 132. In Natural Product Medicine, George F. Stickley Co., Philadelphia, 1988
43. Rieger MM: Oxidative reactions in and on skin: mechanism and prevention. Cosmet Toilet 108:43, 1993
44. Bast A, Haenen GRMM, Doelman CJA: Oxidants and antioxidants: state of the art. Am J Med 91:2S, 1991
45. Darr D, Combs S, Dunston S et al: Topical vitamin C protects porcine skin from ultraviolet radiation-induced damage. Br J Dermatol 127:247, 1992
46. Rackett SC, Rothe MJ, Grant-Kels JM: Diet and dermatology. J Am Acad Dermatol 29:447, 1993
47. Burton GW, Joyce A, Ingold KU: Is vitamin E the only lipid-soluble, chain-breaking antioxidant in human blood plasma and erythrocyte membrances? Arch Biochem Biophys 221:281, 1983
48. Idson B: Vitamins and the skin. Cosmet Toilet 108:79, 1993
49. Mayer P, Pittermann W, Wallat S: The effects of vitamin E on the skin. Cosmet Toilet 108:99, 1993
50. Sies H: Oxidative stress: from basic research to clinical applications. Am J Med 91:31S, 1991
51. Berdick M: Color additives in cosmetics and toiletries. Cutis 21:743, 1978
52. US Food and Drug Administration: Cosmetic color additives: frequency of use. Cosmet Toilet 104:39, 1989
53. Anstead DF: Cosmetic colours. p. 101. In Hibbott HW (ed): Handbook of Cosmetic Science. The Macmillan Company, New York, 1963
54. Sugai T, Takahashi Y, Tagaki T: Pigmented cosmetic dermatitis and coal tar dyes. Contact Dermatitis 3:249, 1977
55. Fulton JE, Pay SR, Fulton JE: Comedogenicity of current therapeutic products, cosmetics, and ingredients in the rabbit ear. J Am Acad Dermatol 10:96, 1984
56. Lautenschlager H: Liposomes in dermatological preparations, part 1. Cosmet Toilet 105:896, 1990
57. Junginger HE, Hofland HEJ, Bouwstra JA: Liposomes and niosomes: interactions human skin. Cosmet Toilet 106:45, 1991
58. Hayward JA: Potential of liposomes in cosmetic science. Cosmet Toilet 105:474, 1990
59. Israelachvili JN: Physics of amphiphiles: micelles, vesicles and microemulsions. North Holland, Amsterdam, 1988
60. Elias PM: Structure of function of the stratum corneum permeability barrier. Drug Dev Res 13:97, 1988
61. Mahjour M, Mauser B, Rashidbaigi Z, Fawzi MB: Effect on egg yolk lecithins and commercial soybean lecithins on in vitro skin permeation of drugs. J Control Rel 14:243, 1990
62. Lautenschlager H: Liposomes in dermatological preparations, part 2. Cosmet Toilet 105:63, 1990
63. Weiner N, Williams N, Birch G et al: Topical delivery of lipsomally encapsulated interferon evaluated in a cutaneous herpes guinea pig model. Antimicrob Agents Chemother 33:1217, 1989
64. Korting HC, Blecher P, Schafer-Korting M, Wendel A: Topical liposome drugs to come: what the patent literature tells us. J Am Acad Dermatol 25:1068, 1991

25

Cosmetics, Comedogenesis, Acnegenesis, Irritancy, and Allergenicity

Dermatologists are constantly struggling to find the perfect skin care products and cosmetics to recommend to patients. Ideally, all product recommendations would be for products that are free of comedogenicity, acnegenicity, irritancy, and allergenicity. Realistically, however, it is impossible for a cosmetics chemist to formulate a product that meets all of these criteria for all patients. Even pure water, the major component of the human body, is responsible for irritancy in individuals with low sebum production.

Nevertheless, dermatologists should strive to make quality recommendations to their patients. But, how does one go about assessing the comedogenicity, acnegenicity, irritancy, and allergenicity of a product? Can one read lists of comedogenic substances and then select the facial moisturizer that contains none of these ingredients? Does the nonacnegenic label on a facial foundation guarantee that the product is suitable for patients with acne? If 10 patients use a cleanser and experience no irritation, can it be assumed that the product has low irritancy? Can body lotions that contain none of the ingredients present on a standard dermatologist's patch test tray be considered free of allergenicity?[1]

These represent important considerations given the tremendous variety of products available to consumers. This chapter presents my opinions regarding cosmetic formulation and comedogenicity, acnegenicity, irritancy, and allergenicity.

COMEDOGENICITY

The issue of comedogenicity in relation to cosmetics arose in 1972 when Kligman and Mills[2] described a low-grade acne characterized by closed comedones on the cheeks of women aged 20 to 25. They labeled this phenomenon "acne cosmetica." Many of these women had not experienced adolescent acne. The authors proposed that substances present in cosmetics products induced the formation of closed comedones and, in some cases, a papulopustular eruption.

Further work led to development of the rabbit ear comedogenicity model, which is still sometimes used by cosmetics companies to test their products. The cosmetic is applied to the ears of New Zealand white albino rabbits. One ear serves as a control while the other ear receives 0.50 ml of the test substance 5 days per week for 2 consecutive weeks. Visual observations of enlarged pores and hyperkeratosis are made daily. At the completion of the study a skin biopsy is examined for hyperkeratosis of the sebaceous follicles.[3]

There are several problems assoicated with the use of this model.[4] First, some studies do not perform a biopsy and rely on visual inspection of the rabbit ear, which is less sensitive than microscopic examination. Microcomedones, now known to be important acne precursor lesions, can only be identified through microscopic examination. Second, some studies have confused follicular dilation with comedone formation. Follicular dilation is a side effect of cutaneous irritation and is not necessarily the same as comedone formation. Third, immature or aged rabbits may not yield accurate data, since sebum production is reduced in rabbits not in their prime. Fourth, the rabbit ear may not accurately simulate the human face: many substances that produce comedones in the rabbit ear model produce pustules and inflammatory papules, not comedones, on the human face.

Because of the aforementioned limitations with the rabbit ear model many cosmetic companies are now using the upper back of predominantly male volunteers for comedogenicity assessment.[5] Occlusive patch tests are used to apply the material to the upper back for 30 days with repeated changings as necessary. Follicular biopsies are made at the beginning and end of the test to evaluate keratin plugging. This too has some inherent problems, since most of the cosmetics tested are for female facial application. Thus, another study uses young individuals with acne who apply a product for 4 to 8 weeks. Lesion counts are made before and after the test period. But, due to problems in evaluation, many companies prefer the upper back study technique.[6] Pre- and postmarketing surveillance have also assumed importance for product comedogenicity evaluation.

Thus, the complex issue of comedogenicity is difficult to assess. There are established lists of substances that are generally believed to be comedogenic when rubbed on the skin repeatedly in concentrations of 100%. Table 25-1 is an example of such as list. It should then be easy to hand patients a list of these substances and tell them to purchase products that do not contain these ingredients. Unfortunately, this is a simplistic approach.

It is practically impossible to find formulations that possess none of these ingredient. The list contains some of the most effective emollients (octyl stearate, isocetyl stearate), detergents (sodium lauryl sulfate), occlusive moisturizers (mineral oil, petrolatum, sesame oil, cocoa butter), and emulsifiers found in the cosmetics industry.[7] A product line that avoided all of these substances

Table 25-1. Standard List of Possible
Comedogenic Substances

Butyl stearate
Cocoa butter
Corn oil
D&C red dyes
Decyl oleate
Isopropyl isosterate
Isopropyl myristate
Isostearyl neopentanate
Isopropyl palmitate
Isocetyl stearate
Lanolin, acetylated
Linseed oil
Laureth-4
Mineral oil
Myristyl ether propionate
Myristyl lactate
Myristyl myristate
Oleic acid
Oleyl alcohol
Olive oil
Octyl pamitate
Octyl stearate
Peanut oil
Petrolatum
Propylene glycol stearate
Methyl oleate
Petrolatum
Safflower oil
Sesame oil
Sodium lauryl sulfate
Stearic acid

would not perform well on the skin and would possess low cosmetic acceptability.

Furthermore, just because a product *does not* contain comedogenic substances from this list *does not* guarantee that it is noncomedogenic. Conversely, if a product *does* contain comedogenic substances, this *does not* necessarily mean that the product is comedogenic. It can, therefore, be safely concluded that lists of comedogenic substances are only of academic interest. Why?

Comedogenicity can only be evaluated in light of the patient's susceptibility to the formation of comedonal plugs. Some individuals have never developed a comedone in their life and use cocoa butter daily as a facial moisturizer. For some reason that is not yet understood, certain patients develop fewer comedones than others.[8,9]

Comedogenicity can also only be evaluated in light of the concentration of the comedogen in the product. Few formulations, except for pure petrolatum, are applied to the skin in a concentration of 100%. Substances that are comedogenic when applied to the skin in concentrations of 100% may not be comedogenic when applied to the skin in more realistic concentrations of 1%.

Individual ingredient analysis of comedogens in a product is also not valuable since it does not account for the interaction of substances. Producing cosmetics is much like baking a cake. Each of the required ingredients is added in the proper amount and order, followed by stirring at the right speed for the correct amount of time and heated at the proper temperature for a certain period followed by cooling. Even though a cake may contain flour, margarine, milk, eggs, and baking soda, it is not possible to separate the physical and chemical characteristics of each ingredient in the final baked product. The finished cake is a new chemical entity with its own distinct characteristics. The finished cosmetic is also a new chemical entity with its own distinct characteristics.

ACNEGENICITY

Acnegenicity is a completely separate phenomenon from comedogenicity. Substances that are comedogenic cause comedones, or blackheads, whereas substances that are acnegenic cause papules and pustules. Comedogenicity is due to follicular plugging, whereas acnegenicity is due to follicular irritation.[10] Thus, substances that are comedogenic are not necessarily acnegenic and vice versa.

At first glance, acnegenicity also may seem rather simple. A list of substances that irritate the follicular ostia could be generated and then used to pick skin care products and cosmetics for patient use. Unfortunately, lists of acnegenic substances are useless since the interaction of ingredients, as well as their concentration, is important. But of more importance is the individual patient's susceptibility to acne formation. Cosmetics that are acnegenic in one patient are not necessarily acnegenic in another patient.

It is interesting to note that, in a general dermatologist's practice, the phenomenon of acnegenicity due to cosmetics is a more common occurrence than comedogenicity due to cosmetics. This makes acnegenicity a more important issue than comedogenicity. However, the incidences of comedone and acne formation due to cosmetics are rare, considering the number of persons who use such products on a daily basis.

IRRITANCY

Another issue of importance to the dermatologist is the irritancy of skin care products and cosmetics. This too is complicated by patient variability. The irritancy of a given product is dependent on the intact state of the stratum corneum. If the stratum corneum barrier is intact, a product may not be irritating. If the stratum corneum barrier is damaged, a product may be irritating.[11] An excellent example is the case of a woman who applies a body lotion without stinging or burning to her legs in the morning, but who experiences stinging or burning in the evening when the lotion is applied to freshly shaved legs. Other considerations in irritancy include the concentration of the irritant and the length of time the irritant is left in contact with the skin.[12]

ALLERGENICITY

The last topic to be considered is allergenicity. This too is more complex than simply evaluating the cosmetic ingredients that are present on the standard patch test tray. Some allergens are present in too low a concentration in the final formulation to cause problems in all but the most sensitive patients.[13] Additionally, a given cosmetic may be tolerated in one facial site, but not in others, such as around the eyes. The incidence of allergic reactions to cosmetics is also rare, considering the number of cosmetics users.

SUMMARY

This discussion has illustrated the complexity of cosmetic ingredient selection. Perhaps more questions have been raised than answered, but several conclusions are clear. First, evaluating lists of comedogenic, acnegenic, irritant, and allergenic substances is of limited use when making product recommendations to patients. Second, the only way to ensure that a patient will not have a problem with a given skin care product or cosmetic is to use the finished product. Only through actual product application can patients confirm that a given skin care item or cosmetic is noncomedogenic, nonacnegenic, nonirritating, and nonallergenic on their skin. Unfortunately, the human body and the skin are dynamic, thus necessitating continual reevaluation.

REFERENCES

1. Jackson EM: Hypoallergenic claims. Am J Contact Dermatitis 4:108–110, 1993
2. Kligman AM, Mills OH: Acne cosmetica. Arch Dermatol 106:843, 1972
3. Kaufman PJ, Rappaport MJ: Skin care products. p. 179. In Whittam JH (ed): Cosmetic Safety a Primer for Cosmetic Scientists. Marcel Dekker, Inc, New York, 1987
4. Frank SB: Is the rabbit ear model, in its present state, prophetic of acnegenicity? J Am Acad Dermatol 6:373, 1982
5. Mills OH, Kligman AM: A human model for assessing comedeogenic substances. Arch Dermatol 118:903, 1982
6. Kaufman PJ, Rappaport MJ: Skin care products. p. 179. In Whittam JH (ed):

Cosmetic Safety a Primer for Cosmetic Scientists. Marcel Dekker, Inc. New York, 1987

7. Fulton JE, Pay SR, Fulton JE: Comedogenicity of current therapeutic products, cosmetics, and ingredients in the rabbit ear. J Am Acad Dermatol 10:96, 1984
8. Fulton JE, Bradley S, Aqundez A, Black T: Non-comedogenic cosmetics. Cutis 17:344, 1976
9. Report of the 1988 American Academy of Dermatology Invitational Symposium on Comedogenicity. J Am Acad Dermatol 20:272, 1989
10. Mills OH, Berger RS: Defining the susceptibility of acne-prone and sensitive skin populations to extrinsic factors. Dermatol Clin 9:93, 1991
11. Dooms-Goossens A: Reducing sensitizing potential by pharmaceutical and cosmetic design. J Am Acad Dermatol 10:547, 1984
12. Leyden JJ: Risk assessment of products used on the skin. Am J Contact Dermatitis 4:158, 1993
13. Simion FA, Rau AH: Sensitive skin: what is it and how to formulate for it. Cosmet Toilet 109:43, 1994

26

Contact Dermatitis

The use of cosmetics and skin care products can occasionally result in contact dermatitis. This is certainly a minor issue, but no discussion of cosmetic dermatology would be complete without addressing this important aspect of patient care. With the tremendous variety of products available for purchase, it is easy for the consumer simply to discard or return any product that has produced an untoward reaction. Occasionally, however, patients finds that they experiences numerous reactions or severe reactions requiring the expertise of a dermatologist. This chapter presents the information necessary to evaluate such patients. Additional information on adverse reactions is given in this text as part of the discussions of each cosmetic or skin care product.

Contact dermatitis can be classified as follows: irritant contact dermatitis, allergic contact dermatitis, contact urticaria, phototoxic contact dermatitis, and photoallergic contact dermatitis.

IRRITANT CONTACT DERMATITIS

Irritant contact dermatitis, the most commonly encountered adverse reaction to cosmetics and skin care products, is manifested as erythematous, burning, pruritic skin that may develop microvesiculation and later desquamation. The dermatitis is characterized by stratum corneum damage without immunologic phenomena. The irritancy may be due to the presence of chemical factors with excessively high or low pH or by volatile vehicles that dissolve protective sebum.[1] Physical factors including the rubbing necessary to apply cosmetics or abrasive particles within cosmetics may cause irritancy. Most importantly, a damaged stratum corneum may not be able to provide a protective barrier so that any cosmetic applied to the damaged skin will cause irritation. This is the case in patients with atopic dermatitis, xerotic eczema, or neurodermatitis. These patients frequently will describe numerous products that produce "allergic" symptoms. In actuality, there is no immunologic basis to the dermatitis, but an irritancy heightened by a damaged stratum corneum. Any cosmetic applied

267

to dermatitic skin may produce irritation; therefore, patients should not wear cosmetics or use personal care items until the dermatitis has resolved.

ALLERGIC CONTACT DERMATITIS

Allergic contact dermatitis can be difficult to differentiate clinically from irritant contact dermatitis, but the distinction is important for good patient care. Both conditions may present as erythematous plaques; however, acute allergic contact dermatitis may exhibit more vesiculation. In some cases, late-stage allergic and irritant contact dermatitis cannot be differentiated clinically or histologically. Allergic contact dermatitis is an immunologic phenomenon requiring antigen-presenting and antigen-processing cells without regard to the condition of the protective stratum corneum. Therefore, an intact stratum corneum cannot prevent development of allergic contact dermatitis in sensitized individuals. The only course is avoidance of the allergen.[2] The most common cosmetic-induced causes of allergic contact dermatitis as determined by the North American Contact Dermatitis Group are listed by product category (Table 26-1) and by ingredient (Table 26-2).[3] Other studies have also been published by the European dermatologic community.[4,5]

CONTACT URTICARIA

Contact urticarias may be an immunologic or nonimmunologic reaction to cosmetics and skin care products. It is characterized by the development of a wheal-and-flare response to a topically applied chemical. The spectrum of clinical presentation ranges form itching and burning to generalized urticaria to anaphylaxis. Nonimmunologic contact urticaria is induced by direct contactant release of histamine, and thus passive transfer is not possible. It is more commonly encountered than immunologic contact urticaria where immunologic mechanisms are involved in histamine release; thus the phenomenon can only be elicited in sensitized individuals, and passive transfer is possible. However, there are some chemicals that produce contact urticaria due to uncertain mechanisms. Table 26-3 lists the nonimmunologic and immunologic causes of contact

Table 26-1. Causes of Allergic Contact Dermatitis Reported by the North American Contact Dermatitis Group

Skin care products	28%
Hair care products	24%
Facial cosmetics	11%
Nail cosmetics	8%
Fragrance products	7%

(Data from Adams and Maibach.[5])

Table 26-2. Ingredients Causing Allergic Contact
Dermatitis in Order of Decreasing Incidence

Fragrances
Preservatives
p-Phenylenediamine (hair dye component)
Lanolin
Glyceryl thioglycolate (permanent wave solution component)
Propylene glycol
Toluenesulfonamide/formaldehyde resin (nail polish component)
Sunscreens

(Data from Adams and Maibach.[5])

Table 26-3. Substances Used in Cosmetics
that Can Cause Contact Urticaria

Nonimmunologic
    Acetic acid
    Alcohols
    Balsam of Peru
    Benzoic acid
    Cinnamic acid
    Cinnamic aldehyde
    Formaldehyde
    Sodium benzoate
    Sorbic acid
Immunologic
    Acrylic monomer
    Alcohols
    Ammonia
    Benzoic acid
    Benzophenone
    Diethyltoluamide
    Formaldehyde
    Henna
    Menthol
    Parabens
    Polyethylene glycol
    Polysorbate 60
    Salicylic acid
    Sodium sulfide
Uncertain
    Ammonium persulfate
    p-Phenylenediamine

---

urticaria to substances encountered in cosmetics.[6] Testing for contact urticaria should be carried out under carefully controlled conditions with nearby resuscitation facilities, since anaphylaxis due to topically applied chemicals has occurred in sensitized individuals.

PHOTOTOXIC AND PHOTOALLERGIC DERMATITIS

Phototoxic and photoallergic dermatitis are limited to areas exposed to light. Phototoxic reactions are based on nonimmunologic mechanisms and usually appear as a sunburn that may be followed by hyperpigmentation and desquamation. The molecules that produce phototoxicity are generally of low molecular weight and possess highly resonant structures that readily absorb mainly UVA radiation.[7] Photoallergic dermatitis, on the other hand, is less common, immunologically mediated, generally requires repeat exposure, and can be passively transferred. It is characterized by erythema, edema, and vesiculation. Photoallergens are generally low-molecular-weight lipid-soluble substances that possess highly resonant structures absorbing energy over a wide range of wavelengths, but again predominantly UVA.[8] The light energy photochemically converts the photosensitizer into its active form.[9] Less ultraviolet radiation energy is required to elicit a photoallergic reaction compared with a phototoxic reaction.[10] Differentiating between the two may be difficult, however, especially if a severe phototoxic reaction results in vesiculation. Substances found in cosmetics that may cause photoallergic reactions include the fragrances methylcoumarin and musk ambrette, antibacterial agents, and the *p*-aminobenzoic acid esters as sunscreening agents.[11]

PATCH TESTING

Patch testing is performed to determine the source of allergic contact dermatitis.[12] Generally, the appropriate substances for patch testing are selected from the dermatologic patch test tray (Table 26-4) and applied to filter paper discs affixed to a strip of polyethylene-coated aluminum foil (A1-test) or placed in 8 mm aluminum chambers (Finn chambers) affixed to a nonwoven textile tape (Scanpor tape).[13] A newer product has the allergens in hydrophilic vehicles already applied to polyester patches (TRUE test). The healthy skin of the upper back is selected and marked for placement of the tape strips, which are worn for 48 hours. During this time, the patient should not get the patches wet or engage in activities that induce heavy sweating. The tests are initially evaluated at 20 minutes after removal and again at 2 to 7 days.[14] Table 26-5 contains the method of evaluation used by the North American Contact Dermatitis Group.

Occasionally, it may be necessary to patch test cosmetic or skin care product

Table 26-4. Substances on AAD Standard Patch Test Tray

1. Benzocaine 5% petrolatum
2. Imidazolidinyl urea 2% aqueous
3. Thiram mix 1% petrolatum
4. Lanolin alcohol 30% petrolatum
5. Neomycin sulfate 20% petrolatum
6. *p*-Phenylenediamine 1% petrolatum
7. Mercaptobenzothiazole 1% petrolatum
8. *p*-Tert-butylphenol formaldehyde resin 1% in petrolatum
9. Formaldehyde 1% aqueous
10. Carba mix 3% petrolatum
11. Rosin (colophony) 20% petrolatum
12. Black rubber mix 0.6% petrolatum
13. Ethylenediamine dihydrochloride 1% petrolatum
14. Quaternium-15 2% petrolatum
15. Mercapto mix 1% petrolatum
16. Epoxy resin 1% petrolatum
17. Balsam of peru 25% petrolatum
18. Poassium dichromate 0.25% petrolatum
19. Nickel sulfate 2.5% petrolatum
20. Cinnamic aldehyde 1% petrolatum

ingredients that are not present on the dermatologic patch test tray. Many times the cosmetics manufacturer may need to supply materials. A list of resource individuals and company addresses can be found in the Cosmetic Industry On Call brochure published by the American Academy of Dermatology and the Cosmetic, Toiletry, and Fragrance Association-(1101 17th Street, NW, Suite 300, Washington, DC, 20036). These substances or products need to be suitably formulated for patch testing so as to avoid an irritant reaction. The reader is referred to two excellent sources for recommendations on the subject.[6,15]

There are two other methods of patch testing that are useful for patients with suspected cosmetics or skin care product sensitivities: open patch tests and provocative use tests. Open patch testing is useful when the test chemical is suspected of being a cutaneous irritant. The chemical is applied to the skin on the outer aspect of the arms above the elbow unoccluded twice daily for 2 or

Table 26-5. Evaluation of Patch Test Reactions

+ ?	=	Doubtful reaction, possibly caused by a weak irritant effect; the reaction shows only a weak erythema without infiltration
+	=	Weak reaction; erythema with infiltration and possibly papules
+ +	=	Strong reaction; erythema, infiltration, papules, vesicles
+ + +	=	Extreme reaction; erythema, infiltration, papules, confluent vesicles or bullae
−	=	Negative reaction
IR	=	Irritant reaction
NT	=	Not patch tested

more days without washing the test site. The site is evaluated in the same manner as illustrated in Table 26-5. False-negative results can occur with this method, however. Provocative use testing is valuable in confirming positive reactions to cosmetics products containing ingredients that were previously found to be sources of allergic contact dermatitis with standard patch testing. The product is applied twice daily to the skin 3 cm in diameter above or below the antecubital fossae for 1 week. A modification of this test for eye cosmetics is application to the skin lateral to the eye twice daily for 1 week. Reactions are also evaluated as illustrated in Table 26-5.

ADDITIONAL TESTS

Testing beyond patch testing may be required to ensure the complete safety of cosmetics and skin care products. Ingredients used in cosmetics are evaluated by the Cosmetic Ingredient Review (CIR) committee, which makes recommendations for use and concentration of the chemcial in question.

Draize Test

The Draize test is an evaluation of dermal irritation using an animal model.[16] Semiocclusive patch tests of the evaluation substance are placed at 100% concentration on both intact and abraded albino rabbit skin. Readings are performed at 24 and 72 hours after leaving the skin uncovered for 30 to 60 minutes to allow local effects to subside. The sites are evaluated for erythema and edema to determine the degree of irritancy.[17] This test is required by law for cosmetics and skin care products under the Federal Hazardous Substances Act[18] to predict the toxicity of chemicals to humans in a manner that overestimates the risk.[19,20]

Guinea Pig Maximization Test

The guinea pig maximization test (GPMT) is designed to assess the sensitizing potential of particular ingredient, such as those found in cosmetics or skin care products.[21] Freund's complete adjuvant, as an immune enhancer, is injected intradermally into the guinea pig followed by topical application of the ingredient under occlusion. The tests are read at 24 hours.

Repeat Insult Patch Test

Repeat insult patch testing (RIPT) evaluates sensitization by repeating chemical exposure at the same site on the body. Ten patches are applied to the same site at 48 hour intervals for a 3 to 4 week period. The skin is allowed to rest for 2 weeks, and then a repeat challenge of the same chemical to the skin is applied for 48 hours and read. This method is commonly used by reputable cosmetics companies in evaluating ingredients and final products for minor sources of sensitization prior to large-scale manufacturing.

Cumulative Irritancy Test

The cumulative irritancy test is designed to assess the irritancy of an ingredient, such as those found in a cosmetic or skin care item or a final product. The test involves daily application of the same substance to the test site under occlusion for 21 days.[22] The repeat application is designed to maximize irritant reactions.

Soap Chamber Test

The soap chamber test was devised since some of the other evaluation methods previously described did not produce the irritation known to occur with certain soap, lotion, and cream products. The test is performed by applying small aluminum chambers containing the test product to the forearm of human volunteers with occlusive tape. The test product is applied daily to the same site and worn continuously for 24 hours. This procedure is repeated each week day for 1 week with a rest period over the weekend. The materials are then reapplied on the following Monday for a few hours, and the final readings are made in terms of erythema, scaling, and fissuring. This test is generally only used for cosmetics and skin care products or individual ingredients that may not have shown their true irritancy with other test methods.

Eye Irritancy Test

The eye irritancy test is important for cosmetics products since accidental introduction of cosmetics into the eye can occur. This test assesses the irritant effects of substances on the conjunctivum, cornea, and iris of albino rabbits. This is similar to patch testing; however, 0.10 ml of the test substance is instilled into the eye. In one group of rabbits the treated eyes are left unwashed, in the second group the treated eye is washed with 20 ml of lukewarm water after 2 seconds, and in the third group the eyes are washed with 20 ml of lukewarm water after 4 seconds. Evaluation of the eyes are performed at 24 hours, 48 hours, 72 hours, 4 days, and 7 days after treatment or for as long as the injury persists.[23] Human subjects are also used to assess the irritant capacity of products introduced into or around the eye. Cosmetics and skin care products should be tested in this manner to ensure human safety.

Photopatch Testing

Photopatch testing is performed when photosensitivity evaluation is required. Two patch tests with the suspected chemical are placed: one on a site to be irradiated and the other on a protected site. The patch tests remain on the skin for 48 hours.[24] One site is subjected to ultraviolet radiation of the wavelength desired and read in 24 to 48 hours. This process may be repeated if desired.

A phototoxic reaction consists of erythema and usually arises within 6 hours. A photoallergic reaction is characterized by erythema, papules, and vesicles. If only the irradiated site is positive, a diagnosis of photoallergy can be made. If both the irradiated and the protected sites are positive, a diagnosis of allergic contact dermatitis can be made. If the irradiated site is more positive than the protected site, then a diagnosis of allergic contact dermatitis and photoallergy can be made. Substances that cause photoallergic dermatitis found in cosmetics are tested as follows: methylcoumarin 5% in petrolatum, musk ambrette 5% in petrolatum and *p*-aminobenzoic acid esters 10% in petrolatum.

Cutaneous Stinging

There is a group of patients who note stinging or burning within several minutes after applying a cosmetic that intensifies over 5 to 10 minutes and then resolves after 15 minutes. These patients are known as ''stingers'' and will not tolerate

Table 26-6. Substances that Can Induce Stinging

Slight stingers
Benzene
Phenol
Salicylic acid
Resorcinol
Phosphoric acid
Moderate stingers
Sodium carbonate
Trisodium phosphate
Propylene glycol
Prolylene carbonate
Propylene glycol diacetate
Dimethylacetamide
Dimethylformamide
Dimethylsulfoxide
Diethyltoluamie
Dimethyl phthalate
2-Ethyl-1,3-hexanediol
Benzoyl peroxide
Severe stingers
Crude coal tar
Phosphoric acid
Hydrochloric acid
Sodium hydroxide
2-Ethoxyethyl p-methoxy-cinnamate

(Adapted from Frosch and Kligman,[25] with permission.)

certain cosmetic products even though patch testing for allergic contact dermatitis is negative and no evidence of irritant contact dermatitis is present. Patients who are stingers can be identified by inducing sweating (100°F and 80% relative humidity or exposure to a desktop facial sauna machine) and applying a 5% to 10% aqueous solution of lactic acid to the nasolabial fold. Those who develop stinging for at least 5 to 10 minutes are identified as "stingers." These individuals can then be used as test panel subjects to evaluate the stinging capacity of cosmetic ingredients or finished products by applying the test substance on one nasolabial fold and a bland control on the other nasolabial fold. Substances that can induce stinging are listed in Table 26-6.[25]

REFERENCES

1. Jackson EM: Irritation and sensitization. p. 23. In Waggoner WC (ed): Clinical Safety and Efficacy Testing of Cosmetics. Marcel Dekker, Inc, New York, 1990
2. Baer RL: The mechanism of allergic contact hypersensitivity. p. 1. In Fisher AA: Contact Dermatitis. 3rd Ed. Lea & Febiger, Philadelphia, 1986
3. Adams RM, Maibach HI: A five-year study of cosmetic reactions. J Am Acad Dermatol 13:1062, 1985
4. De Groot AC, Beverdam EGA, Ayong CT et al: The role of contact allergy in the spectrum of adverse effects caused by cosmetics and toiletries. Contact Dermatitis. 19:195, 1988
5. De Groot AC: Contact allergy to cosmetics: causative ingredients. Contact Dermatitis 17:26, 1987
6. Fisher AA: Contact Dermatitis. 3rd Ed. Lea & Febiger, Philadelphia, 1986
7. Billhimer WL: Phototoxicity and photoallergy. p. 43. In Waggoner WC (ed): Clinical Safety and Efficacy Testing of Cosmetics. Marcel Dekker, Inc, New York, 1990
8. Elmets CA: Drug-induced photoallergy. Dermatol Clin 231:4, 1986
9. Stephens RJ, Bergstresser PR: Fundamental concepts in photoimmunology and photoallergy. In EM Jackson (ed): Photobiology of the Skin and Eye. Marcel Dekker, New York, 1986
10. Epstein JH: Phototoxicity and photoallergy in man. J Am Acad Dermatol 8:141, 1983
11. DeLeo VA, Harber LC: Contact photodermatitis. p. 454. In Fisher AA: Contact Dermatitis. 3rd Ed. Lea & Febiger, Philadelphia, 1986
12. Nethercott JR: Sensitivity and specificity of patch tests. Am J Contact Dermatitis 5:136, 1994
13. Goldner R: Clinical tests. p. 201. In Jackson EM, Goldner R (eds): Irritant Contact Dermatitis. Marcel Dekker, Inc, New York, 1990
14. Fowler JF: Reading patch tests: some pitfalls of patch testing. Am J Contact Dermatitis 5:170, 1994
15. De Groot AC, Weyland JW, Nater JP: Unwanted Effects of Cosmetics and Drugs Used in Dermatology. 3rd Ed. Elsevier, Amsterdam, 1994
16. Draize JH, Woodard G, Calvary HO: Methods for the study of irritation and toxicity of substances applied topically to the skin and mucous membranes. J Pharmacol Exp Ther 82:377, 1944

17. Bronaugh RL, Maibach HI: Primary irritant, allergic contact, phototoxic, and photo-allergic reations to cosmetics and tests to identify problem products. p. 223. In Frost P, Horwitz SN (eds): Principles of Cosmetics for the Dermatologist. CV Mosby Company, St. Louis, 1982
18. Method of testing primary irritant substances, United States Code of Federal Regulations, 16 CFR, 1500.41, 1979, Consumer Product Safety Commission, Washington, DC.
19. Philips L, Steingerg M, Maibach HI, Akers WA: A comparison of rabbit and human skin response to certain irritants. Toxicol Appl Pharmacol 21:369, 1972
20. Gabrial KL: In vivo preclinical tests. p. 191. In Jackson EM, Goldner R (eds): Irritant Contact Dermatitis. Marcel Dekker, Inc, New York, 1990
21. Magnusson B, Kligman AM: The identification of contact allergens by animal assay. The guinea pig maximization test. J Invest Dermatol 52:268, 1969
22. Kligman AM, Wooding WM: A method for the measurement and evaluation of irritants in human skin. J Invest Dermatol 49:78, 1967
23. Wortzman MS: Eye products. p. 205. In Whittam JH (ed): Cosmetic Safety: A primer for Cosmetic Scientists. Marcel Dekker, Inc, New York, 1987
24. DeLeo VA: Photocontact Dermatitis in Photosensitivity. Igaku-Shoin, New York, 1992
25. Frosch PJ, Kligman AM: A method for appraising the stinging capacity of topically applied substances. J Soc Cosmet Chem 28:197, 1977

27

Approach to the Patient with Cosmetic Problems

The previous chapters provide detailed information on the composition, use, and selection of various cosmetic and skin care products. The dermatologist must utilize this knowledge to guide the patient in a systematic manner toward a desired goal. The first step in dealing with a patient's cosmetic problems is to establish realistic goals. This is critical. Patients often have unrealistic expectations and focus more on how they can resemble a friend or celebrity rather than on how they can improve their own appearance. If the dermatologist feels that the patient has an unattainable goal, this should be discussed and more realistic expectations defined. Some patients are not satisfied with realistic expectations and should not be further encouraged.

Many patients seek cosmetic advice or surgical procedures shortly after experiencing a major life change or loss. These patients may need both psychiatric and cosmetic counseling. Only the combination can yield a good result.

Another commonly encountered situation is the patient who has an unstable marriage. This patient may also have unrealistic expectations: he or she may link marital problems with appearance. This may be true, but more often an improved appearance does not solve deeper interpersonal problems. Marriage counseling would benefit this patient more than cosmetics counseling.

Once the patient has identified which area to improve cosmetically and has set a realistic goal, the dermatologist can counsel effectively. The second step is to evaluate whether the defect should be corrected surgically or cosmetically; sometimes a combination of both is optimal. The following discussion focuses on the patient who has completed surgery or needs only cosmetic correction.

The third step is to determine whether the defect should be covered or deemphasized. Discrete defects are generally best covered. A forehead scar can be covered with bangs, a dark congenital nevus on the cheek can be covered with an opaque facial foundation, psoriatic nails can be covered with sculptured nails, omphiasis can be covered with a hair piece, and so on. If the defect is not discrete, it may not be possible to cover it appropriately. For example, the appearance of actinically wrinkled facial skin will not improve with use of a thick foundation. On the contrary, the thick foundation will only accentuate the wrinkling. This situation demands that the defect be deemphasized.

Deemphasizing a defect involves drawing attention away from the negative feature and toward positive features. For example, upper eyelid blepharochalasis cannot be improved by thick application of colored eye shadow. Rather, the patient with intact eyelashes can deemphasize the blepharochalasis by using a fibered lash lengthening mascara followed by curling the thickened, elongated eyelashes. A thin, subdued eye shadow can then be applied to the upper lid. Learning how to deemphasize negative features is part of the art of using cosmetics.

The fourth step is to encourage the patient to practice and experiment. Proper cosmetic application is not easy. Fortunately, a bad result can be removed in a matter of minutes. Even though the patient may choose not to purchase cosmetics counter products, most clerks are more than happy to assist the patient in the use of sample cosmetics. Some physicians may wish to have sample products in their office for demonstration.

The fifth and final step is to have the patient evaluate the success of the cosmetic result. The patient should check the appearance under the lighting conditions present where the cosmetic will be worn. A patient who works in an office should look at the appearance under bright office lighting, while a cosmetic for evening wear should be evaluated under subdued incandescent lighting. A makeup mirror that simulates various lighting conditions is valuable, since color is perceived as reflected light. Subtle changes in lighting may change an attractive cosmetic application into a theatrical result. Patients should be advised that department and drug store lighting is extremely bright and most cosmetics will appear lighter than under natural sunlight. This means that when selecting cosmetics for purchase, a sample should be placed on the skin and then evaluated under natural sunlight.

The physician can optimize patient satisfaction if a systematic approach is taken when advising the patient with cosmetic problems.

28

Approach to the Patient with Diffuse, Nonscarring Hair Loss

The practicing dermatologist frequently encounters patients who express concerns regarding hair loss. Generally, patients state that their usually thick, shiny, and manageable hair has become thin and difficult to style. If this is the dermatologist's first consultation with the patient, verifying the degree of hair loss is difficult. It is estimated that an individual must loose approximately 50% of their hair before an unacquainted observer can examine the scalp and note a reduction in hair shaft number. In the hair cosmetics industry, the following number of hairs are used to give the impression of fullness for each hair color:

Blond: 140,000 hairs
Brown: 110,000 hairs
Black: 108,000 hairs
Red: 90,000

Red hair requires fewer shafts than blond hair to appear full since red hair shafts have the thickest diameter while blond hair shafts are the thinnest. Nevertheless, hair loss is a complex problem mediated by internal and external factors. This chapter describes my approach to the patient with diffuse, nonscarring hair loss. Hair loss caused by scarring is beyond the realm of this text.[1]

EVALUATING EXTERNAL VERSUS INTERNAL HAIR LOSS CAUSATION

It is of utmost importance to begin evaluation of the hair loss patient by differentiating internal versus external factors. Generally, internal causes of hair loss result in shedding of the complete hair shaft, including the bulb. If the bulb is elongated, the hair has been shed during the anagen phase, indicating anagen effluvium. On the other hand, if the bulb is club shaped, the hair has been shed during the telogen phase, indicating telogen effluvium.

External causes of hair loss resulting from grooming practices or cosmetic chemical hair treatments weaken the hair shaft such that breakage occurs. These broken hair shafts do not contain the bulb. However, abnormally formed hair shafts, found sporadically or in association with genodermatoses (trichoschisis, trichorrhexis invaginata, pili torti, monilethrix, and trichorrhexis nodosa), can also result in decreased hair shaft strength and subsequent breakage. Examination of several plucked hairs under the microscope is necessary to ensure normal hair structure.

Hair loss can be easily distinguished from hair breakage by performing 10 hair pulls over various areas of the scalp. The hair pull is performed by grasping the hair shaft close to the scalp with the fingers and firmly pulling over the length of the shaft. Removed hairs are examined for the presence and formation of the bulb. If more than six hairs are removed per pull, excessive hair loss is present. This procedure also provides an opportunity to ascertain that no localized areas of total hair loss are present, allowing elimination of tinea capitas, alopecia areata, and so forth, as the cause.

EVALUATING HAIR LOSS MAGNITUDE

Hair pull tests performed in the office can be misleading, especially if the patient has shampooed before being examined and has removed the loose or broken hairs. It may prove difficult to accurately estimate the magnitude of the hair loss from the patient as a normal individual may lose approximately 100 hairs per day. If grooming of the hair is infrequent, shampooing may yield up to 200 lost hairs.

Information on the magnitude of the loss can best be obtained by having the patient collect all hair lost for 4 consecutive days and place each day's loss in a separate envelope, noting days shampooing was performed. The hair should be brushed or combed over the sink and the hair collected from the sink and also from the brush or comb. Hairs should also be removed from the drain following shampooing. The dermatologist can examine each day's loss, noting both amount and presence or absence of the hair bulb.

INTERNAL CAUSES OF HAIR LOSS

Once it has been determined that the hair loss is indeed in excess of 100 hairs per day and that normally formed hairs are being shed diffusely from a nonscarred scalp with an intact bulb, anagen effluvium and telogen effluvium must be considered. Anagen effluvium is generally due to internally administered medications, such as chemotherapy agents, that act as cell poisons and

Table 28-1. Internal Causes of Diffuse, Nonscarring Alopecia

Hormonal causes: postpartum, oral contraceptives, menopause, hormone supplementation
Physical stress: surgery, illness, anemia, rapid weight change
Emotional stress: psychiatric illness, death of family member
Endocrinopathy: hypothyroidism, hyperthyroidism, hypoparathyroidism, hyperparathyroidism
Oral medications:
    Blood thinning agents: heparin, coumarin
    Retinoids: high-dose vitamin A, isotretinoin, etretinate
    Antihypertensive agents: propanolol, captopril
    Miscellaneous: quinacrine, allopurinol, lithium carbonate, thiouracil compounds

disrupt the growing hair follicle. Telogen effluvium, on the other hand, is due to an increased number of hair follicles prematurely exiting the anagen phase or hair cycle synchronization.[2] Premature anagen exit can be due to medications, such as coumarin or heparin, while hair cycle synchronization occurs during pregnancy and with oral contraceptive use.

The causes of diffuse, nonscarring telogen hair loss to be considered are summarized in Table 28-1. Most of these considerations can be eliminated by a review of systems and some basic laboratory work. Anemia, thyroid abnormalities, and many illnesses can be detected by obtaining a complete blood count with differential, thyroid panel and chemistry panel to include liver function studies. If deemed clinically necessary, an antinuclear antibody (ANA) can also be obtained to rule out any collagen vascular diseases. A complete history can determine the nature of any severe physical or emotional stress and document the ingestion of prescription or over-the-counter medications or vitamin supplements.

Physical or Emotional Stress

Surgeries, febrile illnesses, and severe emotional stresses experienced in the past 6 months must be evaluated by the dermatologist. In many cases, a 3 month delay is present between the actual event and the patient's onset of hair loss. Furthermore, there may be another 3 month delay prior to the return of noticeable hair regrowth. Thus, the total hair loss and regrowth cycle can last 6 months or possibly longer. Patients should be educated as to when reasonable regrowth can be expected.

Diet Considerations

Hair loss caused by rapid weight loss is not uncommon. Many times patients embark on franchised diet programs administered under the direction of a physician with prescribed meals and dietary supplements. Sometimes patients are told that vitamin supplements purchased as part of the weight loss program are necessary to prevent hair loss associated with dieting. From a dermatologist's standpoint, however, the vitamins cannot prevent hair loss associated with rapid, significant weight loss.

Hormonal Considerations

Hormonal causes of hair loss deserve special attention for the female patient. Many women do not realize that hair loss can occur postpartum or following discontinuation of oral contraceptives. It is important to remind the female patient that hair loss may be delayed by 3 months following a hormonal status change, and another 3 to 6 months may be required for regrowth to be fully appreciated.

Menopausal women with decreased ovarian estrogen production may also experience diffuse hair thinning, generally more prominent over the top of the head with bitemporal recession. A thin strip of hair at the anterior hairline is usually spared. An FSH (follicle-stimulating hormone) level can be obtained to document the onset of menopause, although menopausal hair thinning may be present even though FSH levels are not low. Institution of estrogen replacement can prevent further loss, but has not been shown to promote regrowth. Other treatments such as topical minoxidil may be indicated.[3]

Lastly, it is important to rule out any hormonal abnormalities in the female patient. Inquiring as to the regularity of menses and the presence of infertility problems can uncover ovarian hormonal failure or the presence of excess endogenous androgens. Questions should also be directed as to whether the patient is ingesting oral steroids with androgenic effects. If necessary, hormone levels such as a free testosterone and DHEA-S (dehydroepiandrosterone sulfate) can be measured and an endocrinologic evaluation initiated.[4] A more detailed discussion of hormonally induced hair loss is beyond the scope of this text.[5,6]

EXTERNAL CAUSES OF HAIR LOSS

Shed hairs without a hair bulb are considered broken hairs. Hair breakage is generally due to external factors; however, abnormalities in hair shaft formation must be eliminated. Table 28-2 contains the technical terms used to describe hair shaft abnormalities and a definition of the term.[7] Trichoschisis, trichorrhexis invaginata, pill torti, and monilethrix are all abnormalities intrinsic to the hair shaft.[8] Trichoptilosis and trichonodosis may be due to cosmetic manipulation of the hair. Trichorrhexis nodosa may be due to intrinsic abnormalities or cosmetic manipulation. All of these conditions predispose the hair to breakage that can become magnified by extensive grooming, chemical waving procedures, or permanent dyeing.

Table 28-2. Structural Hair Shaft Abnormalities

Intrinsic abnormalities
> Trichoschisis—a clean, transverse fracture across the hair shaft through both cuticle and cortex. Congenital forms seen in trichothiodystrophy characterized by hair with an abnormally low sulfur content
> Trichorrhexis invaginata—a nodular expansion of the hair shaft in which a ball in socket joint is formed, also known as bamboo hair. Congenital forms seen in Netherton's syndrome
> Pili torti—a flattened hair shaft that is twisted through 180 degrees on its own axis
> Monilethrix—elliptical nodal swellings along the hair shaft with intervening, tapering constrictions that are nonmedullated

Extrinsic abnormalities
> Trichoptilosis—a longitudinal splitting or fraying of the distal end of the hair shaft, also known as split ends
> Trichonodosis—knotting of the hair shaft

Intrinsic or extrinsic abnormalities
> Trichorrhexis nodosa—small, beaded swellings associated with a loss of the cuticle. Congenital forms seen in argininosuccinic aciduria and Menke's disease, but may also be due to cosmetic hair shaft manipulation

Gross Hair Shaft Evaluation

Once it has been determined that the primary cause of hair loss is breakage, the patient's scalp hair should be grossly examined to assess the state of the hair shafts. An overall impression should be formed:

Does the hair have shine?
Does the hair feel soft?
Does the hair lay in an orderly fashion?
Is there evidence of hair styling aid use?
Does the hair color appear natural and match the patient's eyebrow, eyelashes, and body hair?
Is the hair curly or straight?
How long is the hair, and when was it last cut?

Hair Shine

Hair possessing an intact cuticle with closely overlapping cuticular scales is shiny, healthy hair. It is the smoothness of the overlapping scales that promotes light reflection, interpreted by the eye as shine. Normal grooming processes such as combing and brushing result in loss of cuticular scales, which is more pronounced at the distal hair shaft.[9] This process is known as "weathering" and is accelerated by overly aggressive grooming and chemical processing.[10,11]

Hair Softness

Hair softness is also due to an intact cuticle, which creates a smooth hair shaft surface. Permanently waved or dyed hair must have a disrupted cuticle in order to allow penetration of the waving lotion or dye. Thus, chemically processed hair never feels as soft as virgin hair, even though hair conditioners attempt to smooth the disrupted cuticle temporarily. Harsh-feeling hair is evidence of cuticular damage.

Hair Frizziness

Hair that has been chemically processed is also prone to static electricity. This allows the hair to appear frizzy and unruly, especially at the distal hair shafts. Generally, chemicals applied to the hair penetrate better at the distal hair shaft due to less cuticular scale. A well-educated cosmetologist is aware of this fact, especially when processing long hair, and will apply the chemicals to the scalp first and then dilute the product prior to applying the solutions to the distal hair shafts. Overprocessed hair appears frizzy and is severely weakened.

Use of Styling Aids

It is important not to be misled, when evaluating hair shine, softness, and frizzines, by the use of hair styling aids such as hair spray, mousse, and styling gels. These products usually contain a polymer that forms a thin film over the hair shafts, imparting shine and stiffness. Combing the hair will remove the polymer film, which will appear as tiny white flakes throughout the hair, but the true state of the hair shafts can be better appreciated.

Use of Hair Coloring

Unfortunately, some patients who dye their hair will not openly admit that they use hair coloring. Furthermore, many patients do not know what kind of dye has been applied to the hair and whether any bleaching has occurred. This means that the dermatologist must rely on his or her powers of observation.

Hair color should be compared with eyelashes, eyebrows, or other body hair. (It is possible to dye the eyelashes and eyebrows.) If the scalp hair color is lighter than other hair, bleaching has occurred. If regrowth is present at the scalp, a permanent hair color has been used. If the color appears to vary gradually from the proximal hair shaft to the distal hair shaft with the presence of some grayish hairs, a semipermanent hair color has been used. If the hair has a yellowish cast, a metallic hair color has been used. These guidelines can be used to initiate conversation when obtaining a patient history.

Degree of Curl

The degree of curl the hair possesses should also be evaluated since tightly curled hair is more prone to breakage. It should also be determined whether the curl is natural or due to permanent waving. Hair that has been chemically waved appears straight at the scalp and curlier at the ends. Hair that is naturally curly will have an even curl throughout the length of the hair shaft. If the hair has been chemically waved, the type of permanent wave and length of processing should be obtained either from the patient or from the salon. These factors cannot be determined by visual examination.

Hair Length

Lastly, it is important to note the length of the hair and ask the patient when it was last cut. Longer hair has been subject to more weathering, and increased breakage is expected. Patients also evaluate hair loss by the amount of hair in the brush or sink; longer hair shafts will create a larger lump than shorter hair shafts even though the same number of hairs have been lost. Thus, patients with longer hair tend to overestimate their actual loss. Hair that has been cut frequently shows less evidence of damage than infrequently cut hair. If the damaged hair shaft ends have been removed prior to visiting the dermatologist, the full extent of hair damage may not be appreciated; however, chemical processing damages the whole hair shaft, and evidence of damage will reappear shortly.

Microscopic Hair Shaft Examination

The gross findings should be confirmed by microscopic examination of a shed hair shaft. The cuticular scales should be examined to note if weathering is present. The decrease or absence of scales can confirm the gross observation that the hair is dull, harsh, and frizzy. If the cuticular scales are greatly decreased at the distal hair shaft, trichoptilosis results from exposure of the soft medulla. If trichonodosis is observed, hair twisting or teasing may be the cause of the knots predisposing the hair to breakage. If trichorrhexis nodosa is present, and not part of a genodermatosis, this suggests extensive cuticular loss.

COSMETIC TECHNIQUES FOR MINIMIZING HAIR LOSS

Hair grooming includes cleansing, drying, combing, brushing, and styling of the hair. While any manipulation of the hair shaft can cause breakage, loss can be minimized by recommending proper grooming practices to the patient.

Hair Cleansing

Cleansing the hair should be done only when required due to dirt in the hair or excess sebum. If sebum production is minimal and the patient has a sedentary lifestyle, daily washing is not necessary for good hygiene. The patient should select a shampoo appropriate for the hair type: normal, oily, dry, fine, damaged, or chemically treated. These types usually appear on the outside of the shampoo bottle. If the patient with normal to minimal sebum production insists on daily shampooing, a dry hair shampoo with less detergent action should be recommended. Aggressive removal of sebum results in hair that tangles readily, appears dull, and attracts static electricity.

Hair Conditioning

An instant conditioner or a cream rinse can be valuable in minimizing hair loss by detangling the hair, especially long hair.[12] Patients who have excess sebum production may prefer a cream rinse over a conditioner. All formulations of instant conditioners are good at detangling hair by smoothing the cuticle and reducing friction. However, if the hair has been severely damaged and the cuticular scales are sparse with the presence of trichoptilosis, only a protein-containing conditioner can penetrate the hair shaft and temporarily mend split ends. This is due to the substantivity of protein conditioners for hair keratin.

Hair Drying

It is best if the hair is allowed to dry without externally applied heat; however, many patients wish to speed up the drying process or style their hair while drying. Heat-damaged hair from improper dryer use appears frizzy and curly at the ends. It may also develop an abnormality known as "bubble hair".[13] Any tension applied to the burned hair shaft will cause the hair to break in tiny fragments, some of which can be crushed between the fingers. Heat damage can be avoided by using the lowest heat setting and holding the nozzle at least 6 inches from the scalp. A specially designed vented blow drying brush should be used to prevent high temperatures along the brush.

Hair Combing and Brushing

Hair shafts are most subject to fracture when wet due to increased elasticity. It is much easier to stretch a wet hair shaft to the breaking point than a dry one. Therefore, hair should be initially detangled with the fingers and slightly dried prior to detangling with a wide-toothed comb. Brushes should not be used for detangling. Combing and brushing should be kept to a minimum. The idea that 100 brush strokes a day is beneficial to the hair is mistaken. Combs should be selected for their smooth, widely spaced teeth so that they glide freely through the hair. Brushes should have widely spaced bristles with rounded tips for the same reasons. Whether the bristles are synthetic or natural is less important than the spacing of the bristles.

Hair Styling

Hair styles that minimize breakage are loose and do not require excessive hair pins or combs. All hair pins should be rubber coated with smooth edges so that the hair is not broken as the clasp is closed. Unfortunately, the clasp must hold the hair tightly or it will not remain in place. Rubber bands should not be used in the hair, as they are difficult to remove.

There are several common presentations by patients who are experiencing hair breakage caused by hair styling. The first is the patient who wears a pony tail or braid and claims decreased hair growth. Examination of the hair shows hair shafts fractured at the same distance from the scalp. This is due to repeated breakage where the hair clasp is placed. A second presentation is the patient who wears braids on the scalp, also known as corn rows, and notes thinning at the front hairline. In this instance, the hair is broken because of maximum tension at the front hairline; traction alopecia may also be present. The third presentation is the patient who has had hair extensions glued or woven into the natural hair. The weight of the extensions can cause hair breakage and traction alopecia. It may be necessary to question patients on hair styling practices, as they may wear their hair differently on the day they visit the dermatologist.

Hair Appliances

Burning of the hair and subsequent breakage can also be caused by heated hair appliances: curling irons, crimping irons, straightening irons, and heated curlers. Most patients prefer to use these appliances at their hottest setting as this produces the tightest, longest lasting curl, but it also induces the most hair damage. This burning is minimized if a lower heat setting is chosen. Hair that is burned with a heated appliance appears frizzy at the ends.

Permanent Hair Coloring

Darkening the natural hair color is less damaging than lightening the natural hair color, as the original eumelanins and pheomelanins are not removed. Any lightening of the hair color requires the use of bleaching to remove existing pigments. In general, the more bleaching required to achieve the final hair color, the weaker the hair shaft at the end of the chemical process. Many patients erroneously think that if bleached blonde hair is redyed to their darker original color, it will be healthier. This is not true. Any further dyeing only contributes to additional weakening of the hair shaft.

Hair Permanent Waving

Permanent waving of the hair is more damaging than dyeing since the protein structure of the hair shaft is actually degraded and reconstructed in a new form. Damage can be minimized, however, by wrapping the hair loosely around larger curlers. This results in a looser, shorter lasting curl, but breakage is minimized.

The processing time can also be shortened, which decreases the degree of bond breaking. The processing time is checked by performing a "test curl." The test curl is one rod, usually selected at the nape of neck, where the hair is periodically unwound to determine if the desired amount of curl has been achieved. Not all cosmetologists use a test curl, but it is highly recommended. It is also recommended that the test curl not be placed at the nape of the neck, but rather at the front hairline. Traditionally, the nape of the neck is chosen because this hair is more difficult to permanently wave than at any other area of the scalp. If the appropriate amount of curl is present at the nape, then the rest of the scalp will also be curled. However, hair at the front hairline curls more readily and may be overprocessed by the time the nape has curled. This accounts for patients noting more breakage at the anterior hairline.

Many patients both permanently dye and permanently wave their hair. While the damage produced by these procedures is additive, it can be minimized by allowing 10 days between procedures and permanently waving the hair first, followed by dyeing the hair.

REFERENCES

1. Bergfeld WF: Scarring alopecia. p. 759. In Roenigk RR, Roenigk HR (eds): Dermatolgic Surgery, Principles and Practice. Marcel Dekker, New York, 1989
2. Headington JT: Telogen effluvium. Arch Dermatol 129:356, 1993
3. Olsen EA, DeLong ER et al: Safe response study of topical minoxidil in male pattern baldness. J Am Acad Dermatol 15:30, 1986
4. Redmond GP, Bergfeld WF: Diagnostic approach to androgen disorders in women. Cleve Clin J Med 57:423, 1990
5. Sperling LC, Heimer WL: Androgen biology as a basis for the diagnosis and treatment of androgenic disorders in women. I. J Am Acad Dermatol 28:669, 1993
6. Sperling LC, Heimer WL: Androgen biology as a basis for the diagnosis and treatment of androgenic disorders in women. II. J Am Acad Dermatol 28:90, 1993
7. Whiting DA: Structural abnormalities of the hair shaft. J Am Acad Dermatl 16:1, 1987
8. Camacho-Martinez F, Ferrando J: Hair shaft dysplasias. Int J Dermatol 27:71, 1988
9. Wolfram L, Lindemann MO: Some observations on the hair cuticle. J Soc Cosmet Chem 2:839, 1971
10. Rook A: The clinical importance of "weathering" in human hair. Br J Dermatol 95:111, 1976
11. Robbins C: Weathering in human hair. Text Res J 37:337, 1967
12. Menkart J: Damaged hair. Cutis 23:276, 1979
13. Detwiler SP, Carson JL, Woosley JT et al: Bubble hair. J Am Acad Dermatol 30:54, 1994

29

Advising the Patient on Cosmetics Selection

The dermatologist is called upon with increasing frequency to give advice on cosmetics selection. Patients are searching for cosmetics that improve skin quality while offering value. Dermatologists, with their understanding of skin physiology and disease, are best suited to render opinions in this area; however, unfamiliarity with available cosmetics and their uses may make physicians unable to give valuable, concrete advice. This text is intended to serve as a basic guide for formulating individual patient recommendations. I now outline my approach to advising the patient on cosmetic selection.

The first step in making cosmetics selection recommendations is to determine where the patient purchases her cosmetics. This is important because point of purchase is related to the cost of the product. It is wise to keep cost in mind when making patient recommendations. Cosmetics manufacturers intentionally produce products to reach consumers through a variety of markets. Some cosmetics are sold in mass merchandisers, such as grocery stores, drug stores, and discount stores. Cosmetics sold through these vendors generally range in price from $2 to $15. Other cosmetics are sold exclusively through cosmetics counters in department stores. Even within the department store market there are products designed for lower price point department stores and higher price point department stores. Lower price point department stores market cosmetics that sell for $8 to $20 as compared with higher price point department store cosmetics that sell for $20 to $60. The most expensive cosmetics are sold through boutiques and spas. These products range from $25 to $90. Interestingly, some of these exclusive products are manufactured by the same companies that produce cosmetics under a different label for sale in mass merchandisers. Generally, boutique lines have more attractive, elaborate packaging accompanied by a greater color selection, more expensive fragrances, and innovative specialty additives.

Another route for cosmetics purchase is through household parties and individuals who sell door-to-door in their neighborhood. These products generally are in the $8 to $25 range. Lastly, private cosmetics are produced on a contract basis generally through small manufacturers. Cosmetics can be customized to the needs of the business or simply be a standard formulation with a customized label. The price variation in this market is tremendous. It is worthwhile noting that cosmetics sold in these manners, which are produced and marketed for intrastate use, do not fall under the guidelines of the Food and Drug Administration. Furthermore, smaller cosmetics manufacturers do not have the capital or the facilities to undertake extensive premarketing and postmarketing consumer research. There are several large cosmetics companies, however, that market quality products worldwide and also reach the consumer through these routes.

The second step is, to determine the patient's skin type: very oily, oily, combination, normal, dry, very dry, and so forth. Moisturizer and facial foundation recommendations must be carefully made with skin type in mind. Interestingly, many patients do not know their skin type or have been erroneously assigned a skin type by a salesperson at a cosmetics counter. In my opinion, skin type can be most easily assigned by asking the patient about the amount of sebum production on the nose throughout the day following morning washing. Sebum production can be assessed by having the patients run a finger down the nose at various times during the day. If the patient has flaking skin on the nose all day and no sebum from morning until 5 pm, the skin is very dry. If the patient has no flaking, but no sebum on the nose at 5 pm, the skin is dry. If the patient has minimal sebum on the nose at 5 pm, the skin is normal. If the patient has sebum on the nose at noon, the skin is oily. And if the patient has sebum on the nose 1 hour following morning washing, the skin is very oily. Combination skin, the most common skin type in both women and men, can be assessed by comparing the amount of sebum present on the nose at 5 pm with the amount present on the cheeks. This is a simplistic, but fairly accurate, method of determining skin type.

Table 29-1A. Cosmetic Colors for Caucasian Skin

Cosmetic	Light Skin	Medium Skin	Dark Skin
Facial foundation	Light beige, pale ivory, light pink	Medium beige, ivory, medium pink, peach	Beige, tan, dark peach
Blush and lipstick	Rose pink, true red	Deep pink, blue red, cherry red, coral	Deep red, cinnamon, burgundy
Eyebrow pencil and mascara	Charcoal gray, dark brown, brown black	Dark brown	Dark brown
Eyeliner	Charcoal gray, brown black	Dark brown	Black
Eye shadow	Light green, purple, pink, light brown, light blue	Deep green, brown, blue	Muted green, brown, muted blue

Table 29-1B. Cosmetic Colors for Black Skin

Cosmetic	Light Skin	Medium Skin	Dark Skin
Facial foundation	Rose, medium beige, medium peach	Medium beige, bronze	Sun bronze, taupe
Blush and lipstick	Medium coral, medium pink, orange red	Deep coral, rose, translucent red	Cinnamon, deep translucent rose, true translucent red
Eyebrow pencil and mascara	Dark brown, charcoal, black	Charcoal, black	Black
Eyeliner	Beige, charcoal, black	Beige, charcoal, black	Beige, charcoal, black
Eye shadow	Beige, lavender, aqua, light blue	Beige, deep lavender, medium blue	Deep violet, deep sea green

Table 29-1C. Cosmetic Colors for Oriental Skin

Cosmetic	Light Skin	Medium Skin	Dark Skin
Facial foundation	Light pink, peach, beige	Medium pink, deep peach, medium beige	Dark pink, dark beige
Blush and lipstick	Light pink, orange	Rose, light red	Rose, red
Eyebrow pencil and mascara	Black, charcoal	Black, charcoal	Black
Eyeliner	Black, charcoal	Black, charcoal	Black
Eye shadow	Beige, pink, violet, blue	Turquoise, aqua, lavender, deep blue, green	Deep violet, deep pink, vivid blue, vivid green

Table 29-1D. Cosmetic Colors for American Indian Skin

Cosmetic	Light Skin	Medium Skin	Dark Skin
Facial foundation	Light beige	Medium beige	Dark beige
Blush and lipstick	Pink, light red	Peach, pink, light red	Deep rose, cranberry red
Eyebrow pencil and mascara	Charcoal, dark brown, black	Black, charcoal	Black
Eyeliner	Black, charcoal	Black, charcoal	Black
Eye shadow	Beige, cool turquoise, green, aqua	Medium beige, turquoise, aqua, green, deep blue	Beige, deep green, deep blue

Table 29-1E. Cosmetic Colors for Asian Skin

Cosmetic	Light Skin	Medium Skin	Dark Skin
Facial foundation	Beige, rose beige	Medium beige, rose beige	Beige, light taupe
Blush and lipstick	Peach, pale orange, rose	Red, rose, pink, coral	Deep red, deep rose, orange
Eyebrow pencil and mascara	Dark brown, charcoal	Black, charcoal	Black
Eyeliner	Black, charcoal	Black charcoal	Black
Eye shadow	Pink, lavender, blue, turquoise, sea green	Deep violet, deep beige, deep pink	Violet, purple, blue

Third, once skin type has been determined, appropriate sections within this text can be consulted for specific cosmetic product recommendations. Some patients, however, also wish to know what color cosmetics should be selected to enhance the appearance of their skin and facial features. This advice may be beyond the realm of what most dermatologists can provide, and questions of this nature may be more appropriately handled by cosmetologists. Nevertheless, for the physician with an interest in this area, color charts based on skin pigmentation have been provided to coordinate facial foundation, blush, lipstick, eyebrow pencil, mascara, and eye shadow color with skin tones (Table 29-1).[1,2]

Finally, there is no doubt that a personal visit to a mass merchandiser cosmetics display or the department store cosmetics counter can provide valuable firsthand experience. Smelling, touching, and applying cosmetics can provide a wealth of information that cannot be fully described in a text.

REFERENCES

1. Soldo BL, Drahos M: The Inside-Out Beauty Book. Fleming H. Revell Company, Old Tappan, NJ, 1978
2. Bruce J, Cohen SS: About Face. G.P. Putnam's Sons, New York, 1984

30

Personal Product Recommendations

Even after reading a discussion of the formulation, use, efficacy, and adverse reactions associated with certain cosmetics and skin care products, practical application of this information may be difficult. Patients generally will not understand if a dermatologist recommends they select a moisturizer with both humectant and occlusive agents. They want the brand name of a product that the dermatologist feels will produce the desired result. But, how does the dermatologist select products to recommend to patients? Do you go to the sample closet and grab a handful of products and tell them to use the one they like? Do you recommend the product your spouse or nurse likes? Do you buy one of each of the nationally marketed brands and use them yourself for 1 month or more? Or, do you tell the patient that anything they select will be fine?

Certainly, with the number and variety of cosmetics and skin care products available for purchase, specific product recommendations can be difficult. This is complicated by the fact that established products are frequently reformulated and new products are introduced monthly. Yet the issue remains important, and patients who request such information from the dermatologist expect a timely answer. After all, who better to ask about cosmetics and skin care products than a phsycian who has spent considerable time and energy studying the skin?

The only method I know with which to determine somewhat scientifically which products perform well is to use them personally. This is a rather extensive undertaking since the products must be used for at least 1 week and preferrably 1 month or longer. Patient evaluations are also helpful, but personal experience is far more valuable. This chapter contains my personal recommendations for products I use with my patients. The information is to be taken as my opinion and does not represent an endorsement of the product. I do not have a financial interest in any of the products that are discussed. Certainly, there are many

Table 30-1. Facial Cosmetics: Personal Recommendations

Facial Cosmetics	Recommendation
Facial foundations	See Chapter 1
Facial powders	Transparent Face Powder, Clinique or Almay
Blush, powdered	Clinique
Bronzing gels and gel blush	Blushing Gel or Sun Bronzer, Bonnie Bell
Facial highlighters and buffers	Clinique
Facial cover sticks	Invisible Concealer, Cover Girl
Undercover creams	Color Primer Undercover, Estee Lauder or Beauticontrol
Eye shadow, powdered	Merle Normal or Maybelline
Eye shadow setting cream	Eye Fix, Elizabeth Arden
Mascara, rub resistant	Super Rich Mascara, Almay
Eyeliner, pencil	Lancome
Eyebrow pencils	Maybelline
Eyebrow sealers	Merle Norman
Lipstick, long wearing crayon	Lip Pencil Plus, Merle Norman
Lip sealant	Stop It!, Coty; or Lip Fix, Elizabeth Arden

Table 30-2. Nail Cosmetics: Personal Recommendations

Nail Cosmetics	Recommendation
Nail polish	Revlon or Almay
Fibered nail polish	Sally Hansen
Nail polish remover	Cutex

Table 30-3. Hair Cosmetics: Personal Recommendations

Hair Cosmetic	Recommendation
Normal hair shampoo	Ivory Shampoo, Procter & Gamble
Dry hair shampoo	Flex Shampoo, Revlon or Pantene Shampoo, Procter & Gamble
Oily hair shampoo	Pert Shampoo, Procter & Gamble
Sensitive skin hair shampoo	DHS Clear Dermatological Hair and Scalp Shampoo, Person & Covey
Damaged hair shampoo	Finesse Shampoo, Helene Curtis; or Jhirmack Shampoo, Playtex; or Silkience Shampoo, Gillette

(continued)

Table 30-3. *(continued)*

Hair Cosmetic	Recommendation
Medicated shampoo	T-Gel, Neutrogena
Instant conditioner	Flex, Revlon
Leave-in conditioner	Styling Glaze, Vidal Sassoon
Deep conditioner	Kolestral, Wella
Cream rinse	Advanced Salon Formula Conditioning Rinse, Vidal Sassoon; or Conditioning Rinse, Person & Convey
Hair spray	Shpritz Forte, Sebastian International
Conditioning hair spray, black hair care	TCB Hi-Lite and Hold, Alberto-Culver; or Curly Look Control, Lustrasilk
Hair mousse	Condition Mousse, Clairol
Styling gel	Styling Gel, L'Oreal
Sculpturing gel	Sculpturing Gel, Vidal Sassoon
Liquid brilliantine, black hair care	Ultra Sheen Conditioner and Hair Dressing, Johnson Products; or TCB Comb Out Conditioner and Oil Sheen, Albert-Culver; or Right On, Lustrasilk
Glycerin hair dressing, black hair care	Glycerin Curl, Activator, Pro-Line; or TCB Easy Comb, Alberto-Culver
Hair wax removal	Zip, Colorado Chemical; or Natural Cold Was Hair Remover, Sally Hansen
Hair bleach	Extra Strength Creme Bleach, Sally Hansen
Depilatory	Neet, Whitehall Laboratories
Gradual hair coloring	Grecian Formula, Combe
Temporary hair coloring	Come Alive Gray, Clairol; or Fanci-Full Rinse, Roux
Semipermanent hair coloring	Loving Care Color Lotion, Clairol; or Advantage, L'Oreal
Semipermanent hair coloring black hair care	Color Accents, Soft Sheen
Permanent hair coloring	Nice 'N Easy, Clairol; or Performing Preference, L'Oreal
Permanent hair coloring black hair care	Dark and Lovely, Carson; or Satin Doll, Roux
Permanent hair highlighting	Brush-On Soft Color Highlights; L'Oreal; or Frost and Tip, Clairol
Hair color remover	Metalex, Clairol; or Delete Color Remover, Roux
Acid permanent hair wave	Quantum, Helene Curtis; or One N' Only, Jheri Redding
Self-regulated permanent hair wave	Feels So Lively, Zotos; or Post-Impressions, Helene Curtis
Exothermic permanent hair wave	Warm and Gentle, Zotos; or Even Heat, Helene Curtis
Alkaline permanent hair wave	Lasts So Long, Helene Curtis
Home permanent hair wave	Toni, Gillette; or Home Permanent, Ogilivie; or Toni, Procter & Gamble
Hair straightener, thioglycolate	Wellastrate, Wella; or Smooth Away, Helene Curtis
Hair straightener, ammonium bisulfite	Curl Free, Gillette; or Uncurl, Clairol
Hair straightener, sodium hydroxide (lye)	Ultrasheen Creme Relaxer, Johnson Products; or Conditioning Creme Relaxer, Revlon Realistic

Table 30-4. Skin Care Products: Personal Recommendations

Skin Care Product	Recommendation
Hand cream	Norwegian Formula Hand Cream, Neutrogena
Facial moisturizer, normal to combination skin	Eucerin Facial Moisturizing Lotion SPF 25, Beiersdorf
Facial moisturizer, dry mature skin	Eucerin Plus Cream, Beiersdorf
Body moisturizer, normal skin	Nutraderm 30, Owen/Galderma; or Moisturel Lotion, Westwood; or DHS Lotion, Person & Covey
Body moisturizer, dry skin	Moisturel Cream, Westwood; or Eucerin Cream, Beiersdorf
Lip moisturizer	Lip Moisturizer, Neutrogena; or Catrix Lip Cream, Savage Laboratories
Facial cleanser, oily skin	Dial Soap, Dial
Facial cleanser, normal skin	Ivory Soap, Procter & Gamble; or Purpose Cleanser, Johnson & Johnson; or Moisturel Cleanser, Westwood
Facial cleanser, dry skin	Nondrying Facial Cleanser, Neutrogena
Facial cleanser, sensitive skin with acne	Cleansing Wash, Neutrogena
Lipid free cleanser	Aquanil, Person & Covey
Cleansing cream	Cold Cream, Chesebrough-Ponds; or Deep Cleansing Cold Cream, Almay
Antiperspirant and deodorant	Dry Idea, Gilette
Antiperspirant and deodorant, sensitive skin	Stick, Almay
Shaving cream	Edge Gel, SC Johnson & Son
Sunscreen, sensitive skin	Chemical-Free Sunblocker SPF 17, Neutrogena
Sunscreen, waterproof	Sunscreen SPF 30, Neutrogena

good products on the market that are not mentioned. This is because I have not personally tested them. This chapter is divided into charts listing facial cosmetics (Table 30-1), nail cosmetics (Table 30-2), hair cosmetics (Table 30-3), and skin care products (Table 30-4). These products may not work well for every patient. This chapter is included for dermatologists who want specific product recommendation suggestions. It is far better for dermatologists to use the products and arrive at their own conclusions, but the information is provided for those physicians who cannot use this approach.

31

Glossary of Terms

abrasive scrubber a mechanical exfoliant that uses an abrasive sponge or abrasive scrubbing granules in a creamy base to remove skin scale.

acid permanent wave permanent curling of the hair employing thioglycolic acid at a pH of 7 to 8.5.

acne cosmetica acne due to the use of cosmetics.

acnegenesis the formation of pustular and papular acne lesions.

aerosol a suspension of fine solid or liquid particles in a gas.

alkaline permanent wave a permanent hair curling procedure occurring at a pH of 9 to 10 employing ammonium thioglycolate.

allergenic evoking an immunologic response.

allergic contact dermatitis an immunologic reaction to a substance placed on the skin.

alpha-hydroxy acids organic carboxylic acids in which there is a hydroxy group at the alpha position, such as glycolic acid, malic acid, mandelic acid, and tartaric acid.

amphoteric a substance having two different characteristics, such as hydrophilic and hydrophobic.

anhydrous containing no water.

anionic containing ions possessing a negative electrical charge.

antioxidant a substance designed to prevent a chemical reaction with oxygen.

antiperspirant a product designed to prevent sweating at the application site.

aqueous formed from water.

aquiline nose hooked nose.

aromatherapy the use of herbal extracts, rare oils, and massage to enhance the body.

astringent a drying substance applied to the skin.

automatic emulsion a suspension of one substance in another encased in a cylindrical tube with a sponge-tipped applicator wand.

base coat an unpigmented transparent or translucent nail enamel applied to the nail plate to increase adherence of a pigmented nail polish.

bleaching the process of removing color.

bleeding the movement of a pigmented cosmetic to a site other than where it was originally placed.

bloom the absorption of sebum by a cosmetic, which can change its color or finish.

blotter a substance that absorbs sebum.

blow drying lotion a conditioner applied to the hair after towel drying that is not removed.

blush a pigmented cosmetic applied to the cheeks.

booster a substance added to the standard ammonia and hydrogen peroxide hair bleaching solution to intensify color removal.

brassy an undesirable orange hue that appears following permanent dyeing in hair containing red, pheomelanin pigments.

brilliantine a liquid pomade.

bronzing gel a gel designed to impart transparent color to the skin.

buffer a pigmented powder used for facial contouring or color blending.

cake compressed powder.

cascade a hair piece of curls or a bun designed to rest on the posterior scalp.

cationic containing ions with a positive electrical charge.

chemical sunblock a substance that absorbs light energy.

cloth wrap linen or silk cloth imbedded within acrylic nail sculptures to add strength to sculptured nails.

cold processing a permanent hair wave that does not require externally applied heat for the chemical reaction to proceed.

colorant a pigment.

color drift a shift in the color of a pigmented cosmetic during wearing.

coloring the process of dyeing the hair.

color wash a pigmented liquid applied to the face to impart transparent color.

combination skin facial skin that is dry on the periphery and oily in the central facial area.

comedogenesis the formation of comedones.

comedogenic capable of inducing comedones.

comedogenicity the ability to produce comedones.

conditioner a product generally applied to the hair to improve its cosmetic appearance and feel.

contouring the application of facial cosmetics to create the illusion of a well-proportioned face.

corrective cosmetic any cosmetic designed to correct a facial pigmentary or contour defect.

cosmetic a product designed to enhance appearance.

cosmetic color all nonpermanent methods of hair coloring.

cover cosmetic an opaque cosmetic designed to mask an underlying cutaneous defect.

coverage the amount of opacity provided by a facial cosmetic.

crayon a thick, firm, extruded rod usually encased in wood.

cream an emulsified cosmetic preparation that must be scooped from a jar.

cream/powder a cosmetic than can be applied with a dry sponge to act as a powder or applied with a water-moistened sponge to form a cream.

deep conditioner a product applied to the hair for 20 to 30 minutes followed by shampooing designed to improve the cosmetic appearance and texture of the hair.

demilashes sparse artificial eyelashes designed to supplement existing natural eyelashes.

demiwig an artificial hair piece designed to cover the entire head except the front hairline.

deodorant a fragrance designed to mask axillary odor.

depilatory a thioglycolated-based chemical hair remover.

dye a coloring agent.

electrolysis the use of galvanic current to destroy germinative cells of the hair follicle electrochemically.

emollient a product that soothes or softens the skin.

emulsifier a surface-active agent, usually a soap, that promotes the formation of an emulsion.

emulsion the suspension of one substance in another.

epilate hair removal by plucking.

exfoliant a substance that removes the upper layer of the stratum corneum.

exfoliate desquamate.

exothermic permanent wave a permanent hair curling technique occurring at an acidic pH that produces heat as a by-product of the chemical reaction.

eye shadow a colored cosmetic applied to the upper and sometimes lower eyelid.

eyeliner a colored cosmetic applied in a thin line along the upper and/or lower eyelashes.

fall a hair piece formed of long locks designed to rest on the crown.

fibered containing textile filaments.

filler a hair conditioner designed to aid in the even uptake of hair dye.

filling the process of adding additional acrylic to the proximal nail fold in a patient with existing nail sculptures to cover new natural nail growth.

film a thin polymer layer.

finish the surface characteristics of a cosmetic spanning a spectrum from matte to shiny.

floured a dusty facial appearance imparted by the use of loose powder that is not well-adhered to the underlying facial foundation.

foundation a pigmented cosmetic applied to the entire face to impart color and cover underlying pigment or contour defects.

fragrance perfume.

fragrance free the absence of any added perfume.

French manicure a series of nail polishes designed to mimic the appearance of a natural nail, including a pink nail bed and a white hyponychium.

frosted a pearled finish.

gleamer a transparent colored facial cosmetic.

gloss a shiny, transparent lip cosmetic.

gradual hair coloring metallic hair coloring that darkens the natural hair color with successive applications.

greasies limp, dull hair due to excessive hair shaft conditioner residue.

hair glaze a hair conditioning agent applied to towel-dried hair to improve manageability and impart shine.

hair straightening the act of removing curls and kinks from hair shafts.

hair thickener a leave-in hair conditioner applied to towel-dried hair.

hardening the act of reforming hair disulfide bonds with a neutralizer following permanent waving.

heat processing the use of eternally applied heat from a hair dryer to promote a permanent hair wave chemical reaction.

henna a vegetable dye derived from the *Lawsonia alba* plant.

highlighter a deeply pigmented cosmetic used to contour the face.

highlighting the process of selectively bleaching strands of hair.

hold the ability to maintain the hair in its styled position.

home product a product sold over the counter for home use.

hot combing the use of a heated metal comb to straighten hair.

humectant a substance that attracts moisture.

hydrolyzed split into fragments by the addition of water.

hydrophilic having an affinity for water.

hydrophobic repulsing water.

hypoallergenic having reduced allergenic potential.

instant conditioner a hair product applied immediately after shampooing followed by rinsing designed to improve the cosmetic appearance and texture of the hair.

ionic possessing an electrical charge.

iridescent having a metallic shine.

irritant contact dermatitis a dermatitis resulting from the caustic nature of a substance placed on the skin.

lightening decreasing the degree of color.

lip liner a pigmented cosmetic used to apply a thin line inside, on, or outside the upper and lower lips.

lipophilic having an affinity for fat.

lipstick a molded tube of pigmented cosmetic stroked over the lips.

lotion a combination of water and oil that is poured from a bottle.

lubricant a substance capable of reducing friction.

lubricity the capacity to reduce friction.

makeup cosmetic.

manageability the ability to style hair with ease.

manicure grooming of the fingernails.

mascara a pigmented cosmetic applied to the eyelashes.

matte dull finish.

metallic hair coloring metal oxides, suboxides, and sulfides that are deposited on the hair to produce gradual color production.

moist semimatte a minimally shiny finish.

moisturization the process of adding moisture.

moisturizer a product that adds moisture.

mousse an aerosolized foam.

nail hardener a product that increases the resistance of the nail to breakage.

nail polish a pigmented or unpigmented liquid enamel designed to adorn the nail.

nail polish remover a solvent designed to remove nail enamel from the nail plate.

neutralizer an oxidizing liquid designed to stop the action of a permanent waving solution.

noncomedogenic does not produce comedones.

nonglossy not possessing shine.

off-shades an undesirable, unintended color resulting from chemical dyeing of hair.

oil-based a cosmetic with oil as the primary ingredient.

oil control a product designed to absorb oil.

oil-free a product that contains no animal, vegetable, or mineral oils, but may contain silicone oils.

oil-in-water emulsion a preparation of oil distributed in small globules throughout water.

ointment a semisolid preparation for external application.

one-step processing permanent dyeing of the hair to a darker color.

on-shade the achievement of the desired, intended hair color upon chemical dyeing.

opacifier a substance that renders a liquid impervious to light rays.

opaque impervious to light rays; neither transparent nor translucent.

optical whitening make an off-white color appear closer to a true white color.

overdyeing attaining a deeper color than desired.

oxidant the electron receptor in an oxidation-reduction reaction.

pearl light reflective particles.

pearlesence the presence of pearl.

pearlized pearlesence.

pencil a thin, firm, extruded rod usually encased in wood.

permanent hair coloring hair dye that is not removed with shampooing.

permanenting permanently waving the hair.

permanent wave curling of the hair that is not removed with shampooing.

physical sunscreen a substance that reflects light energy.

pigment color.

plasticizer a substance added to make a product soft and flexible.

playtime the time during which a facial foundation can be spread over the face prior to drying or setting.

pomade an oily hair dressing.

porosity the presence of holes or pores that allow the passage of substances in or out of the hair shaft.

powder matter in a finely ground state.

pressing cream an oily cream applied to the hair to aid in heat transfer during heat straightening of kinky hair.

professional cosmetics products sold only to licensed cosmetologists.

quats quaternary ammonium compounds.

recontour to redefine a shape.

redye to change color.

reprocess to perform another chemical reaction on the hair.

rinse a thin liquid applied to the hair after shampooing to impart color or to act as a conditioning agent.

rouge a cream blush.

salon products product lines sold only through franchised salons.

sculptures custom-made artificial nails that are built or "sculpted" over the natural nail plate.

sealant a product applied to the lips or eyelids to increase adherence of a pigmented cosmetic.

sealer an impervious covering.

self-regulated permanent wave an acid chemical curling process employing dithioglycolic acid and thioglycolic acid designed to cease bond breakage at chemical equilibrium.

semimatte a minimally shiny finish.

semipermanent dye a textile dye hair coloring that is removed in four to six shampooings.

sequestering agent a substance that chelates magnesium and calcium ions so that other salts or insoluble soaps are not formed.

shake lotion powder in a vehicle that must be mixed by shaking to produce a suspension.

shampoo a soap or detergent designed for cleansing hair.

sheer a thin, transparent layer.

shiny a reflective finish that appears moist.

singlets individual artificial eyelashes.

softening an alteration of the hair to allow increased penetration of a permanent dye or a permanent waving solution.

softness a pleasing hair texture.

solute a substance dissolved in a solvent.

solvent the liquid in which a solute is dissolved.

solvent-based a cosmetic using a nonaqueous solvent, such as a petroleum distillate.

soufflé a whipped cream.

split ends separation of the distal hair shaft into two or more pieces due to absence of the cuticle and cortex with exposure of the fragile medulla, known medically as trichoptilosis.

spray an aerosolized liquid.

spritz synonymous with spray.

stain a transparent pigment that cannot be removed by rubbing.

stick a molded wax pigmented cosmetic encased in wood, plastic, or a metal tube.

substantivity the ability to adhere to another substance.

surfactant a soap or synthetic detergent.

switch long strands of hair in the form of braids or ponytails secured together at one end.

syndet bar a synthetic detergent soap formed into a bar.

take successful completion of chemical hair processing, either hair dyeing or permanent waving.

temporary hair coloring textile type dyes applied to the hair and removed in one shampooing.

thermolysis a method of hair removal employing high frequency electrocoagulation to destroy germinative hair cells.

tint a permanent dye used in one-step processing to darken hair color.

tips molded, preformed plastic pieces that are glued to the distal natural fingernails to extend nail length.

toner a permanent dye used in two-step processing to color hair following bleaching.

top coat a clear nail enamel applied on top of the pigmented polish layer to prevent chipping.

toupee a hair piece for men designed to cover the top of the balding head.

translucent used in cosmetology to describe a cosmetic that both colors and provides sheer coverage.

transparent used in cosmetology to describe a cosmetic that colors without providing coverage.

trichoclasis breakage of the hair.

trichoptilosis the condition in which the hairs split; split ends.

trichorrhexis invaginata telescoping of the hair shaft.

trichorrhexis nodosa nodelike swellings on the hair shaft where the cortex of the shaft has fractured and split into strands, weakening the hair so that breakage occurs at these nodes.

trichotherapy the application of substances to the hair shafts accompanied by massage to enhance the appearance of the hair.

trueness used in cosmetology to describe how closely the final dyed hair color resembles the sample hair swatches.

tweezing plucking.

two-step processing a permanent hair lightening technique in which the natural hair color is first bleached and subsequently redyed to a lighter shade.

undercover a cosmetic applied under a foundation to mask a pigmentation defect.

unpigmented without color.

unscented no smell, but may contain a masking fragrance to cover the natural odor of the ingredients.

volume in cosmetology, the number of liters of oxygen released by a liter of hydrogen peroxide hair bleaching solution.

wand a slender brush or sponge-tipped applicator.

water-based a product in which water is the solvent.

waving lotion a thioglycolate containing liquid used in the permanent curling of hair.

waxing a method of hair removal where the unwanted hairs are embedded in wax and subsequently epilated with wax stripping.

weartime the time a cosmetic remains on the application site.

wearability the ability of a cosmetic to perform its desired function on the application site.

weathering the loss of cuticle scales from the hair shaft.

wefted woven.

wig hair piece.

Index

Note: Page numbers followed by f indicate figures, and those followed by t indicate tables.